Inducible Gene Expression, Volume 1

Environmental Stresses and Nutrients

Progress in Gene Expression

Series Editor:

Michael Karin
Department of Pharmacology
School of Medicine
University of California, San Diego
La Jolla, CA 92093-0636

Books in the Series:

Gene Expression: General and Cell-Type-Specific
M. Karin, editor
ISBN 0-8176-3605-6

Inducible Gene Expression, Volume I: Environmental Stresses
and Nutrients
P.A. Baeuerle, editor
ISBN 0-8176-3728-1

Inducible Gene Expression, Volume II: Hormonal Signals
P.A. Baeuerle, editor
ISBN 0-8176-3734-6

Inducible Gene Expression, Volume 1

Environmental Stresses and Nutrients

P.A. Baeuerle
Editor

Birkhäuser
Boston • Basel • Berlin

P.A. Baeuerle
Institute of Biochemistry
Albert-Ludwigs-University Freiburg
Hermann-Herder-Str. 7
D-79104 Freiburg i.Br.
Germany

Library of Congress Cataloging-in-Publication Data

Inducible gene expression/P.A. Baeuerle, editor.
     p.   cm. – – (Progress in gene expreesion)
    Includes bibliographical references and index.
    Contents: v. 1.   Enviromental stresses and nutrients – – v.
2. Hormonal signals.
    ISBN 0-8176-3800-8 (set). – – ISBN 0-8176-3728-1 (v. 1). – – ISBN
0-8176-3734-6 (v. 2)
    1. Genetic regulation. 2. Gene expression. I. Baeuerle, P.A.
(Patrick Alexander), 1957- . II. Series.
QH450.I53 1994
574.87'322– –dc20   94-27957
                                      CIP

Printed on acid-free paper

©1995 Birkhäuser Boston   *Birkhäuser*

ISBN 0-8176-3728-1
ISBN 3-7643-3728-1

Typeset by Alden Multimedia, Northampton, England.
Printed and bound by Quinn-Woodbine, Woodbine, NJ.
Printed in the United States of America

9 8 7 6 5 4 3 2 1

Dedicated to
Anette, Katharina and Alexander

Contents

Preface   ix
     P.A. Baeuerle

List of Contributors   xi

1   Prokaryotic Control of Transcription: How and Why Does It Differ
     From Eukaryotic Control?
     Stefan Oehler and Benno Müller-Hill   1

2   The Heat Shock Transcriptional Response
     Paul E. Kroeger and Richard I. Morimoto   25

3   The Role and Regulation of the Jun Proteins in Response to
     Phorbol Ester and UV Light
     Peter Angel   62

4   NF-κB: A Mediator of Pathogen and Stress Responses
     Ulrich Siebenlist, Keith Brown and Guido Franzoso . .   93

5   PPAR: A Key Nuclear Factor in Nutrient/Gene Interactions?
     Béatrice Desvergne and Walter Wahli 142

6   Mechanism of Signal Transduction by the Basic Helix-Loop-Helix
     Dioxin Receptor
     Lorenz Poellinger 177

7   Transcriptional Regulation by Heavy Metals, Exemplified at the
     Metallothionein Genes
     Rainer Heuchel, Freddy Radtke and Walter Schaffner . 206

8   Post-Transcriptional Regulation of Gene Expression by Iron
     Matthias W. Hentze 241

Index 267

Preface

Cells have evolved multiple strategies to adapt the composition and quality of their protein equipment to needs imposed by changes in intra- and extracellular conditions. The appearance of proteins transmitting novel functional properties to cells can be controlled at a transcriptional, posttranscriptional, translational or posttranslational level. Extensive research over the past 15 years has shown that transcriptional regulation is used as the predominant strategy to control the production of new proteins in response to extracellular stimuli. At the level of gene transcription, the initiation of mRNA synthesis is used most frequently to govern gene expression. The key elements controlling transcription initiation in eukaryotes are activator proteins (transactivators) that bind in a sequence-specific manner to short DNA sequences in the proximity of genes. The activator binding sites are elements of larger control units, called promoters and enhancers, which bind many distinct proteins. These may synergize or negatively cooperate with the activators. The do novo binding of an activator to DNA or, if already bound to DNA, its functional activation is what ultimately turns on a high-level expression of genes. The activity of transactivators is controlled by signalling pathways and, in some cases, transactivators actively participate in signal transduction by moving from the cytoplasm into the nucleus.

In this first volume of *Inducible Gene Expression*, leading scientists in the field review six eukaryotic transactivators that allow cells to respond to various extracellular stimuli by the expression of new proteins. Common to these activators is that they control gene expression in response to stresses, which, from an evolutionary point of view, belong to the oldest threats to life: heat, UV light, reactive oxygen species, heavy metals and xenobiotics. The various transactivators are used as emergency switches that coordinately turn on the production of a set of novel proteins which protect the cell from the damaging effect of the stimuli.

As an introduction to the eukaryotic systems, the first chapter by Oehler and Müller-Hill works out the differences between prokaryotic and eukaryotic control of gene expression. Kroeger and Morimoto describe transcription factors responding to an increase in temperature. Angel reports on Jun, a factor involved in the UV response of organisms ranging from yeast to man. Siebenlist and colleagues review the inducible transcription factor NF-κB, which can respond to a great variety of pathogenic conditions, including oxidative stress, energy-rich radiation and viral and bacterial infections. Desvergne and Wahli describe a member of the steroid hormone super family (see also Volume 2) which controls the expression of peroxisomal proteins in response to toxic xenobiotics. These appear to mimic fatty acids, the physiological inducers. A factor which turns on genes in response to the environmental pollutant dioxin is reviewed by Poellinger. The last two chapters deal with gene regulation in response to toxic metal ions. Radtke and Schaffner describe a heavy metal-binding transcriptional activator of the metallothionein gene. The last chapter by Hentze underscores the fact that translational events also can efficiently control gene expression in response to metal ions; it review that upon binding iron can increase the stability of one mRNA species and at the same time prevent translation of another mRNA species.

One central idea behind bringing together these different systems in one book is to invite readers to compare the various molecular mechanisms used for intracellular signalling and induction of gene expression. Another exciting aspect of this first volume of *Inducible Gene Expression* is that the "archaic" gene-inductory stimuli discussed here have gained considerable attention because, as a consequence of environmental pollution, they have experienced a revival as "modern" threats to human life. Hence, it is very important to medical researchers, biologists, and chemists who study the effects of UV, heavy metals, oxygen radicals and xenobiotics to understand the molecular mechanisms underlying inducible gene expression in response to adverse environmental stimuli.

Patrick A. Baeuerle

List of Contributors

Peter Angel, Kernforschungszentrum Karlsruhe, Institut für Genetik, Postfach 3640, D-76021 Karlsruhe 1, Germany

Keith Brown, Laboratory of Immunoregulation, National Institute of Allergy and Infectious Diseases, National Institutes of Health, Building 10, Room 11B-16, Bethesda, MD 20892, USA

Béatrice Desvergne, Institut de Biologie Animale, Université de Lausanne, Bâtiment de Biologie, CH-1015 Lausanne, Switzerland

Guido Franzoso, Laboratory of Immunoregulation, National Institute of Allergy and Infectious Diseases, National Institutes of Health, Building 10, Room 11B-16, Bethesda, MD 20892, USA

Rainer Heuchel, Institut für Molekularbiologie II, Universität Zürich, Winterthurerstr. 190, CH-8057 Zürich, Switzerland

Matthias W. Hentze, European Molecular Biology Laboratory, Meyerhofstrasse 1, D-69117 Heidelberg, Germany

Paul E. Kroeger, Department of Biochemistry, Molecular Biology and Cell Biology, Northwestern University, 2153 North Campus Drive, Evanston, Illinois 60208-3500, USA

Richard I. Morimoto, Department of Biochemistry, Molecular Biology and Cell Biology, Northwestern University, 2153 North Campus Drive, Evanston, Illinois 60208-3500, USA

Benno Müller-Hill, Institut für Genetik, Universität Köln, Weyertal 121, D-50931 Köln, Germany

Stefan Oehler, Institute of Genetics, University of Cambridge, Downing Street, Cambridge CB2 3EH, United Kingdom

Lorenz Poellinger, Department of Medical Nutrition, Karolinska Institute, Huddinge University Hospital F60, NOVUM, S-141 86 Huddinge, Sweden

Freddy Radtke, Institut für Molekularbiologie II, Universität Zürich, Winterthurerstr. 190, CH-8057 Zürich, Switzerland

Walter Schaffner, Institut für Molekularbiologie II, Universität Zürich, Winterthurerstr. 190, CH-8057 Zürich, Switzerland

Ulrich Siebenlist, Laboratory of Immunoregulation, National Institute of Allergy and Infectious Diseases, National Institutes of Health, Building 10, Room 11B-16, Bethesda, MD 20892, USA

Walter Wahli, Institut de Biologie Animale, Université de Lausanne, Bâtiment de Biologie, CH-1015 Lausanne, Switzerland

1

Prokaryotic control of transcription: How and why does it differ from eukaryotic control?

STEFAN OEHLER AND BENNO MÜLLER-HILL

Introduction

Escherichia coli and all other prokaryotes have developed elaborate mechanisms to adapt their metabolism to a rapidly changing environment. Some of these mechanisms allow the bacteria to approach or to flee particular chemicals (Adler, 1975; Boyd and Simon, 1982). We will not discuss such mechanisms here. Other mechanisms adapt the transcription rates of genes whose products are needed or not needed in a particular environment. Genes which deal with the catabolism of chemicals which suddenly appear in the environment have to be rapidly turned on. We have to recall that the inner bacterial membrane does not allow the entry of most organic chemicals. There has to be a permease, a specific pump, present which transports the chemical into the cell.

The cases of the *lac* and Lambda systems are illuminating. Lactose can not enter an *E. coli* cell through the inner membrane. It needs the presence of a specific permease (Rickenberg et al, 1956). In cells which have not seen lactose for several generations about one molecule of Lac permease per cell is present. Its presence allows equilibration with the outside lactose. Lactose itself is no inducer of the *lac* system. In fact, it is a weak antiinducer. But β-galactosidase, which upon induction rapidly breaks down large amounts of lactose, is present at a basal level of about 3 tetrameric molecules per cell. It converts some of the lactose (1-4-glucosido-β-D-galactoside) into its isomers, particularly allolactose (1-6-glucosido-β-D-galactoside). In contrast to lactose, allolactose is able to induce expression of the *lac* system. In its presence, the transcription rate of the Lac system (i.e. of the Z, Y and A genes coding for β-galactosidase, Lac permease and Lac transacetylase) is increased about 1000-fold (Müller-Hill, 1971).

INDUCIBLE GENE EXPRESSION, VOLUME 1
P.A. Baeuerle, Editor
© 1995 Birkhäuser Boston

Lambda repressor keeps those genes shut off that have to be expressed to multiply the phage DNA and to shield it with a coat i.e. to produce phage. When *E. coli* is exposed to UV radiation, many cells die. *E. coli* tries to save itself by producing a set of enzymes which repair the UV radiation damage (Walker, 1984). This induction has been called the SOS response. The production of the SOS enzymes is repressed by the LexA repressor, which is inactivated upon UV irradiation. When DNA is damaged, the RecA protein gains the ability to catalyse autoproteolysis of the LexA protein. The same happens with Lambda repressor. If enough activated RecA protein is present, Lambda repressor cuts its own reading head from its core (Roberts and Roberts, 1975; Little, 1984). The reading heads need the core to assemble to dimers. As monomers they do not act as repressor since they cannot bind efficiently to their operators. The silent passenger Lambda uses the repair system of *E. coli* to escape the sinking ship.

If we compare the *lac* and Lambda stories, we see that the response to the challenging stimulus in both cases is quite direct. It is not lactose itself that induces, but rather allolactose, a product of lactose, and it is not the thymine-dimer itself that induces Lambda repressor, but here again the action is quite direct. There is no long signalling cascade involved between the stimulus and the eventual response.

If we summarize the difference between *E. coli* and mouse cells, we see that *E. coli* cells almost invariably react on stimuli from the outside world in a rather direct manner. Most mouse cells in contrast interact with stimuli created by other mouse cells which promote or maintain differentiation. These processes of early development are not well understood in the mouse. In contrast they are well analysed in *Drosophila* (Lawrence, 1992). Only some specialized cells of *Drosophila* or the mouse interact with stimuli from the outside world, such as mouse B and T cells with viral or bacterial proteins. And viral proteins are often similar in structure and function to endogenous mouse proteins.

Major Differences Between Transcription in *E. coli* and in the Mouse

The recent flood of papers dealing with eukaryotic transcription factors has led to the notion that the problem of prokaryotic transcription is essentially solved and moreover that it has little application to the eukaryotic problems. What is true for *E. coli* seems irrelevant to the mouse. We think this is a profound misunderstanding. We think that to understand the principles of prokaryotic transcription will help to understand eukaryotic transcription and vice versa. In order to make this clear, we will concentrate on general principles and differences between prokaryotic and eukaryotic systems (Figure 1.1). We will concentrate on a very few prokaryotic systems, i.e. those in which our understanding is most advanced. We will also point out the large areas in which both the prokaryotic and the eukaryotic systems are still not well

	E.coli	Mouse
Volume of a cell (nucleus)	2×10^{-12} cm^3	4×10^{-9} cm^3 (3×10^{-10} cm^3)
Organisation of genome	semi-naked DNA	nucleosome
Size of genome	4.7×10^6 bp	3×10^9 bp
Structure of genome	90% coding for protein. No junk.	10% coding for protein. Junk?
Length of unique DNA sequence	11 bp	16 bp
Structure of DNA recognizing proteins	modular	modular
Predominant mode of protein DNA recognition	alpha helix in major groove	alpha helix in major groove
Maximal number of bp recognized by one recognition unit of one protein subunit	5-6 bp	5-6 bp
Minimal necessary number of particular protein dimer per cell capable of interacting specifically with DNA	20	20.000
Maximal size of chromosomal DNA-Protein-DNA loop	500 bp	30.000 bp
Number of subunits of main RNA polymerase	5	about 10
Number of protein factors interacting with RNA polymerase	1-3	up to 10
Genes transcribed from one start	up to 10	1
Predominant mode of control	negative	positive
Predominant function of control	adaptation in a changing environment	development from egg to organism
Type of analysis	Bacterial and phage genetics. Reverse genetics	Reverse genetics

Figure 1.1 Similarities and differences between bacteria (*E. coli*) and cells of higher organisms (mouse) with respect to gene regulation.

understood. For the reader who wants to know more about the subject, we provide here a list of books (Beckwith, Davies and Galland, 1983; Losick and Chamberlin, 1976; McKnight and Yamamoto, 1992; Miller and Reznikoff, 1978; Ptashne, 1992) and articles (Johnson and McKnight, 1989; Struhl, 1989; Renkawitz, 1990; Guarente and Bermingham-McDonogh, 1992; Grunstein, 1990; Cowel, 1994), and we warn the reader that our list is far from complete.

The transcriptional machinery of *E. coli* is much more compact than the transcriptional machinery of the mouse (Figure 1.1). First of all, the *E. coli* chromosome contains only 4.7×10^6 base pairs (bp), i.e. about one thousandth of the haploid mouse genome. More than 90 percent of the *E. coli* DNA codes for protein. The DNA sequences which can be exclusively used as recognition sites for transcriptional factors are rather limited. If they do not lie within coding sequences as for example the operators of O2 the *lac* system (Reznikoff et al, 1974) and O_I of the *gal* system (Irani et al, 1983; Fritz et al, 1983), they have to be positioned very close to the binding site of RNA polymerase.

The different sizes of the *E. coli* and mouse genomes have consequences for the number of protein subunits which are necessary to recognize a particular DNA region to activate or repress RNA polymerase at a particular promoter. A sequence of 11 bp occurs only once by chance on the *E. coli* chromosome ($4^{11} \sim 4 \times 10^6$). Most transcription factors which recognize *E. coli* or mouse DNA use alpha helices which are positioned in the major groove of the DNA to be recognized (Pabo & Sauer, 1984; Gehring et al, 1990; Ellenberger et al, 1992; Ferré-d'Amaré et al, 1993). In all cases where these factors have been well analysed, it can be seen that five or maximally six base pairs can be specifically recognized by such an alpha helix and its surroundings. Thus, two protein subunits are sufficient to bind specifically to one or possibly a very few additional binding sites which are present by chance on the *E. coli* chromosome. As far as we know, *E. coli* has only developed proteins with one such DNA binding site per subunit.

Furthermore, *E. coli* has followed the simple and economic principle of creating subunit interfaces which allow dimer formation. Dimer formation is not necessary, but it facilitates the binding of the two subunits to their binding sites (Ogata and Gilbert, 1978; Khoury et al, 1991). Most DNA targets of prokaryotic and of some eukaryotic repressors and activators are obviously palindromic and not direct repeats. This reflects the aggregation of two protein monomers to a closed dimer, in which the two subunits face each other with the same surface. This mode of aggregation efficiently precludes polymerization of monomers along the DNA. It is revealing that Lac and Gal repressors form tetramers or dimers respectively (we will come back to the tetramer), but that the homologous periplasmic ribose and galactose binding proteins are monomeric (Mowbray and Cole, 1992; Vyas et al, 1988). A protein dimer may thus recognize a palindrome of 10 to 12 base pairs. Dimeric DNA binding proteins often protect about 20 bp against DNAase attack, but not all of the covered bases are specifically recognized. In summary, two protein subunits are sufficient to recognize a DNA sequence which occurs only once on the *E. coli* chromosome.

In the mouse genome, with its 3×10^9 bp, a sequence of 16 base pairs occurs only once by chance ($4^{16} \sim 3 \times 10^9$). It is immediately clear that one dimer of a DNA recognizing monomer carries not enough specificity to bind only at the required position. At least three binding sites for three monomers are necessary. In *E. coli* usually only one or two transcription factors, a specific repressor or activator and possibly a general activator like CAP (Zubay et al, 1970; Emmer et al, 1970), are involved. There are a few cases where the expression of prokaryotic genes is subjected to a threefold transcriptional control. An example is the *deo* operon which is positively regulated by the CAP protein and repressed by both the Deo and the Cyt repressors (Hammer-Jespersen and Munch-Petersen, 1975).

In mouse development as many as ten different transcription factors are involved to regulate transcription of one gene (Mitchell and Tjian, 1989). Half a dozen such factors, which cooperate in binding, combine enough specificity to bind exclusively near the relevant RNA polymerase. Together, they are able to specifically enhance transcription (see below). The cooperative interaction of these numerous factors removes the necessity for them to form homodimers to gain sufficient specificity. Consequently most mouse transcription factors are monomers.

There are a few proteins that occur in large amounts and bind nonspecifically to DNA in *E. coli* (Drlica and Rouviere-Yaniv, 1987; Pettijohn, 1988). However, they do not have the quality to create a solid structure similar to the nucleosome. Whereas DNA which is present as nucleosome is incapable of being transcribed, which is most of the mouse DNA, no such region is known to exist in growing *E. coli*. It follows that specific negative control, the simplest type of control, is prevalent in *E. coli* but not in the mouse. Negative control, where a repressor competes with RNA-polymerase for binding, is most common in *E. coli*; it occurs in the *lac* (Reznikoff and Abelson, 1978) and Lambda systems (Takeda, 1979; Meyer et al, 1980) and also in many other systems (Miller and Reznikoff, 1978).

Positive control in the mouse may mean two things. It may mean opening up the tight nucleosome structure that bars all transcription, or it may mean activation of RNA polymerase. In *E. coli* it means the latter.

Here, we observe two types of activating transcription factors: some very few which act on many systems, such as the CAP protein (de Crombrugghe et al, 1984), and many which each act on a very few specific genes, such as AraC (Englesberg et al, 1965), or MalT (Schwartz, 1967). We will come back to mechanistic studies in *E. coli* later.

As the last major difference between the *E. coli* and the typical mouse cell, we would like to point out their different size or volume. An *E. coli* cell has a volume of $2 \times 10^{-12}\,cm^3$. This implies that in one cell one molecule is present in a $10^{-9}\,M$ solution. Twenty dimers of Lac repressor per cell suffice for maximal repression of the *lac* system (Gilbert and Müller-Hill, 1966). If a mouse cell wants to reach the same concentration of dimers in the nucleus, it has to synthesize about 20,000 dimers per cell and must transport all of them through the nuclear membrane. The dimer concentration in the cell nucleus remains the same, but the number of protein molecules which have to be synthesized per cell has been drastically increased.

Modular Structure of the Transcription Factors of *E. coli*

The repressors and activators of *E. coli*, wherever they have been properly analysed, have a modular structure like the transcription factors of the mouse. Lac repressor, for example, consists of three such modules.

(1) Residues 1–59 form the DNA reading head (Adler et al, 1972). It consists of an N-terminal helix-turn-helix (HTH) motif followed by two alpha helices which stabilize it (Kaptein et al, 1985).

(2) Residues 60 to 330, the core, carry the methyl-β-D-galactoside binding domain. Several sugar binding proteins, which are homologous with the entire Lac repressor core, have been analyzed (Vyas et al, 1991). This sugar binding core has developed the additional capability to dimerize (Müller-Hill, 1983). Here, an interesting, unsolved problem arises: Lac repressor belongs to a family of homologous repressors. For example, Gal repressor is one member of this family, but it does not form mixed dimers with Lac repressor. We do not know how this specificity comes about.

(3) Finally, Lac repressor differs from all other members of its family by carrying two leucine heptad repeats as a third module at its C-terminus. Two dimers of Lac repressor can aggregate to a tetramer by forming a four helical bundle with these heptad repeats (Alberti et al, 1993). Here the question arises: is Lac repressor the only protein in *E. coli* which uses this simple trick for tetramer formation? If it is not the only protein in *E. coli* carrying C-terminal heptad repeats, how does it retain its specificity?

Lambda repressor has, as Lac repressor, a modular structure. Its residues 1–92 form the DNA reading head (Pabo et al, 1979). Like Lac repressor, it carries an HTH motif at its N-terminus. The recognition helix recognizes the same DNA sequence as does Lac repressor (Kolkhof et al, 1992). Its residues 132–236 form the core, which is able to dimerize (Pabo et al, 1979). This core also has a proteolytic activity, which in the presence of RecA protein leads to autoproteolysis between residue 111 and 112 (Pabo et al, 1979). We note that dimerization of the core is, with respect to the HTH-motif, opposite to Lac repressor. This places the recognition helix of Lambda repressor in the opposite orientation to the Lac repressor/operator complex over the major groove (Kolkhof et al, 1992). We note that we are still amazed about the structural similarity of both paradigms of the Jacob-Monod theory (Jacob and Monod, 1961).

In contrast to the exclusive homodimer and -tetramer formation of the *E. coli* regulatory proteins, eukaryotic transcription factors form predominantly heterodimers. These interactions are determined by subtle differences in mutual affinity of the monomers. Examples are the Jun-Fos family of bZip proteins (Nicklin and Casari, 1991; Ransone et al, 1990) or the Myc-Max transcription factors (Blackwood and Eisenman, 1991). Furthermore, phosphorylation or glycosylation may change the activity of some transcription factors. This difference from bacteria is obviously due to the need for more differentiated regulation of many more target promoters by many more regulatory pathways in multicellular organisms.

Most Pro- and Eukaryotic Transcription Factors Use an Alpha Helix for DNA Recognition

The vast majority of those repressors and activators of *E. coli* which have been properly analysed use an alpha helix for DNA recognition. How the alpha helices enter the major groove of DNA varies among the different recognition modules. In all but one case (see below), the side chains of the contacting residues of the alpha helix form hydrogen bonds or van der Waals contacts with specific bases in the major groove of DNA (Harrison and Aggarwal, 1990). In most cases, the alpha helix lies directly across the major groove (Brennan, 1992). This is the case with the HTH-bearing Lac and Lambda repressors.

It seems strange that the various DNA recognizing motifs are not common to pro- and eukaryotes. They are either found only in *E. coli*, its phages and, of course, in other bacteria, or exclusively in eukaryotic organisms. In both we find several families that present the alpha helix in different manners. In the case of the homeodomain, the presentation of the recognition helix differs from the HTH domain by being longer. Therefore not residue six but residue nine of the alpha helix touches the bases (Hanes and Brent, 1989). It is the mode of presentation which marks the difference between the alpha recognition helices of the HTH motif and the homeo domain. The general type of interaction is similar in both cases.

There is one peculiar exception among the prokaryotic HTH motifs: Trp repressor. According to the X-ray analysis, one dimer of Trp repressor binds to a 19 bp *trp* operator (Otwinowski et al, 1988). Its recognition helix does not lie across the major groove but enters it perpendicularly. The X-ray structure shows no direct interactions between the side chains of the recognition helix and the base pairs in the major groove. This has been interpreted as the first example of indirect readout (Otwinowski et al, 1988). We and others think this is an artifact (Staacke et al, 1990; Nichols et al, 1993). It remains to be seen whether indirect readout, which will be totally unpredictable, is indeed a reality or an artifact.

Finally, we note that there are two repressors that are encoded by bacteriophage P22 of *Salmonella* (Knight et al, 1989; Berg et al, 1990) and Met repressor from *E. coli* (Somers and Phillips, 1992) which recognize DNA in the major groove with a beta sheet. Examples of this mode of recognition so far have not been found among eukaryotic transcription factors.

The Advantage of Two DNA Binding Sites

In all *E. coli* systems which have been analysed in depth, at least two DNA binding sites for two repressor dimers have been found. We will discuss this in some detail and suggest that this is not a curious artifact but the result of the economic design of Darwinian evolution (Adhya, 1989). In the Lambda system (Figure 1.2), the evidence is old and undisputed. Two Lambda operators, O_R2 and O_R1, are placed 24 bp apart (Pirrotta, 1975; Maniatis et al, 1975) and serve for two Lambda repressor dimers to repress the P_R promoter which initiates the Cro message (Ptashne et al, 1976). If one of these operators is destroyed, repression of P_R drops drastically (Meyer et al, 1980). It has been shown that the two Lambda repressor dimers interact with each other and stabilize their DNA complex through this cooperativity (Johnson et al, 1979). We note that this interaction is strongly favoured by the closeness of the two dimers which is realised by binding to two adjacent target sites.

It took longer to identify the corresponding cooperativity in regulation of the *lac* operon (Oehler et al, 1990). To the best of our knowledge, all

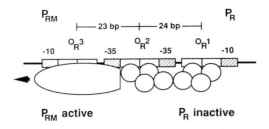

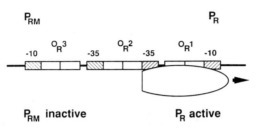

Figure 1.2 Top: Two dimers of Lambda repressor strengthen binding to O_R1 and O_R2 by an interaction of their C-terminal domains. P_R is repressed and P_{RM} is active. Bottom: When no repressor binds, polymerase transcribes from P_R and P_{RM} is inactive.

textbooks still carry the old and misleading view that tetrameric Lac repressor acts by binding to only one operator (O1) directly downstream from the *lac* promoter. In fact, the *lac* system carries two auxiliary *lac* operators (O2 and O3), both of which have to be destroyed before an effect upon repression can be seen (Figure 1.3). O2 lies within the *lac Z* gene (Reznikoff et al, 1974) 401 bp downstream from O1 (we measure from center of symmetry to center of symmetry). O3 lies 92 bp upstream from 01, upstream of the *lac* promoter (Gilbert et al, 1976). If one of the auxiliary operators is destroyed, repression drops about threefold. However, if we destroy both O2 and O3 and insert one copy of the construct back into the chromosome, a 70-fold decrease of repression is observed (Oehler et al, 1990). We explain this large effect by proposing that one of two alternative loops is formed, either a loop O1-Lac repressor-O2, or a loop O3-Lac repressor-O1.

Cooperatively between multiple target sites, as is obvious from these two examples, enhances both tightness and specificity of protein/target interactions. Because of the great excess of non-target-DNA in eucaryotes, cooperativity between transcriptional regulators should predominate by far. Indeed, extensive interactions between eukaryotic transcription factors have been reported (Janson and Pettersson, 1990; Kristie et al, 1989; Schüle et al, 1990). A general lesson which may be learned for eukaryotic system is that where two or more alternative

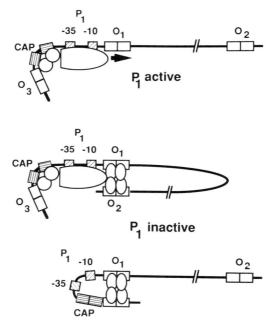

Figure 1.3 Top: Transcription from the *lac* promoter is constitutive when Lac repressor is absent or interacts with inducer. The dimeric CAP protein strongly bends its target site and activates RNA polymerase. Bottom: In the absence of inducer, tetrameric wt Lac repressor binds simultaneously to either O1 and O2, where it is likely that CAP binds, or to O1 and O3, where it is unlikely that CAP binds. The operon is thousandfold repressed. The figure does not intend to make a claim about the topology of the Lac repressor tetramer.

cooperative interactions exist, the inactivation of one auxiliary binding site will have little or no effect and may thus be misinterpreted.

Local Protein Concentration and DNA-protein-DNA Loop Formation

We compared in vivo the Lac repressor binding constant (i.e. the repression values) of O2 with the binding constant of O1, and found that the binding constant of O2 is lower by a factor of 10. The binding constant of O3 is lower by a factor of 300 (Oehler et al, 1994) than the binding constant of O1. Consequently, the question arises as to how these weak auxiliary operators are able to promote efficiently the occupation of O1? The explanation is simple. In a wt I^+ cell ten tetramers of Lac repressor are present on average per cell. If one tetramer is bound to O2, the local concentration of the repressor around O1 increases about 20-fold. The volume of a sphere whose center is O1 and whose radius is the distance between O1 and O2 is 0.5 percent of the volume of *E. coli*. This calculation seems realistic since the 401 bp DNA is easily bendable (Figure 1.4).

If we consider the same situation between O3 and O1, bending of the short intervening DNA needs a lot of energy (Shore et al, 1981). Thus, even though the histone-like protein HU may facilitate the bending (Flashner and Gralla, 1988), the extreme increase in local concentration of Lac repressor predicted from a similar calculation as above is not observed. However, the increase in local concentration is still sufficient to increase repression substantially, although O3 is occupied only part of the time by Lac repressor. The closer the distance, the higher the effect, at least in this simplistic theory. One may ask the question of how phasing influences the action of O3. We actually did the experiment and found that O3 is positioned right in an optimum (Müller, 1994). Cooperation between two or more operators and tetrameric repressor increases repression in a rather efficient way. There are alternative ways to further increase the occupation of an operator. The affinity of repressor for its target, or the amount of repressor protein could be increased. In both cases, rapid and full release of repression can become a problem. Neither overproduced wt Lac repressor (Gilbert and Müller-Hill, 1970) nor tight binding mutant Lac repressors (Chamness and Willson, 1970) are fully inducible.

The distance between O1 and O2 is 401 base pairs. What happens if we increase the distance? A simple calculation shows that at a distance of one thousand bp, only a twofold increase in local concentration of Lac repressor can be obtained. There are statistically 10 molecules of Lac repressor in one cell, and the volume of the sphere almost equals one tenth of the volume of the *E. coli* cell (Figure 1.4). We made the experiment (for practical reasons we used the distance of about

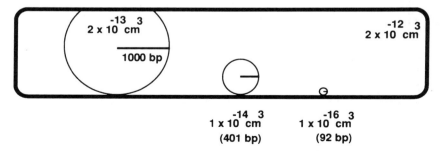

Figure 1.4 A schematic cross section through an *E. coli* cell and the centers of three spheres with the radius of 1000 bp, 401 bp and 92 bp. An *E. coli* cell is assumed to be a cylinder of about 3 μm length with a diameter of 0.6 μm.

3600 bp) and found, as expected, no effect. This is reassuring and in line with other findings in *E. coli*. There are no repressors that work over such long distances, and there is just one activator, NR_I, which works over more than 1000 bp (Reitzer and Magasanik, 1986). How does it work? The same question may be asked for the 30,000 bp loops that have been observed to work in mouse cells (Müller et al, 1988). We propose that multiple, different binding sites may do the trick, but this remains to be shown experimentally.

How Does Lac Repressor Find its Target?

The typical transcription factor of mouse has no problem in finding its target on mouse DNA. If the target is, as in general, 6 bp long, it occurs once every 4000 bp. This is different for Lac repressor and the other prokaryotic repressors. They recognize twelve base pairs, i.e. a DNA sequence which occurs statistically only once and in reality only very few times on *E. coli* DNA. It has been shown that at least nine of the ten Lac repressor molecules which are present in *E. coli*, are bound somewhere to the *E. coli* DNA (Lin and Riggs, 1975; Kao-Huang et al, 1977). We have not found other strong *lac* repressor binding sites besides O1 and O2 (Simons, 1984). Where are the Lac repressor molecules bound? A mutant of Lac repressor (X86) exists which binds about 50 times tighter to *lac* operator (Jobe and Bourgeois, 1972), and about five times tighter to nonspecific DNA than wt Lac repressor (Pfahl, 1976). The binding specificity of X86 remains unaltered (Kolkhof, 1992). This mutant Lac repressor gets lost in the *E. coli* DNA. Repression by X86 is low, but increases in the presence of the inducer IPTG (Jobe and Bourgeois, 1972). Since inducer lowers specific, but not unspecific binding of Lac repressor, this suggests that X86 is retained by weak operator-like sequences on the *E. coli* chromosome (Pfahl, 1976). Thus nonspecific and specific binding of wt Lac repressor have been perfectly balanced in respect to size and composition of the *E. coli* chromosome.

In vitro kinetic measurements have led to a paradox. The association rate constant of Lac repressor to *lac* operator buried in the 49,000 bp of Lambda DNA is found to be ten times larger than when *lac* operator is inserted in a 3000 bp piece of DNA, or is present as a synthetic DNA piece of 30 bp. How does Lambda DNA help Lac repressor to find its real target? We and others have speculated that tetrameric Lac repressor may use its two separate reading heads to touch transiently DNA which resembles vaguely in its sequence *lac* operator, i.e. sequences to which Lac repressor binds very weakly but specifically (Berg et al, 1981; Fickert and

Müller-Hill, 1992). The local increase of Lac repressor concentration inside the Lambda DNA may allow the other reading head to scan the rest of the Lambda DNA molecule much faster than would be possible if it were free in solution. This seems plausible but remains to be shown.

The Molecular Mechanisms of Repression of Transcription

The molecular mechanism of repression is simple as is all negative control. Repressor either competes with RNA polymerase or an activator of transcription for the actual occupation of their places, or it acts through steric hindrance in which case RNA polymerase or the activator are still able to bind to their DNA sites, but their function is blocked. In the case of Lambda repressor, the situation is clear. The -35 box of the P_{RM} promoter, which lies immediately adjacent to the divergently transcribed P_R promoter is flanked by the operators O_R1 and O_R2 (Figure 1.2). The -10 box partly overlaps with O_R1 and the -35 box partly overlaps with O_R2. The presence of Lambda repressor on O_R1 and O_R2 precludes binding of RNA polymerase at P_R, while it does not inhibit RNA polymerase to sit on P_{RM} (Meyer et al, 1980).

In the case of Lac repressor, the answer is not straightforward. One has to consider two cases: first the loop between O3 and O1, and second the loop between O2 and O1 (Figure 1.3). All in vivo experiments should be performed with low (ideally I^+) amounts of Lac repressor (10 tetramers per cell). The same holds true for in vitro experiments. Furthermore, different sets of experiments should be done, one in the absence of O2 and the other in the absence of O3. This has not yet been done properly. So far the experiments seem to indicate that RNA polymerase but not CAP may be bound in an inactive form in presence of Lac repressor (Schmitz and Galas, 1979; Strainey and Crothers, 1987). There is one additional weak binding site for RNA polymerase close to, but upstream of the *lac* promoter (Malan and McLure, 1984). It is not clear whether or how it is involved in RNA polymerase binding when O1 is occupied by Lac repressor.

The repression of the *deo* system by Cyt repressor is noteworthy. Here the presence of CAP is required for Cyt repressor binding to P2 (Sogaard-Anderson et al, 1991). Finally, we would like to comment on a simple mode of repression which has been much discussed, the roadblock (Sellitti et al, 1987; Deuschle et al, 1986). Here, RNA polymerase is not hindered in binding to its promoter. It is also not kept inactive at the promoter. Instead, the operator lies far downstream of the promoter. We have compared the efficiency of O2 as a roadblock or as an operator at the position of O1. We find that it works at least 200 times less efficiency as a roadblock than at the proper position adjacent to the promoter (Oehler et al, 1994). This does not imply that the roadblock story is wrong. Either there are additional surrounding sequences which drastically increase the efficiency of the roadblock, or the efficiency is in general rather bad. This remains to be resolved.

The Molecular Mechanisms of Activation of Transcription

There are two activators of transcription in *E. coli* which have been analyzed in detail, Lambda repressor and CAP protein. Yet in both cases the molecular mechanisms of activation have not been elucidated. There are two possible types of activation. One of them is exceedingly simple, the other exceedingly complicated. In the simple case, activation is actually repression of repression. A particular repressor is precluded from binding by a different repressor, which itself does not interact with the original target of repression. It has been argued that activation of Gal4 is of this type (Croston et al, 1991). The negative charges of Gal4 may interact with the histones and dissolve the nucleosomes. The DNA may become naked and may thus be reached by RNA polymerase (Laybourn and Kadonaga, 1991). This could be true, if not in this case, in other cases of apparent activation. If this were generally true, it would indeed be a triumph of Leo Szilard and the Jacob-Monod repression theory (Jacob and Monod, 1961).

On the other hand, the activator may indeed stimulate RNA polymerase in an unknown manner. Wonderful metaphors have been used to describe this process. For example Mark Ptashne called this "tickling" of RNA polymerase in a seminar. One immediately understands what is meant, but unfortunately is still in doubt about the molecular interaction. Identification of a strong suppressor would be experimental proof for activation by protein-protein interaction. Starting with a mutant protein, which no longer activates because of a particular amino acid exchange but still binds to DNA, a mutant RNA polymerase should be found which is activated by this mutant protein but not any other activator. This suppression would prove the interaction of both molecules during activation, but one would still not understand the activation process itself.

What is the situation with Lambda repressor and CAP, the two best analyzed activators of *E. coli*? Two dimers of Lambda repressor bind cooperatively to the operators O_R1 and O_R2 (Figure 1.2). One subunit of the Lambda repressor bound to O_R2 interacts with RNA polymerase at P_{RM} and activates it. Three positive control (PC) mutant Lambda repressors have been found which abolish activation of transcription of the CI gene from the P_{RM} promoter (Guarente et al, 1982; Hochschild et al, 1983). Paradoxically one of them (Gly43-Arg) is so positioned that it can not easily reach RNA polymerase (Jordan and Pabo, 1992). One of the other positive control (PC) mutants Asp38-Asn (Hochschild et al, 1983) is suppressed by the mutation Arg596-His of the sigma70 factor (Li et al, 1994). In this case, positive control seems to be mediated at least partly by the sigma subunit of RNA polymerase. However, the spectre of repression of repression has been also raised as a partial explanation for the P_{RM} activation. RNA polymerase situated on P_R which is close to P_{RM} may inhibit the action of RNA polymerase on P_{RM} (Figure 1.2) (Hershberger and de Haseth, 1991; Hershberger et al, 1992).

The other activator which is well analysed is the CAP protein (Aiba et al, 1982; Cossart and Gicquel-Sanzey, 1982; Ebright, 1993; Kolb et al, 1993). The X-ray structure of the complex with its DNA target is known (Schultz et al, 1991). It can be seen that CAP bends the target DNA to which it is bound. This raises the first problem. It has been shown that if the CAP binding site is replaced by intrinsically bent DNA, the transcription rate increases about 20-fold (Bracco et al, 1989). Is the CAP-induced DNA bending sufficient for the activation? Does it explain all of the activation? The natural CAP-cAMP-DNA complex increases the rate of transcription in the *lac* and *gal* systems by about 50-fold. The distance between the CAP site and the start site of transcription differs in the *gal* and *lac* systems. In the *gal* system it is 41 bp upstream of the P1 starting point, whereas in the *lac* system it is 61 bp from the starting point. In the *gal* system, the CAP protein is thus placed directly next to the RNA polymerase. It has been shown that the CAP site has to be properly phased (Aiba et al, 1990; Gaston et al, 1990). The highest effect is seen at 41 bp. With increasing distance, activation becomes smaller. The next maxima are at 52, 61 and 72 bp. It should be noted that the effect at 72 bp distance is rather small. The resulting activation is only about fivefold. The fact that CAP has to be positioned very close to RNA polymerase indicates that the interaction between the two proteins, if there is any, is rather weak. Indeed, CAP and RNA polymerase are found to interact in solution with a dissociation constant of the complex of about $3 \times 10^{-7}\,M$ (Heyduk et al, 1993). This is close to the concentration of RNA-polymerase in *E. coli*.

The regions of the CAP protein and of RNA polymerase which putatively interact with each other have been defined (Williams et al, 1991; Ebright, 1993). In the CAP protein a loop between residues 156 and 163 is involved. The exchange of the single residue His 159 totally abolishes activation from both −61 and −41 bp (Bell et al, 1990).

Furthermore, in an elegant experiment, the subunit of the dimeric CAP protein which lies proximal to RNA polymerase has been shown to be solely responsible for activation (Zhou et al, 1993). In the α subunit of RNA polymerase, the 73 C-terminal residues have been defined to be responsible for interaction with CAP protein (Igarashi and Ishihama, 1991; Igarashi et al, 1991). A deletion of the C-terminal 73 or 94 codons of the α subunit reduces in vitro activation from position −61 at least 14-fold. Since a mutant of the sigma subunit has been identified as a suppressor for Lambda repressor activation, this implies that not only one subunit of RNA polymerase may be involved in activation. What is lacking is a suppressor mutation in the α subunit of RNA polymerase which suppresses a particular point mutation in the CAP loop which abolishes activation. This would define the interacting partner. However we may add that even if this is found, the actual mechanism of activation is still not understood.

Repressors from *E. coli* in Eukaryotic Cells and Eukaryotic Transcriptions Factors in *E. coli*

In order to study developmental processes, it would be helpful to experimentally control the expression rates of proteins of interest. For this purpose, it is desirable to introduce prokaryotic control systems, which can be easily turned on and off at will, into eukaryotic cells. The Lac repressor/operator system has been used for this purpose (Hu and Davidson, 1987; Brown et al, 1987; Figge et al, 1988). *lac* operator has been placed close to a viral TATA box, and Lac repressor has been overexpressed (Fuerst et al, 1989). It can be seen immediately that these constructs raise several problems. First, it is not known what the optimal distance is between *lac* operators for loop formation in mouse chromosomal DNA. In fact this problem has not been faced even superficially. Second, intensive overproduction of Lac repressor is necessary to get strong repression without DNA loop formation, and third, induction by IPTG requires that the inducer freely enters the cells one analyzes. Furthermore, IPTG will only partially induce if the concentration of Lac repressor is very high. The full induction which is observed with the wt *lac* system is due to the low amounts of Lac repressor (10^{-8} M) and the effective loops.

It can be understood that with these difficulties unresolved, other systems have been examined. In fact, the *tet* repressor/operator system seems most promising. Here, the repressor forms no DNA loops in *E. coli*. One dimer is enough to bind efficiently and with high specificity (Kleinschmidt et al,

1987). The first attempts to install this system in plant and yeast cells look most promising (Gatz et al, 1992; Faryar and Gatz, 1992).

Finally we may briefly ask the question, do eukaryotic transcription factors function in *E. coli*? Little has been published on this problem. Judging from our own experience with Gal4 (Paulmier et al, 1987) and glucocorticoid-receptor (Teichmann, 1991), we have come to the conclusion that it is almost impossible to use common *E. coli* strains as a background for measuring the effective binding of eukaryotic factors. Why is this so? One reason may be that many eukaryotic factors have essential disulfide bonds which are not formed in the cytoplasm of wt *E. coli*. The recent isolation of an *E. coli* mutant which allows disulfide bond formation in the cytoplasm without harming growth (Derman et al, 1993) is challenging in this context.

Conclusions

The difference between transcriptional control in the mouse and *E. coli* appears not to be determined by an exclusive use of a particular kind of module or mode of control. Rather, the overall architectures of their control machineries differ. Both organisms predominantly use alpha-helices as DNA-recognition units, and in both, positive and negative control can be found. The difference lies in how the cells make use of the protein-DNA recognition units. In *E. coli*, regulation means mainly a response to environmental stimuli which involves one or a few promoters. To achieve specific targeting of a promoter, one homodimeric DNA binding protein and one palindromic target site are sufficient. To increase the specificity of the interaction, cooperativity is often involved, which employs additional DNA-binding sites and the aggregation of dimeric regulatory proteins to at least tetramers. Regulation is direct, and regulatory cascades are the exception. On the other hand, the requirements are more complex for gene regulation in mouse cells. Here, developmental processes and cellular communication have to be controlled. There is 1000-fold more DNA, and the number of genes is about twenty times greater than in *E. coli* cells. Genes are often part of several different regulatory networks. One homodimeric transcription factor is incapable of binding exclusively to a unique sequence in the genome. Instead, multiple transcription factors, which alone bind only with low affinity to their target sites, form stable higher complexes by extensive cooperation with each other. Transcription factors are involved in the formation of several different regulatory complexes, which allows the achievement of complex control patterns in different tissues and during development, with relatively few regulatory proteins. Consequently, monomeric DNA-binding proteins (which recognize non-palindromic target sites) as well as heterodimeric association of transcription factors, both rare in bacteria, are commonly used in eukaryotes. Clearly, evolution has provided bacteria, with their relatively small amount of genetic material, as well as higher eukaryotes, with their about 1000-fold greater genome, with the optimal strategies of transcriptional control.

Acknowledgments

We would like to thank Ruth Ehring and Andrew Barker for discussion and Deutsche Forschungsgemeinschaft and the Bundesministerium für und Technologie for support of our experimental work.

References

Adhya S (1989): Multipartite genetic control elements: communication by DNA loop. *Ann Rev Gent* 23: 227–250

Adler J (1975): Chemotaxis in bacteria. *Ann Rev Biochem* 44: 341–356

Adler K, Beyreuther K, Fanning E, Geisler N, Gronenborn B, Klemm A, Müller-Hill B, Pfahl M, Schmitz A (1972): How *Lac* repressor binds to DNA. *Nature* 237: 322–327

Aiba H, Fujimoto S, Ozak N (1982): Molecular cloning and nucleotide sequencing of the gene for E. coli cAMP receptor protein. *Nucl Acids Res* 10: 1363–1378

Alberti S, Oehler S, v Wilcken-Bergmann B (1993): Genetic analysis of the leucine heptad repeats of Lac repressor: evidence for a 4-helical bundle. *EMBO J* 12: 3227–3236

Beckwith J, Davies J, Gallant JA, eds. (1983): *Gene Function in Procaryotes*. Cold Spring Harbor: Cold Spring Harbor Laboratory Press

Bell A, Gaston K, Williams R, Chapman K, Kolb A, Buc H, Minchin S, Williams J, Busby S (1990): Mutations that alter the ability of the *Escherichia coli* cyclic AMP receptor protein to activate transcription. *Nucl Acids Res* 18: 7243–7250

Berg JN, von Opheusden JHJ, Burgering MJM, Boelens R, Kaptein R (1990): Structure of Arc repressor in solution: Evidence for a family of β-sheet DNA-binding proteins. *Nature* 346: 586–589

Berg OG, Winter RB, von Hippel PH (1981): Diffusion-driven mechanisms of protein translocation on nucleic acids. 1. Models and theory. *Biochemistry* 20: 6929–6948

Blackwood EM, Eisenman RN (1991): Max: A helix-loop-helix zipper protein that forms a sequence-specific DNA-binding complex with myc. *Science* 251:1211–1217

Boyd A, Simon M (1982): Bacterial chemotaxis. *Ann Rev Physiol* 44: 501–517

Bracco L, Kotlarz D, Kolb A, Dieckmann S, Buc H (1989): Synthetic curved DNA sequences can act as transcriptional activators in *Escherichia coli*. *EMBO J* 8: 4289–4296

Brennan RG (1992): DNA recognition by the helix-turn-helix motif. *Curr Op Str Biol* 2: 100–108

Brown M, Figge J, Hansen U, Wright C, Jeang K-T, Khoury G, Livingston DM,

Roberts TM (1987): *Lac* repressor can regulate expression from a hybrid *SV40* early promoter containing a *lac* operator in animal cells. *Cell* 49: 603–612

Chamness GC, Willson CD (1970): An unusual *lac* repressor mutant. *J Mol Biol* 53: 561–565

Cossart P, Gicquel-Sanzey B (1982): Cloning of the *crp* gene of *Escherichia coli* K12. *Nucl Acids Res* 10: 1363–1378

Cowell IG (1994): Repression versus activation in the control of gene transcription. *TIBS* 19: 38–42

Croston GE, Kerrigan LA, Lira LM, Marshak DR, Kadonaga JT (1991): Sequence-specific antirepression of histone H1-mediated inhibition of basal RNA polymerase II transcription. *Science* 251: 644–649

Derman AI, Prinz WA, Belin D, Beckwith J (1993): Mutations that allow disulfide bond formation in the cytoplasm of *Escherichia coli*. *Science* 262: 1744–1747

Deuschle U, Gentz R, Bujard H (1986): *Lac* repressor blocks transcribing RNA polymerase and terminates transcription. *Proc Natl Acad Sci USA* 83: 4134–4137

de Crombrugghe B, Busby S, Buc H (1984): Cyclic AMP receptor protein: Role in transcription activation. *Science* 224: 831–838

Drlica K, Rouviere-Yaniv J (1987): Histonelike proteins of bacteria. *Microb Rev* 51: 301–319

Ebright R. (1993): Transcription activation at Class I CAP-dependent promoters. *Molecular Microbiology* 8 (5): 797–802

Ellenberger TE, Brandl CJ, Struhl K, Harrison SC (1992): The GCN4 basic region leucine zipper binds DNA as a dimer of uninterrupted α-helices: crystal structure of the protein-DNA complex. *Cell* 71: 1223–1237

Emmer M, de Chrombrugghe B, Ractan I, Perlman R (1970): Cyclic AMP receptor protein of *E. coli*: Its role in the synthesis of inducible enzymes. *Proc Natl Acad Sci USA* 66: 480–487

Englesberg E, Irr J, Power N, Lee J (1965): Positive control of enzyme synthesis by gene C in the L-arabinose system. *J Bact* 90: 946–957

Faryar K, Gatz C (1992): Construction of a tetracycline-inducible promoter in *Schizosaccharomyces pombe*. *Curr Genet* 21: 345–349

Ferré-d'Amaré A-R, Prendergast GC, Ziff EB, Burley SK (1993): Recognition by Max of its cognate DNA through a dimeric b/HLH/Z domain. *Nature* 363: 38–45

Fickert R, Müller-Hill B (1992): How Lac repressor finds *lac* operator *in vitro*. *J Mol Biol* 226: 59–68

Figge J, Wright C, Collins CJ, Roberts TM, Livingston DM (1988): Stringent regulation of stably integrated chloramphenicol acetyl transferase genes by E. coli *Lac* repressor in monkey cells. *Cell* 52: 713–722

Flashner Y, Gralla JD (1988): DNA dynamic flexibility and protein recognition: differential stimulation by bacterial histone-like protein HU. *Cell* 54: 713–721

Fritz H-J, Bicknäse H, Gleumes B, Heibach C, Rosahl S, Ehring R (1988): Characterization of two mutations in the *Escherichia coli galE* gene inactivating the second galactose operator and comparative studies of repressor binding. *EMBO J* 2: 2129–2135

Fuerst TR, Fernandez MP, Moss B (1989): Transfer of the inducible *lac* repressor/ operator system from *Escherichia coli* to a vaccinia virus expression vector. *Proc Natl Acad Sci USA* 86: 2549–2553

Gaston K, Bell A, Kolb A, Buc H (1990): Stringent spacing requirements for transcription activation by CAP. *Cell* 62: 733–743

Gatz C, Frohberg C, Wendenburg R (1992): Stringent repression and homogeneous de-repression by tetracycline of a modified CaMV 35S promoter in intact transgenic tobacco plants. *Plant J* 3: 397–404

Gehring WJ, Müller M, Affolter M, Percival-Smith A, Billeter M, Qian YQ, Otting G, Wüthrich K (1990): The structure of the homeodomain and its functional implications. *TIG* 6: 323–329

Gilbert W, Müller-Hill B (1966): Isolation of the Lac repressor. *Proc Natl Acad Sci USA* 56: 1891–1898

Gilbert W, Müller-Hill B (1970): The lactose repressor. In: *The Lactose Operon*, Beckwith JR, Zipser D, eds. Cold Spring Harbor: Cold Spring Harbor Laboratory Press

Gilbert W, Majors J, Maxam A (1976): How proteins recognize DNA sequences. In: *Organization and Expression of Chromosomes, Dahlem Konferenzen*, Allfrey VG, Bautz EKF, McCarthy BJ, Schimke RT, Tissières A, eds. Berlin: Abakon Verlagsgesellschaft

Grunstein M (1990): Nucleosomes: regulators of transcription. *TIG* 6: 395–400

Guarente L, Birmingham-McDonogh O (1992): Conservation and evolution of transcriptional mechanisms in eucaryotes. *TIG* 6: 395–400

Guarente L, Nye JS, Hochschild A, Ptashne M (1982): Mutant phage repressor with a specific defect in its positive control function. *Proc Natl Acad Sci USA* 79: 2236–2239

Hammer-Jespersen K, Munch-Petersen A (1975): Multiple regulation of nucleoside catabolizing enzymes: Regulation of the *deo* operon by the *cytR* and *deoR* gene products. *Mol Gen Genet* 137: 327–335

Hanes SD, Brent R (1989): DNA specificity of the Bicoid Activator Protein is determined by Homeodomain recognition helix residue 9. *Cell* 57: 1275–1283

Harrison SC, Aggarwal AK (1990): DNA recognition by proteins with the helix-turn-helix motif. *Ann Rev Biochem* 59: 933–969

Hershberger PA, deHaseth PL (1991): RNA polymerase bound to the P_R promoter of bacteriophage λ inhibits open complex formation at the divergently transcribed P_{RM} promoter. *J Mol Biol* 222: 479–494

Hershberger P, Mita BC, Tripatara A, deHaseth PL (1992): Interference by P_R-bound RNA polymerase with P_{RM} function *in vitro*. *J Biol Chem* 268: 8943–8948

Heyduk T, Lee JC, Ebright YW, Blatter EE, Zhou Y, Ebright RH (1993): CAP interacts with RNA polymerase in solution in the absence of promoter DNA. *Nature* 264: 548–549

Hochschild A, Irwin N, Ptashne M (1983): Repressor structure and the mechanism of positive control. *Cell* 32: 319–325

Hu MC-T, Davidson N (1987): The inducible *lac* operator-repressor system is functional in mammalian cells. *Cell* 48: 555–566

Igarashi K, Hanamura A, Makino K, Aiba H, Aiba H, Mizuno T, Nataka A, Ishihama A (1991): Functional map of the α subunit of *Escherichia coli* RNA polymerase: Two models of transcription activation by positive factors. *Proc Natl Acad Sci USA* 88: 8958–8962

Igarashi K, Ishihama, A (1991): Bipartite functional map of the E. coli RNA polymerase subunit: Involvement of the C-terminal region in transcription activation by cAMP-CRP. *Cell* 65: 1015–1022

Irani MH, Orosz L, Adhya S (1983): A control element within a structural gene: the *gal* operon of *Escherichia coli*. *Cell* 32: 783–788

Jacob F, Monod J (1961): Genetic regulatory mechanisms in the synthesis of proteins. *J Mol Biol* 3: 318–356

Janson L, Pettersson U (1990): Cooperative interactions between transcription factors Sp1 and OFT-1. *Proc Natl Acad Sci USA* 87: 4732–4736

Jobe A, Bourgeois S (1972): The *Lac* repressor-operator interaction VII. A repressor with unique binding properties: the X86 repressor. *J Mol Biol* 72: 139–152

Johnson AD, Meyer BJ, Ptashne M (1979): Interactions between DNA-bound repressors govern regulation by the λ phage repressor. *Proc Natl Acad Sci USA* 76: 5061–5065

Johnson PF, McKnight SL (1989): Eucaryotic transcriptional regulatory proteins. *Annu Rev Biochem* 58: 799–839

Jordan SR, Pabo CO (1988): Structure of the Lambda complex at 2.5 Å resolution: Details of the repressor-operator interactions. *Science* 242: 839–899

Kao-Huang Y, Revzin A, Butler A, O'Conner P, Noble D, von Hippel P (1977): Nonspecific DNA binding of genome-regulating proteins as a biological control mechanism: Measurement of DNA-bound *E. coli lac* repressor *in vivo*. *Proc Nat Acad Sci USA* 74: 4228–4232

Kaptein R, Zuiderweg ERP, Scheek RM, Boelens R, van Gunsteren WF (1985): A protein structure from nuclear magnetic resonance data. *Lac* repressor headpiece. *J Mol Biol* 182: 179–182

Khoury AM, Nick HS, Lu P (1991): *In vivo* interaction of *Escherichia coli Lac* repressor N-terminal fragments with the *lac* operator. *J Mol Biol* 219: 623–634

Kleinschmidt C, Tovar K, Hillen, W, Porschke D (1987): Dynamics of repressor-operator recognition: The Tn*10*-encoded tetracycline resistance control. *Biochemistry* 27: 1094–1104

Knight KL, Bowie JV, Vershon AK, Kelley RD, Sauer RT (1989): The Arc and Mnt repressors. A new class of sequence-specific DNA-binding protein. *J Biol Chem* 264: 3639–3642

Kolb A, Busby S, Garges S, Adhya S (1993): Transcriptional regulation by cAMP and its receptor protein. *Ann Rev Biochem* 62: 749–795

Kolkhof P (1992): Specificities of three tight-binding Lac repressors. *Nucl Acids Res* 20: 5035–5039

Kolkhof P, Teichmann D, Kisters-Woike B, Wilcken-Bergmann Bv, Müller-Hill B (1992): Lac repressor with the helix-turn-helix motif of cro binds to *lac* operator. *EMBO J* 11: 3031–3038

Kristie TM, LeBovitz JH, Sharp PA (1989): The octamer-binding proteins form multi-protein complexes with the HSV α TIF regulatory protein. *EMBO J* 8: 4229–4238

Lawrence, PA (1992): *The making of a fly. The genetics of animal design.* London: Blackwell Scientific Publications

Laybourn PJ, Kadonaga JT (1991): Role of nucleosomal cores and histone H1 in regulation of transcription by RNA polymerase II. *Science* 254: 238–245

Li M, Moyle H, Susskind MM (1994): Target of the transcriptional activation function of phage λcI protein. *Science* 263: 75–77

Lin S-Y, Riggs AD (1975): The general affinity of *lac* repressor for E. coli DNA: Implications for gene regulation in procaryotes and eucaryotes. *Cell* 4: 107–111

Little JW (1984): Autodigestion of *lexA* and phage lambda repressors. *Proc Natl Acad Sci USA* 81: 1357–1359

Losick R, Chamberlin M (1976): *RNA Polymerase.* Cold Spring Harbor: Cold Spring Harbor Laboratory Press

Malan TP, McLure WR (1984): Dual promoter control of the Escherichia coli Lactose operon. *Cell* 39: 173–180

Maniatis T, Ptashne M, Backman K, Kleid D, Flashman S, Jeffrey A, Maurer R (1975): Recognition sequences of repressor and polymerase in the operators of bacteriophage lambda. *Cell* 5: 109–113

Meyer BJ, Maurer R, Ptashne M (1980): Gene regulation at the right operator (O_R) of bacteriophage λ II. O_R1, O_R2, and O_R3: their roles in mediating the effects of repressor and cro. *J Mol Biol* 139: 163–194

McKnight SL, Yamamoto KR (1992): *Transcriptional Regulation*. Vol. 1 and 2. Cold Spring Harbour: Cold Spring Harbor Laboratory Press

Miller JH, Reznikoff WS, eds. (1978): *The Operon*. Cold Spring Harbor: Cold Spring Harbor Laboratory Press

Mitchell PJ, Tjian R (1989): Transcriptional regulation in mammalian cells by sequence-specific DNA-binding proteins. *Science* 245: 371–378

Mowbray SL, Cole LB (1992): 1.6 Å X-ray structure of the periplasmic ribose receptor from *Escherichia coli*. *J Mol Biol* 225: 155–175

Müller (1994): unpublished observation

Müller MM, Gerstner T, Schaffner W (1988): Enhancer sequences and regulation of gene transcription. *Eur J Biochem* 176: 485–495

Müller-Hill B (1971): Lac Repressor. *Angew Chem Int Ed* 10: 160–172

Müller-Hill B (1983): Sequence homology between Lac and Gal repressors and three sugar-binding periplasmatic proteins. *Nature* 302: 163–164

Nichols JC, Vyas NK, Quiocho FA, Matthews KS (1993): Models of Lactose repressor core based on alignment with sugar-binding proteins is concordant with genetic and chemical data. *J Biol Chem* 268: 17602–17612

Nicklin MJH, Casari G (1991): A single mutation in a truncated Fos protein allows it to interact with the TRE *in vitro*. *Oncogene* 6: 173–179

Oehler S, Amouyal M, Kolkhof P, Wilcken-Bergmann Bv, Müller-Hill B (1994); Quality and position of the three *lac* operators of E. *coli* define efficiency of repression. *EMBO J* 13; 3348–3355

Oehler S, Eismann ER, Krämer H, Müller-Hill B (1990): The three operators of the *lac* operon cooperate in repression. *EMBO J* 9: 973–979

Ogata RT, Gilbert W (1978): An amino-terminal fragment of *Lac* repressor binds specifically to *lac* operator. *Proc Natl Acad Sci USA* 75: 5851–5854

Otwinowski Z, Schevitz RW, Zhang R-G, Lawson CL, Joachimiak A, Marmorstein RQ, Luisi BF, Sigler PB (1988): Crystal structure of *trp* repressor/operator complex at atomic resolution. *Nature* 335: 321–329

Pabo CO, Sauer RT (1984): Protein-DNA recognition. *Ann Rev Biochem* 53: 293–321

Pabo CO, Sauer RT, Sturtevant, JM, Ptashne M (1979): The λ repressor contains two domains. *Proc Natl Acad Sci USA* 76: 1608–1612

Paulmier N, Yaniv M, von Wilcken-Bergmann B, Müller-Hill B (1987): *gal4* transcription activator protein of yeast can function as a repressor in *Escherichia coli*. *EMBO J* 6: 3539–3542

Pettijohn DE (1988): Histone-like proteins and bacterial chromosome structure. *J Biol Chem* 263: 12793–12796

Pfahl M (1976): *Lac* repressor-operator interaction. Analysis of the X86 repressor mutant. *J Mol Biol* 106: 857–869

Pirrotta V (1975): Sequence of the O_R operator of phage λ *Nature* 254: 114–117

Ptashne M (1992): *A genetic Switch*. Cambridge: Blackwell Scientific Publications & Cell Press

Ptashne M, Backmann K, Humayun MZ, Jeffrey A, Maurer R, Meyer B, Sauer RT

(1976): Autoregulation and function of a repressor in bacteriophage lambda. *Science* 194: 156–161

Ransone LJ, Wamley P, Morley KL, Verma A (1990): Domain swapping reveals the modular nature of Fos, Jun, and CREB proteins. *Mol Cell Biol* 10: 4565–4573

Reitzer LJ, Magasanik B (1986): Transcription of *glnA* in *E. coli* is stimulated by activator bound to sites far from the promoter. *Cell* 45: 785–792

Renkawitz R (1990): Transcriptional repression in eucaryotes. *TIG* 6: 192–196

Reznikoff WS, Abelson JN (1978): The *Lac* promoter. In: *The Operon*, Miller JH, Reznikoff WS, eds. Cold Spring Harbor: Cold Spring Harbor Laboratory Press

Reznikoff WS, Winter RB, Hurley CK (1974): The location of the repressor binding sites in the *lac* operon. *Proc Natl Acad Sci USA* 79: 2314–2318

Rickenberg HV, Cohen GN, Buttin G, Monod J (1956): La galactoside-permease d'*Escherichia coli*. *Ann Inst Pasteur* 91: 829–857

Roberts JW, Roberts CW (1975): Proteolytic cleavage of bacteriophage Lambda repressor in induction. *Proc Natl Acad Sci USA* 72: 147–151

Schmitz A, Galas DJ (1979): The interaction of RNA polymerase and lac repressor with the lac control region. *Nucl Acids Res* 6: 111–137

Schüle R, Muller M, Kaltschmidt C, Renkawitz R (1988): Many transcription factors interact synergetically with steroid receptors. *Science* 242: 1418–1420

Schultz SC, Shields GC, Steitz TA (1991): Crystal structure of a CAP-DNA complex: The DNA is bent by 90°. *Science* 253: 1001–1007

Schwartz M (1967): Sur l'existence chez *Escherichia coli* K12 d'une régulation commune à la biosynthèse des receptors du bactériophage et au métabolisme du maltose. *Ann Inst Pasteur* 113: 685–704

Sellitti MA, Pavco PA, Steege DA (1987): *Lac* repressor blocks *in vivo* transcription of *lac* control region DNA. *Proc Natl Acad Sci USA* 84: 3199–3203

Shore D, Langowski J, Baldwin RL (1981): DNA flexibility studied by covalent closure of short fragments into circles. *Proc Natl Acad Sci USA* 78: 4833–4837

Simons (1984): unpublished observation

Sogaard-Anderson L, Pedersen H, Holst B, Valentin-Hansen P (1991): A novel function of the cAMP-CRP complex in Escherichia coli: cAMP-CRP repressor an adaptor for the CytR repressor in the *deo* operon. *Mol Microbiol* 5: 969–975

Somers WS, Phillips SEV (1992): Crystal structure of the *met* repressor-operator complex at 2.8 Å resolution reveals DNA recognition by β strands. *Nature* 359: 387–393

Staacke D, Walter B, Kisters-Woike B, Wilcken-Bergmann Bv, Müller-Hill B (1990): How Trp repressor binds to its operator. *EMBO J* 9: 1963–1967

Straney SB, Crothers DM (1987): Lac repressor is a transient gene activating protein. *Cell* 51: 699–707

Struhl K (1989): Molecular mechanism of transcriptional regulation in yeast. *Annu Rev Biochem* 58: 1051–1077

Takeda Y (1979): Specific repression of *in vitro* transcription by the Cro repressor of bacteriophage λ. *J Mol Biol* 127: 177–189

Teichmann (1991): unpublished observation

Vyas NK, Vyas MN, Quiocho FA (1988): Sugar and signal-transducer binding sites of the *Escherichia coli* galactose chemoreceptor protein. *Science* 242: 1290–1295

Vyas NK, Vyas MN, Quiocho FA (1991): Comparison of the periplasmic receptors for L-arabinose, D-glucose/D-galactose, and D-ribose. *J Biol Chem.* 266: 5226–5237

Walker GC (1984): Mutagenesis and inducible responses to deoxyribonucleic acid damage in *Escherichia coli*. *Microbiol Rev* 48: 60–93

Williams R, Bell A, Sims G, Busby S (1991): The role of two surface exposed loops in transcription activation by the *Escherichia coli* CRP and FNR proteins. *Nucl Acids Res* 19: 6705–6712

Zhou Y, Busby S, Ebright RH (1993): Identification of the functional subunit of a dimeric transcription activator protein by use of oriented heterodimers. *Cell* 73: 375–379

Zubay G, Schwartz D, Beckwith J (1970): Mechanism of activation of catabolite-sensitive genes: A positive control system. *Proc Natl Acad Sci USA* 66: 104–110

2

The Heat Shock Transcriptional Response

PAUL E. KROEGER AND RICHARD I. MORIMOTO

Introduction

The heat shock response represents one of the most dramatic changes in gene expression and has served as a paradigm for inducible transcriptional responses. The response to temperature elevation, exposure to toxic agents, or other physiological stresses is universal and mediated through the induction of a highly conserved set of genes referred to as heat shock (HS) genes (Lindquist, 1986; Lindquist and Craig, 1988; Morimoto and Milarski, 1990; Morimoto, 1993; Morimoto et al, 1994). Studies in the early 1970's had revealed that the elevation of temperature induces the synthesis of new polypeptides. It had been recognized early that these newly synthesized HS proteins (HSPs) are important to the survival response mounted by the cell. Perhaps the most significant effect of HS is on transcription. As the severity of the HS increases, the transcription of most genes is repressed and the genes coding for HSPs are transcriptionally induced 50 to 100-fold within minutes. HS has additional effects on mRNA stability and translational control which contribute to the preferential expression of HSPs (Lindquist, 1980; Storti et al, 1980; Banerji et al, 1984; Lindquist and Craig, 1988).

The heat shock response represents a safeguard mechanism that the cell employs for survival following exposure to physiological stress. Because of their rapid induction, studies on HSPs have emphasized the inducible response; yet many of the HS proteins are also constitutively expressed. The function of constitutive and inducible HSPs is to regulate the folding of newly synthesized proteins in the cell and to protect or assist in the refolding of proteins during heat shock (Gething and Sambrook, 1992; Craig et al, 1993; Hendrick and Hartl, 1993). Because of their role in these pathways the heat shock proteins are often referred to as chaperones (Rothman, 1989; Hightower, 1991; Gething and Sambrook, 1992; Craig et al, 1993; Hendrick and Hartl, 1993). Consistent with a role for HSPs in protein folding the

INDUCIBLE GENE EXPRESSION, VOLUME 1
P.A. Baeuerle, Editor
© 1995 Birkhäuser Boston

Saccaromyces cerevisiae chaperones Ssb (HSP70) and SIS1 (DnaJ homolog) have been found in association with nascent polypeptide chains and are required for translation (Nelson et al, 1992; Zong and Arndt, 1993). The concentration of certain HSPs such as HSP70 in the nucleolus of stressed cells presumably reflects the need for these proteins in ribosome biogenesis and the sensitivity of this process to heat (Welch and Feramisco, 1984). The general function of heat shock proteins is of great interest but beyond the scope of this review so we refer readers to some recent reviews on the subject (Gething and Sambrook, 1992; Hartl et al, 1992; Craig et al, 1993; Georgopoulos and Welch, 1993; Hendrick and Hartl, 1993).

This chapter will describe the current state of knowledge on the activation of heat shock responsive genes. We will emphasize studies on the regulation of the HSP70 gene and the role of the inducible heat shock transcription factor (HSF) in HS gene transcription. Since HSF is the activator responsible for inducible HSP gene transcription, we will focus on the activation pathway of HSF from its latent state; interaction with the heat shock element (HSE) in the promoter of responsive genes; and the biochemistry and molecular biology of the HSF protein. The role of the HSP70 protein in autoregulation of HSP70 gene transcription through interaction with HSF will be discussed. Additionally, since the HSF protein is now known to be a family of factors in larger eukaryotes, a comparative approach has been employed to understand the contribution of each factor in the response to heat and other stresses.

Historical Background

The first reported studies on the genetic response of organisms to heat was in the early 1900s when *Drosophila melanogaster* larvae were subjected to heat shock at various stages of development (Goldschmidt, 1935). These and subsequent studies have revealed that heat shock or other treatments applied during the growth of an organism can adversely affect the developmental program (Capdevila and Garcia-Bellido, 1974; Pleet et al, 1981; Webster et al, 1985). These changes induce developmental defects or phenocopies that represent morphological alterations with phenotypic similarities to known homeotic mutations. Notably, it has been found that the HS-induced phenocopies can be protected against by prior exposure to a mild heat shock.

How can a mild heat shock protect against a subsequent lethal exposure to heat? This question and others regarding the specific response of organisms to environmental and metabolic stress remained unanswered until the early 1960s. In 1962, Ritossa observed that exposure of *Drosophila* polytene chromosomes to heat shock or other stresses results in the appearance of specific chromosomal puffs (Ritossa, 1962). This was the first suggestion that the response to heat shock is genetically regulated. Subsequent studies have demonstrated, by metabolic labeling, that heat shock results in the enhanced and in some cases de novo synthesis of a new set of polypeptides in Drosophila larvae and tissue culture cells (Tissieres et al, 1974; Lindquist-McKenzie et al, 1975; Spradling et al, 1975). Further studies have demonstrated, by the use of in situ hybridization, that the chromosomal puffs correspond to the selective transcriptional activation of heat shock genes. Messenger RNA isolated from polysomes of heat shocked cells have demonstrated that translation in vitro yields the same set of proteins that are observed upon metabolic labeling of heat shocked cells in vivo (Lindquist-McKenzie and Meselson, 1977; Spradling et al, 1977). These results established that the chromosomal puffs correspond to genes whose activity is induced in response to heat. The subsequent cloning of the genes for the heat shock proteins has been aided through this enrichment of HS mRNAs on polysomes. In the ensuing years the cloning of HS genes from a variety of organisms has demonstrated that the heat shock response is, nearly universal and that the genes encoding the HSPs are conserved at the nucleotide level (Livak et al, 1978; Craig et al, 1979; Holmgren et al, 1979; Moran et al, 1979; Corces et al, 1980; Voellmy et al, 1981; Lowe et al, 1983; Hunt and Morimoto, 1985; Voellmy et al, 1985; Wu et al, 1985; Morimoto et al, 1986).

Inducers Of The Heat Shock Response

An understanding of the heat shock response requires an appreciation of the myriad of conditions that lead to elevated levels of HSPs. Initial studies of inducers of the heat shock response in *Drosophila* have not been restricted to temperature and include exposure to salicylate, dinitrophenol, ethanol, and anoxia, all of which induce the same chromosomal puffs as have been induced by HS (Ritossa, 1962; Ashburner, 1970; Tissieres et al, 1974; Lindquist-Mckenzie et al, 1975). Thus, the expression of HSPs can be induced by many conditions which can be divided into three general classes: environmental stress, physiological stress, and nonstressful conditions (Figure 2.1).

Environmental stress

This type of stress is typified by the exposure of cells to heat shock, heavy metals, and amino acid analogs. These treatments have been shown to

CELLULAR STRESS RESPONSE

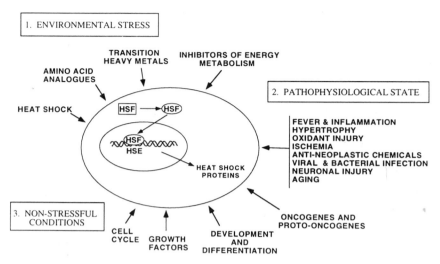

Figure 2.1 Conditions that can induce the expression of heat shock proteins. The three general classes known to induce stress proteins are shown including: (1) environmental stress; (2) pathophysiological conditions; and (3) non stressful conditions such as cell cycle and developmental pathways. Although the activation of Heat Shock Factor (HSF) from a latent to activated state is portrayed schematically, this is only relevant to environmental and pathophysiological stresses. There are other mechanisms for the induction of heat shock genes that do not involve HSF and these are discussed in the text. HSE = Heat Shock Element.

cause protein denaturation and result in the synthesis of malfolded proteins thus triggering the need for increased levels of chaperones such as HSP70 (Goff and Goldberg, 1985; Anathan et al, 1986; Beckmann et al, 1990; Baler et al, 1992; Nelson et al, 1992). Is there a correlation between the rapidity of the HS response and effects on the folded state of nascent or pre existing proteins? Heat shock has immediate effects on protein conformation, whereas other inducers of the HS response, such as the amino acid analog azetidine, must be incorporated into nascent polypeptide chains and are consequently slower to induce the heat shock response (Mosser et al, 1988). Therefore the kinetics, duration and magnitude of the response to environmental stress is dependent on the type of insult.

The severity of the stress can determine the degree to which the cell responds and suggests that the cell is capable of measuring the level of stress (DiDomenico et al, 1982; Mosser et al, 1988; Abravaya et al, 1991a). When the temperature of human HeLa cells grown at 37°C has been raised to 42°C (ΔT = 5°C), the HSP70 gene is transcriptionally induced through the activation of HSF. The activation of HSP70 transcription at 42°C is sensitive to cycloheximide suggesting that it is the malfolding of nascent polypeptide chains that the cell senses (Amici et al, 1992). However, even in the presence of continuous HS the response is transient and attenuates after approximately 2 hr (Figure 2.2). In contrast, if the heat shock temperature is 43°C ($\Delta T = 6°C$) then transcription of the HSP70 gene does not attenuate and is insensitive to cycloheximide suggesting a more generalized effect on protein conformation (Abravaya et al, 1991b). Presumably at 42°C, after sufficient HSPs have been synthesized, the transcriptional response is down regulated. However, at 43°C the cell is incapable of synthesizing sufficient HSPs to overcome the effect of this severe stress. The transcriptional attenuation of the HSP70 gene at 42°C has been proposed to occur through an auto regulatory mechanism which will be discussed in detail below.

The temperature at which the HS response is activated is dependent on the optimal growth temperature for the organism, and generally HS occurs when the ambient temperature is raised ≈5° to 6°C above this optimum. The normal growth temperature for *Drosophila* is ≈25°C and when human HSF1 (see section below on multiple HSFs in large eukaryotes) is expressed in *Drosophila* cells it is activated at ≈10°C below its normal activation temperature of 42°C (Clos et al, 1993). Conversely, when *Drosophila* HSF is expressed in human cells it becomes constitutively active at non-heat-shock temperatures for human cells,

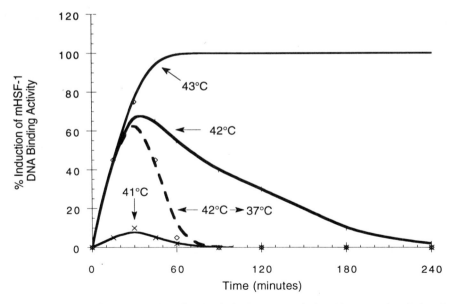

Figure 2.2 Schematic representation of the level of HSP70 transcription. Shown are the relative of HSP70 transcription in human HeLa cells during a continuous 42°C heat shock; the attenuation of transcription when cells are shifted from 42°C to 37°C; and the level of transcription during a continuous 43°C heat shock.

37°C. Additionally, when human HeLa cells are grown at 35°C, a lower then normal temperature, HSF1 is activated at a lower heat shock temperature of 41°C (Abravaya et al, 1991b). Therefore, it can be concluded that the temperature at which an HSF is activated is not strictly intrinsic to the factor, but can be reprogrammed dependent on the environment in which the HSF is expressed.

The ability of the cell to sense the type and severity of stress and respond appropriately is reflected in the overlapping pathways for the activation of HSP genes. Certain family members (e.g. HSP70) are induced strongly by heat and heavy metals and other members (e.g. GRP78) are primarily metal inducible or responsive to malfolded proteins in the endoplasmic reticulum (Morimoto and Milarski, 1990; Vogel et al, 1990; Watowich et al, 1991; Wooden et al, 1991; Dorner et al, 1992). The yeast GRP78/Bip gene, which has an HSE, is heat inducible (several fold) whereas the mammalian GRP78/Bip gene has no HSE yet is also somewhat HS inducible (Watowich et al, 1991; Kohno et al, 1993; Li et al, 1994). Whether the induction of mammalian GRP78/Bip is mediated through HSF remains to determined. Studies in yeast have suggested that HSF need not necessarily be bound to the DNA to activate transcription (Jakobsen and Pelham, 1991). There are likely intersecting pathways for the response to environmental stress because cadmium can induce HSP70 transcription in cells that are attenuating during a continuous heat shock (Morimoto et al, 1990). Analysis of HSP70 promoter mutants has demonstrated that the HS and metal responsive elements map to the binding site for HSF (Williams and Morimoto, 1990). This suggests that the cadmium induction of HSP70 transcription during HS attenuation occurs through an alternative activation pathway for HSF. Additionally, there are other stress induced genes, such as mammalian metallothionein I and II that are metal inducible, but unaffected by heat (Skroch et al, 1993). Heat shock does induce expression of the *S. cerevisiae* metallothionein gene (*CUP1*), and HSF has been shown to mediate this effect through HSE-like sequences in the binding sites for the *CUP1* regulatory protein, *ACE1* (Silar et al, 1991). Together these results suggest that cells have developed the capacity to sense environmental stress in different ways and may utilize multiple regulatory pathways to induce the appropriate genes required for survival.

Physiological stress

Knowledge regarding the induction of HSPs by physiological stress has been broadened greatly over the last several years through studies on the cellular response to viral infection, and traumas such as ischemia (Figure

2.1). The physiological stress perhaps most associated with the induction of heat shock proteins is ischemia. The blockage of blood flow results in anoxia, and the resulting induction of heat shock proteins have been correlated with cell survival (Marber et al, 1993). The induction of HSPs contributes to the cellular response to tissue damage, oxygen and nutrient deprivation. Also, reperfusion following ischemia can result in oxidant damage (Currie and White, 1993). Cell culture models utilizing myocardial cells can mimic the ischemic response and suggest that HSP70 can prevent ischemic damage if induced by a prior ischemic event or if HSP70 has been overexpressed by transient transfection (Benjamin et al, 1992; Williams and Benjamin, 1993). The stress response in the brain has also been a significant area of study as certain populations of neuronal cells are more sensitive to the effects of stress (Nowak and Abe, 1994). The brain responds to global and isolated ischemic events by synthesizing HSP70, and there is evidence that preischemic tolerance can be protective against neuronal damage (Pulsinelli et al, 1982; Blake et al, 1990a, Liu et al, 1992; Aoki et al, 1993). Why do neuronal cells exhibit varying sensitivity to heat? Recent studies have suggested that the sensitivity to heat of some neuronal cells may be due to a selective block in HSP70 expression that originates at the chromatin level (Mather et al, 1994). In these studies the induction of the HSP70 and HSP90 genes have been compared in Y79 retinoblastoma cells (of neuronal origin) and T98G glial cells. The HSP90 gene is heat inducible in both cell lines, whereas the induction of the HSP70 gene in the Y79 cells is significantly lower, and this correlates with a lack of basal transcription factor and HSF interaction in the HSP70 promoter. These results reveal tissue specific differences in the stress response. The role of chromatin and accessibility of HSE sequences will be addressed in more detail in a later section.

Several studies have demonstrated that the heat shock response can be activated in a tissue specific manner by certain physiological stresses (Blake et al, 1990b; Blake et al, 1991; Udelsman et al, 1993). Physical restraint of an animal results in the selective induction of HSP70 in the aorta and adrenal glands (Blake et al, 1991; Udelsman et al, 1993). Interestingly, this response was specific for only some HSPs as the HSP90 family was not induced in either the aorta or adrenals. Further studies of this phenomenon have demonstrated a direct link between the production of adrenocorticotropic hormone (ACTH) in the pituitary and the induction of HSP70 in the inner cortex of the adrenal glands (Blake et al, 1991). The induction of HSP70 in the aorta is not affected by ACTH but is blocked by an a_1-adrenergic blocking agent, prazosin (Udelsman et al, 1993). This result suggested that the neuroendocrine system can modulate the selective induction of HS genes in a tissue specific manner.

Unlike chronic disease states that affect specific tissues, aging is a pleiotropic decline in cellular function which has been characterized by an inability to respond appropriately to various stimuli. As a measure of the response to stress the induction of HSPs has been examined in a variety of model aging systems including primary fibroblasts of young and old animals as well as established tissue culture cell lines with limited doubling capacity. These studies have demonstrated a decrease in the inducibility of the heat shock response during aging and this correlates with a decrease in HSF DNA binding activity (Liu et al, 1989; Choi et al, 1990; Heydari et al, 1993). Recent studies have suggested that there are no differences in HSF levels due to aging thus implicating other mechanisms, perhaps the loss of a critical signaling molecule(s), for the decline in heat shock gene expression (Holbrook and Udelsman, 1994).

Nonstressful inducers

The variety of events that can affect the expression of the HSP genes is not surprising considering the fundamental role of these proteins. HSP70 transcription is modulated during progression through the cell cycle by various growth factors, developmental and differentiation pathways, and certain oncogenes (Figure 2.1) (Wu et al, 1986a; Wu et al, 1986b; Morimoto 1991; Phillips and Morimoto, 1991; Sistonen et al, 1992). Growth regulated expression of the HSP70 gene has been demonstrated in growth arrested HeLa cells and E1a transformed human embryonic kidney cells (293 cells) following the addition of fresh serum (Wu et al, 1985). Serum deprivation reduces basal transcription of the HSP70 gene and subsequent addition results in a 20-fold stimulation with HSP70 mRNA attaining maximal levels at 8 to 12 hr post-stimulation. Activation of HSP70 expression also occurs following the stimulation of resting T lymphocytes with IL-2 (Ferris et al, 1988). Transcription of the HSP70 gene is also regulated during the cell cycle (Milarski and Morimoto, 1986). There is a significant increase in the level of HSP70 mRNA at the G1/S boundary which correlates with the synthesis of HSP70 protein during early S-phase and its translocation to the nucleus. This, along with other studies, suggests that HSP70 is a growth regulated gene.

The activation of the HSP70 gene by serum and other nonstressful conditions is regulated by the basal promoter of the HSP70 gene (Figure 2.3). The identity and the role of the cis-acting elements that comprise the HSP70 basal promoter have been demonstrated (Wu et al, 1986b; Greene et al, 1987; Williams et al, 1989; Greene and Kingston, 1990; Williams and Morimoto, 1990). The CCAAT box at −74 basepairs is important for the function of the basal promoter and known to interact with two

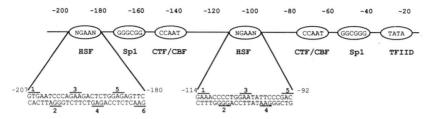

Figure 2.3 Transcription factor binding sites located in the proximal promoter of the human HSP70 gene. The elements are labeled and the critical sequence elements that compose the binding sites are displayed. These include the TATA box, CCAAT boxes, Sp1 sites, and proximal and distal HSEs.

factors, CBF and CTF (Morgan et al, 1987; Lum et al, 1990). CBF activates transcription from the HSP70 promoter and is regulated through direct interaction with p53 protein (Lum et al, 1990; Agoff et al, 1993). There are also binding sites for several other common basal factors such as Sp1 which can positively activate HSP70 gene transcription (Morgan, 1989). The basal promoter complex is also the target for the adenovirus E1a protein which activates HSP70 transcription during infection (Wu et al, 1986a; Williams et al, 1989). Taken together, the complex structure of the HSP70 promoter and the many inducers of the heat shock response demonstrate the diversity of conditions that can modulate and activate HSP70 transcription.

Isolation Of Heat Shock Transcription Factor And Characterization Of The Heat Shock Element

Based on the alignment of 5′ flanking regions from various cloned HSP genes it has been noticed that certain sequence motifs perhaps involved in the regulation of HSP genes are conserved (Holmgren et al, 1981). Among the homologous regions is the dyad symmetrical element (5′-CnnGAAnnTTCnnG-3′) referred to as the heat shock element or HSE (Pelham, 1982). When linked to the promoter of a heterologous reporter gene, this HSE is capable of rendering the reporter heat inducible (Corces et al, 1981; Mirault et al, 1982; Pelham and Bienz, 1982; Bienz and Pelham, 1986. Studies from the Lis and Voellmy laboratories have subsequently demonstrated that the HSE can be more accurately described as a series of pentameric units arranged as inverted adjacent arrays of the sequence 5′-nGAAn-3′ (Amin et al, 1988; Xiao and Lis, 1988; Perisic et al, 1989). A functional HSE is composed of a minimum of three pentamers, and reiteration of the pentamer results in higher affinity interactions between HSF and the HSE (Xiao et al, 1991; Kroeger et al,

1993). Comparison of the nucleotide composition of the HSE indicates that the guanine residue in the second position of each pentamer (5'-nGAAn-3') is absolutely conserved. The adjacent adenine residues are also highly conserved, but may be substituted by other bases. In the mammalian HSP70 and HSP90 promoters the HSE is composed of multiple pentameric units, five and six respectively, in close proximity to the basal promoter elements (Williams and Morimoto, 1990). The activity and interdependence of the HSE in the context of the basal promoter elements has been examined (Greene and Kingston, 1990; Williams and Morimoto, 1990). These studies have demonstrated that the HSE is rotationally independent; however, the degree of induction by heat is dependent on the distance between the HSE and the basal promoter and cooperation with basal factors.

An important step in the understanding of HS gene regulation has been the in vivo detection of DNase 1 hypersensitivity in the 5' flanking region of the *Drosophila* HSP70 gene (Wu, 1980). It was proposed that the HSP70 promoter region is in an accessible configuration with access to trans-acting factors. Subsequent experiments, using exonuclease III footprinting, detected the binding of a protein to the HSE upon temperature elevation and demonstrated that factors are constitutively bound to the TATA box before and after heat stress (Wu, 1984). This suggests that a basal factor in cooperation with an inducible factor are required for the rapid transcriptional activation of the HSP genes of *Drosophila*.

Since the studies in *Drosophila* have demonstrated the appearance of a DNA binding activity that correlates with the induction of the HS genes, there has been considerable effort to identify this regulatory factor. The *S. cerevisiae* and *D. melanogaster* HSFs, induced by heat shock, have been purified and characterized (Sorger et al, 1987; Wu et al, 1987). Notably, the mature proteins are of different sizes (*S. cerevisiae* = 130 kDa; *D. melanogaster* = 110 kDa); they bind to the HSE sequence in vitro, and in the case of *Drosophila* HSF, has been shown to stimulate transcription. The heat induced HSE binding activity also has been detected in crude extracts of mammalian cells using a gel shift assay (Kingston et al, 1987). The HSF protein from *Drosophila* and mammalian cells has been shown to be latent in the cell and inducible with heat treatment (Zimarino and Wu, 1987; Larson et al, 1988; Mosser et al, 1988). The latent HSF can be activated by a variety of treatments that affect protein structure including in vitro heat shock, detergent, or mild denaturant treatment (Larson et al, 1988; Mosser et al, 1990). In contrast to the HSFs of larger eukaryotes, *S. cerevisiae* HSF has been shown to bind DNA constitutively (Sorger et al, 1987; Jakobsen and Pelham, 1988). Even though *S. cerevisiae* HSF is bound to DNA constitutively, heat shock is required to activate transcription, and this correlates well with HSF phosphorylation (Sorger and Pelham, 1988). Not all yeasts exhibit this type of HSF regulation as the fission yeast *Schizosaccharomyces pombe* requires heat shock to activate both HSF DNA-binding and phosphorylation (Gallo et al, 1991). The role of phosphorylation in HSF function will be discussed below. Together these results demonstrate that the factor responsible for induction of HS genes in a number of organisms is functionally conserved and regulated posttranslationally as protein synthesis is not required for HSF induction.

The cloning of the *S. cerevisiae* and *D. melanogaster* HSF molecules reveals a number of important features regarding HSF structure and provides the tools for the isolation of homologues from a variety of organisms (Wiederrecht et al, 1988; Clos et al, 1990). Alignment of the cloned HSFs from yeasts, *Drosophila*, tomato, chicken, mouse, and humans demonstrates that there is a conserved ≈100 amino acid DNA-binding domain located in the N-terminus (Figure 2.4). Immediately adjacent to the DNA-binding domain is a second conserved region that contains three leucine zipper repeats responsible for trimerization of HSF in response to stress (Sorger and Nelson, 1989; Peteranderl and Nelson, 1992). Antibodies specific to each HSF are key tools in the analysis of structure and have been used to demonstrate that all HSFs are trimeric when activated (Sorger and Nelson, 1989; Rabindran et al, 1991; Kroeger et al, 1993; Sarge et al, 1993). In *D. melanogaster* and the larger eukaryotic HSFs an additional leucine zipper has been observed in the C-terminus, and it has been suggested to function in the negative regulation of HSF (Rabindran et al, 1993).

Cloning Of HSFs: Larger Eukaryotes Have A Family Of Factors

The most surprising result from the cloning of HSFs has been the isolation of multiple distinct factors from individual species (Figure 2.4). Two HSFs have been isolated from the human and mouse genome, and three from chicken and tomato (Scharf et al, 1990; Rabindran et al, 1991; Sarge et al, 1991; Schuetz et al, 1991; Nakai and Morimoto, 1993). At first approximation, all of these HSFs have a related structural organization; however, within a species multiple HSFs are ≈40% related at the level of the amino acid sequences largely due to the conservation of the DNA binding and oligomerization domains (Clos et al, 1990; Scharf et al, 1990; Rabindran et al, 1991; Sarge et al, 1991;

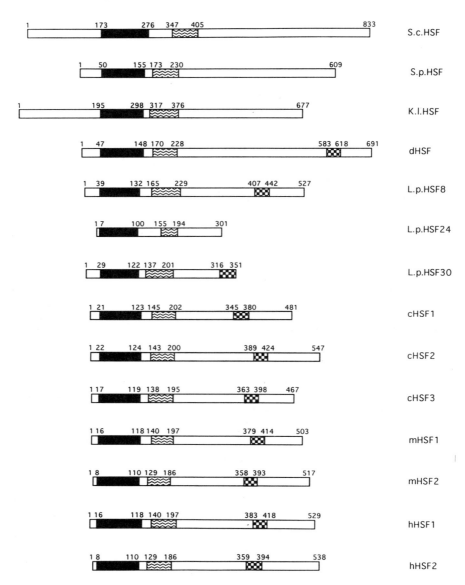

Figure 2.4 Comparison of the basic structural features of HSFs. The HSFs are aligned relative to the position of the conserved DNA-binding domain (shaded box). Adjacent to the DNA-binding domain there are a series of conserved leucine zippers responsible for HSF trimerization (striped box). In the metazoan HSFs there is a fourth leucine zipper motif at the C-terminus of the protein (checkered box). The length of each conserved region and protein is denoted in amino acids. The HSFs are denoted with abbreviations of genus and species as follows: S.c. HSF, *Saccharomyces cerevisiae* (yeast); K.l. HSF, *Kluyveromyces lactis* (yeast); S.p. HSF, *Schizosaccharomyces pombe* (yeast); dHSF, *Drosophila melanogaster* (insect); L.p. HSF8, L.p. HSF24, L.p. HSF30, *Lycopersicon peruvianum* (tomato plant); cHSF1, cHSF2, cHSF3, *Gallus domesticus* (chicken); mHSF1, mHSF2, *Mus musculus* (mouse); hHSF1, hHSF2, *Homo sapiens* (human).

Schuetz et al, 1991; Nakai and Morimoto, 1993). Between homologues from different species there is an 85% to 95% conservation at the sequence level (i.e., mHSF1 and hHSF1). Comparison of the three chicken HSFs with other cloned HSFs suggests that there is a common ancestor from which they diverged (Nakai and Morimoto, 1993). By comparison, the tomato HSFs (L.p. HSF8, HSF24, and HSF30), although similar in structure, have been isolated independently through binding site screening, and their nomenclature does not imply that they are related to the HSF1, 2 and 3 that have been isolated in other eukaryotes (Scharf et al, 1990).

Why have more than one HSF? The fact that only one HSF has been isolated from the yeasts and *Drosophila* suggests that the multiple HSFs of larger eukaryotes developed to fulfill the requirements of more complex organisms or for the expression of HS genes in response to a wider range of developmental and environmental cues. Studies have demonstrated that *S. cerevisiae* HSF is an essential gene with at least two transcriptional activation domains that can respond to sustained or transient heat stress (Nieto-Sotelo et al, 1990; Sorger, 1990). Perhaps the appearance of multiple HSFs in the larger eukaryotes signaled the division of these requirements among multiple factors.

The existence of multiple HSFs also raises the issue of their role in the HS response. Do all factors respond to the same stress signals, perhaps activating different target genes, or are they differentially activated in response to diverse signals? Specific antiserum to mHSF1 and mHSF2 has been used to demonstrate that the factor which is rapidly activated within minutes of temperature increase corresponds to only HSF1 (Sarge et al, 1993). If HSF1 is the factor that responds to heat, what is the role of HSF2? One answer comes from a reexamination of earlier studies which have demonstrated that hemin treatment of K562 erythroleukemia cells, which results in their nonterminal differentiation, also activates HSF DNA binding (Theordorakis et al, 1989). However, in contrast to the rapid induction of HSF1 in response to heat, hemin induced HSF is activated with slower kinetics with full activation requiring 16 to 24 hours. Also, in contrast to the heat activated HSF1, whose activity attenuates after several hours of continuous heat shock, the hemin induced HSF has been maintained in the active DNA-binding state for several days. Antibody perturbation experiments in conjunction with gel mobility shift assays have demonstrated conclusively that hemin induced HSF is composed of HSF2 (Figure 2.5). This provides a model system for the differential activation of multiple HSFs as the K562 cells can be heat-shocked and/or hemin treated. Simultaneous activation of HSF1 and HSF2 in K562 cells leads to a synergistic transcriptional activation of the

HSP70 gene suggesting that HSF1 and HSF2 interact (Sistonen et al, 1994). Other studies on mouse tissues have revealed that HSF2 mRNA is developmentally regulated and accumulates at high levels in the testis at the spermatocyte and round spermatid stages of development which suggests that HSF2 could be involved in the activation of testis specific HSP genes (Sarge et al, 1994). Additionally, several embryonic cell lines (F9, MEL) have a constitutive HSF2 binding activity although the function of this HSF activity has remained elusive as there is no apparent activation of HS genes in these cells in the absence of stress (Murphy and Phillips, 1994).

The cloning and characterization of a third distinct HSF from chickens (cHSF3) has suggested that there may be even more pathways for the

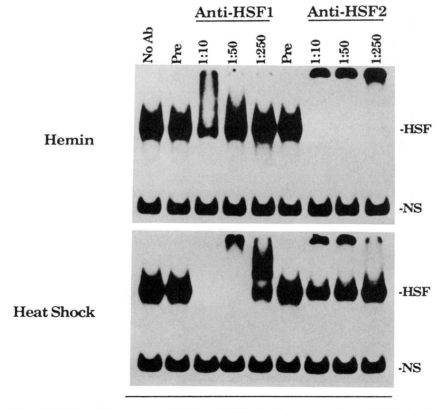

Figure 2.5 Differential activation of HSF1 and HSF2. Antibody recognition of HSF in hemin-treated (20 h; upper panel) and heat-shocked (45 min at 42°C, lower panel) K562 cells. Whole cell extracts were incubated either alone (No Ab), with a 1:10 dilution of preimmune serum, or with a 1:10, 1:50, or 1:250 dilution of HSF1 or HSF2 antiserum at room temperature for 20 min before being subjected to gel mobility shift analysis. (Reprinted with permission of American Society for Microbiology, from Sistonen et al, 1992.)

activation of heat shock factors (Nakai and Morimoto, 1993). Chicken HSF3 is expressed in erythrocytes and a number of other cells types, but appears to acquire heat shock inducibility only in chicken erythroblastic cells (HD6) (Nakai et al, 1994). Chicken HSF3 has many characteristics similar to that of cHSF1 such as DNA binding specificity and negative regulation of DNA binding in rabbit reticulocyte extracts. As with cHSF1, deletion of the 4th leucine zipper has demonstrated that this sequence is involved in the negative regulation of cHSF3 DNA-binding activity (Nakai and Morimoto, 1993). In HD6 cells cHSF3 can be activated by heat but the response is delayed and appears to follow the initial activation of cHSF1 (Nakai et al, 1994). Is cHSF3 involved in the regulation of HSP gene transcription? When cotransfected into cells with an HSE driven reporter construct, cHSF3 is a positive activator. Chicken HSF3 also positively regulates cHSF1 DNA binding activity suggesting interaction in vivo although there is no evidence for the formation of heterooligomers.

A Reexamination Of The HSE In The Context Of Multiple HSFs

Studies in the K562 cell system have demonstrated that both HSF1 and HSF2 can be activated and bind to DNA. These studies also have demonstrated that heat-induced HSF1 appears to be a substantially better activator of HSP70 transcription than hemin-induced HSF2 (Sistonen et al, 1992). One explanation for these results is the difference in binding site occupancy by HSF1 and HSF2. The proximal HSE of the human HSP70 gene, which is required for HS induced transcription, is composed of five pentameric repeats of which the first, third and fourth match the current consensus (5'-nGAAn-3') and the second and fifth sites are divergent (Figure 2.3). Studies from our laboratory have demonstrated with genomic footprinting that HSF1, when activated by heat, rapidly binds to the HSE and protects all five consensus guanine residues from methylation by dimethyl sulfate (Abravaya et al, 1991a). Subsequent studies have demonstrated that while heat induced HSF1 contacts all five pentameric repeats, hemin induced HSF2 recognizes a subset of the binding sites corresponding to repeats 2 to 5 (Figure 2.6) (Sistonen et al, 1992). Can this difference in interaction account for the higher level of transcriptional activation exhibited by HSF1? Consistent with these observations, in vitro studies with the purified recombinant mHSFs have demonstrated that mHSF1 is a more potent activator in a nuclear extract transcription system than mHSF2 (Kroeger et al, 1993). DNase 1

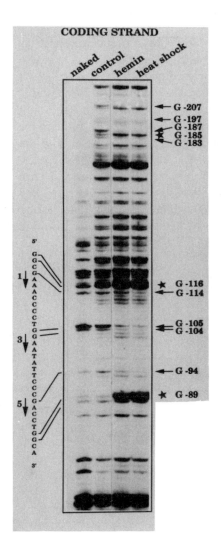
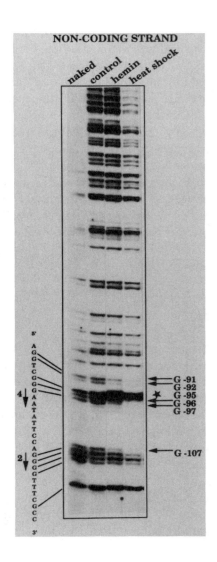

Figure 2.6 Genomic footprinting of the human HSP70 promoter. Methylation patterns of the guanine (G) residues within the HSE regions for the coding and noncoding strands. Genomic DNAs were isolated from control, hemin-treated (20 h), and heat-shocked (20 min) cells that were treated with DMS in vivo. The lane marked "naked" contained protein-free DNA that was DMS treated in vitro. The sequence of the proximal HSE binding sites are denoted at the left of each panel. The G residues that are protected from methylation are denoted with arrows, and stars indicate G residues hypersensitive to methylation. For differences in HSF1 and HSF2 affinity at HSP70 HSE site 1 compare the protection at G-114 in hemin and heat-shocked cells. (Reprinted with permission of American Society for Microbiology, from Sistonen, 1992.)

footprinting, in vitro, has confirmed the in vivo observations that only mHSF1 can bind to all five repeats of the HSP70 HSE (Figure 2.7). Additional footprinting studies have revealed that mHSF1 has a preference for certain repeats within the HSE and have provided an explanation for how two trimers of mHSF1 interact with a five repeat binding site (Kroeger et al, 1993). The first mHSF1 timer binds to repeats 3 to 5, of which 3 and 4 compose a perfect dyad symmetrical sequence. The second trimer of mHSF1 binds to sites 1 and 2, and this interaction is stabilized by cooperative interactions between mHSF1 trimers.

To further explore this differential interaction with the HSE, the DNA binding preference of mHSF1 and mHSF2 has been examined in an unbiased manner through the selection of new binding sites from a pool of random oligonucleotides (Blackwell and Weintraub, 1990; Pollack and Treisman, 1990). This analysis has revealed that both HSFs recognize nearly identical consensus sites composed of inverted pentamers and that the nucleotides at the "n" positions are not random (Kroeger and Morimoto, 1994). The dimeric consensus sites determined for mHSF1 and mHSF2 are $5'$-aGAA$^c/_t$gTTCg-$3'$ and $5'$-$^a/_g$GAAnnTTC$^g/_t$-$3'$ respectively. Notably, in the mHSF1 consensus sequence, adenine and cytosine residues are alternatively preferred at the first position of each nGAAn repeat, and pyrimidines are preferred at the fifth. The similarity in consensus sequences for both factors suggests that the differential recognition of the HSP70 HSE likely is due to other factors such as differences in cooperativity between trimers. In this regard, HSF1 selects oligonucleotides that contain more pentameric repeats per binding site (4 to 5) than HSF2 (2 to 3) and suggests that the binding of multiple HSF1 trimers to a selected oligonucleotide results in increased stability of the DNA-protein complex. DNase 1 footprinting with probes prepared from selected oligonucleotides has demonstrated that some sites exhibit the same differential interaction of mHSF1 and mHSF2 as observed on the HSP70 HSE. This observation is reinforced by the analysis of the HSF1 selected binding site 1B5-13 (Figure 2.8) in which mHSF1 binds to a greater extent than HSF2 due to increased cooperative interaction between HSF1 trimers. The appropriate juxtaposition of potential binding sites (see schematic at bottom of Figure 2.8) suggests that HSF1 trimers bound at the region of the selected oligonucleotide can stabilize the interaction of an adjacent trimer, even across a 5 bp gap (striped box) that does not contain a bonafide binding site. Additional experiments with chimeric mHSF proteins have demonstrated that the amino acid sequences in or near the HSF1 DNA binding domain are likely responsible for the increased cooperative interactions. Perhaps this lack of stable cooperative interaction by HSF2 trimers is in part

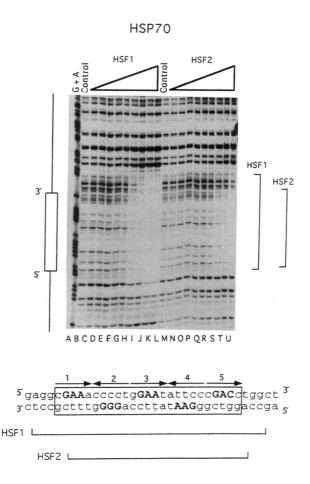

Figure 2.7 DNase I footprinting of the human HSP70 proximal HSE with recombinant mHSF1 and mHSF2. Equilibrium DNase I footprinting of mHSF1 (lanes C–K) and mHSF2 (M–U) binding to the NSP70 HSE was done as described previously (Kroeger et al, 1993). The concentration of HSP70 HSE probe in all reactions was 0.1 nM and the probe was labeled at the 5′ end on the bottom strand. The concentration of mHSF1 in lanes C–K was: 0.026 nM, 0.052 nM, 0.103 nM, 0.206 nM, 0.413 nM, 0.826 nM, 1.65 nM, 3.3 nM, and 6.6 nM. The concentration of mHSF2 in lanes M–U was: 0.03 nM, 0.06 nM, 0.06 nM, 0.12 nM, 0.24 nM, 0.48 nM, 0.96 nM, 1.92 nM, 3.84 nM, and 7.68 nM. Lanes A, B, and L contain the G + A sequencing ladder and control DNase I footprinting reactions respectively. The extent of mHSF1 and mHSF2 binding is indicated at the right with baskets. Below, the sequence of the HSP70 HSE is shown schematically and the boundaries of mHSF1 and mHSF2 interaction are denoted with brackets. The box at the left is marked with the orientation of the sequence and is also overlaid on the sequence below for additional assistance. The orientation of sites 1–5 are indicated with arrows and the core HSE motifs have been bolded.

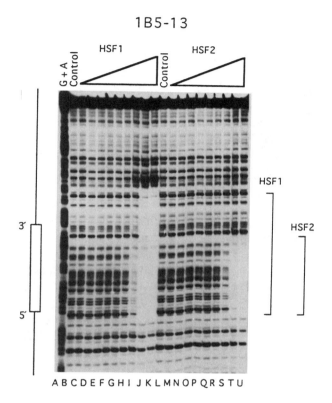

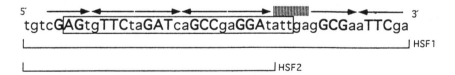

Figure 2.8 DNase I footprinting of mHSF1 and mHSF2 reveals differences in trimer cooperativity. The binding and footprinting reactions were performed as in Figure 2.7 except that the substrate DNA was the HSF1 selected binding site 1B5–13. The concentration of mHSF1 in lanes C–K was: 0.026 nM, 0.052 nM, 0.103 nM, 0.206 nM, 0.413 nM, 0.826 nM, 1.65 nM, 6.6 nM and 12 nM. The concentration of mHSF2 in lanes M–U was: 0.03 nM, 0.06 nM, 0.12 nM, 0.24 nM, 0.48 nM, 0.96 nM, 1.92 nM, 7.68 nM and 15.4 nM. The labeling of the figure is as in Figure 2.7. The sequence of the 1B5–13 binding site and the boundaries of mHSF1 and mHSF2 interaction are denoted. The striped box above the 1B5–13 sequence schematic designates the pentameric sequences 5′-attga-3′ that does contain an HSE pentamer but is contacted by mHSF1.

responsible for the lower level of transcriptional activation observed in vitro and in vivo. In support of this hypothesis, there is evidence from the *S. cerevisiae* system that the ability to bind multiple HSF trimers to an HSE correlates with increased levels of transcription (Bonner et al, 1994).

Transcriptional Activation And Access To The HSE; Regulation Of HSF By Chromatin Structure

As described earlier the local disruption of chromatin structure in the promoter of the HSP70 gene provides access to the HSE for HSF. Our understanding of the consequences of HSF binding is perhaps best understood in the *Drosophila* system. The promoter of the *Drosophila* HSP70 gene, and a number of other *Drosophila* genes, is known to contain a paused polymerase (Rougive and Lis, 1988, 1990). Specifically, a molecule of RNA polymerase II, which has bound and initiated transcription, is paused approximately 30 nucleotides into the transcribed region of the HSP70 gene. Heat shock results in the release of the paused polymerase molecule which continues to synthesize RNA, and there is recruitment of new polymerase molecules to the promoter. Mutational analyses of the HS promoters has demonstrated that the GAGA elements (see below) and transcription initiation region are necessary for the formation of the paused polymerase (Lee et al, 1992). The binding of HSF to the open chromatin region of the HS gene promoter results in the release of polymerase, and it has been suggested that HSF might accomplish this by influencing the phosphorylation status of the RNA polymerase II C-terminal domain (Lis and Wu, 1993). If the rate of polymerase escape from the promoter is the limiting event in HSP70 transcription, then HSF could facilitate this process and thereby increase the rate of transcription.

The ability of transcription factors to locate their cognate binding sites is remarkable given the complexity and number of potentially incorrect sites that may exist in a genome. The binding sites for transcription factors may be constrained by the packaging of DNA into nucleosomes, and there is evidence that the binding of HSF to an HSE under these circumstances is inhibited (Becker et al, 1991; Taylor et al, 1991). In order for HSF to bind the HSE under these circumstances, TFIID has to be present during the formation of the nucleosomal DNA complex, and this is in agreement with the observation that the promoter region of the HSP70 genes are in an open chromatin conformation (Wu, 1980). How is the promoter of HSP70 genes maintained in a open conformation? In *Drosophila*, a constitutive DNA binding protein (referred to as GAGA) has been shown to recognize the repeating dinucleotide motif 5'-GA-3' found in the *Drosophila* HS gene promoters, and it is this interaction that results in the open chromatin configuration (Lee et al, 1992; Lu et al, 1993). Recent in vivo studies in *S. cerevisiae* have demonstrated that yeast HSF can bind to HSEs packaged in nucleosomes (Pederson and Fidrych, 1994). However, this result is not in conflict with previous studies as there is likely an association of TFIID with the yeast promoter prior to HSF binding. What regulates the formation and maintenance of open chromatin in regions will continue to be of interest, and recent results with the HSP70 promoter region and GAGA factor suggest that there is an active ATP-requiring process necessary for the disruption of nucleosomal DNA (Tsukiyama et al, 1994).

Analysis Of HSF1 and HSF2 Structure

Studies on the trimerization of HSF

As noted above, *S. cerevisiae* HSF is already trimerized and localized to the nucleus prior to heat shock. *Drosophila* HSF is localized to the nucleus prior to heat shock, but is maintained in a latent monomeric form (Westwood et al, 1991). The mammalian HSFs are latent monomers found primarily in the cytoplasmic compartment, and the conversion to a trimeric state and translocation to the nucleus represents a major point of regulation. This conversion has been examined by a variety of biochemical methods, for example crosslinking by chemical agents and hydrodynamic studies. The latent HSF Molecule in *D. melanogaster* is a very elongated monomer with a frictional ratio (f/f_0) of ≈ 1.9 (Westwood and Wu, 1993). Studies with human HSF1 and HSF2 have demonstrated that the f/f_0 for monomeric HSF1 ≈ 1.7 and for HSFr is also ≈ 1.7 (Sistonen et al, 1994). Upon conversion to the trimeric form during shock the frictional ratio for *Drosophila* HSF increases ($f/f_0 = 2.6$) suggesting an unfolding event in conjunction with the trimerization. The studies of human HSF1 have demonstrated that heat induction results in HSF1 trimerization but no apparent change in frictional ratio. This is perhaps a reflection of the difference in size of human HSF1 and HSF2 (54 and 58 kDa) and *Drosophila* HSF (100 kDa).

Investigation of the physical parameters for HSF2 from K562 cells has revealed, surprisingly, that it is a dimer in the latent form and converts into an active DNA-binding trimer upon activation by hemin treatment (Sistonen et al, 1994). The dimeric form of HSF2 was unexpected, and whether it is a homodimer or heterodimer remains to be determined. However, the conversion of a heterodimer into a trimer seems more likely. The difference in the oligomeric state of latent HSF1 and HSF2 corroborates the observed differences in activation in response to different signaling pathways. A major objective of future studies will be to determine the composition of the HSF2 dimer and determine the mechanism of conversion to the trimeric state.

A related issue in the activation of mammalian HSF1 is to understand whether the conversion from monomer to trimer occurs in the cytoplasm or nucleus. Current evidence suggests that upon HS the latent monomer is imported into the nucleus where upon it trimerizes (Cotto, 1994). This is surprising as in vitro studies using S-100 extracts from control cells have shown that HSF can trimerize and bind DNA following in vitro heat shock (Larson et al, 1988; Mosser et al, 1988). The fact that, in vivo, trimerization is restricted to the nucleus suggests the possibility of factor(s) that retain HSF1 in the monomeric conformation in the cytoplasm. Subsequently, HSF1 may be imported into the nucleus via interactions with a chaperone complex that controls oligomerization.

As mentioned above, a central question has been to discover how HSF is maintained in the latent state. Studies of *Drosophila* HSF have demonstrated that it may be the association of leucine zipper 4, at the C-terminus of the protein, with the leucine zippers of the oligomerization domain that prevents trimerization (Rabindran et al, 1993). In these studies, mutation of the 4th leucine zipper has resulted in constitutive DNA-binding activity. Additionally, analysis of cHSF3 has demonstrated that deletion of leucine zipper 4 also results in constitutive DNA-binding activity (Nakai and Morimoto, 1993). These studies suggest the interesting possibility that intramolecular interactions between the N- and C-terminal leucine zippers regulate HSF1 activity and are consistent with the observed unfolding events during HS activation. The actual mechanics of how the HSF1 protein unfolds and then associates to form a trimer will require further study.

Heat shock induced modification of HSF

The activation of transcription by *S. cerevisiae* HSF has been associated with a high degree of heat induced serine phosphorylation which results in a significant mobility shift on SDS-PAGE gels (Sorger and Pelham, 1988). Studies with mouse and human HSF1 have demonstrated that they are constitutively and inducibly phosphorylated (Sarge et al, 1993). Recent studies have determined that the inducible phosphorylation of mammalian HSF1 in response to heat shock and cadmium treatment also occurs at serine residues (Kline, 1994). Treatment of cells with other inducers of HSF1, such as salicylate and azetidine, activates HSF1 trimerization and DNA–binding; however, HSF1 is not inducibly phosphorylated and this correlates with a decrease in the induction of HSP70 transcription (Jurivich et al, 1992; Sarge et al, 1993). Current hypotheses suggest that phosphorylation of HSF1 is involved in the transcriptional activation processes; however, a lack of phosphorylation does not completely abolish transcriptional activation. In comparison, hemin treatment of K562 cells results in activation of HSF2, but does not induce HSF2 phosphorylation (Sistonen et al, 1994). Whether the observed differences in HSF1 and HSF2 phosphorylation are related to their relative strength as transcription factors remains to be determined.

Transcriptional activation domains of HSF

Trimerization of HSF is essential to its function and likely provides the necessary DNA binding affinity and specificity required for accurate interactions with the HSE. When bound to the DNA through the N-terminal DNA binding domain, HSF is likely to affect transcriptional activation via sequences in the C-terminus. The activation domains of the yeast HSFs (*S. cerevisiae* and *Kluyveromyces lactis*) and the tomato HSFs have been dissected, and interestingly there appear to be differences in structure between these organisms (Chen et al, 1993; Treuter et al, 1993). As noted earlier there are multiple transcriptional activation domains in yeast HSF that mediate the response to sustained and transient stress. The N-terminal activator of *S. cerevisiae* is responsible for activation of transcription during sustained stress (Nieto-Sotelo et al, 1990; Sorger, 1990). The C-terminal activator of yeast responds to transient stress, and in *K. lactis* this corresponds to a 30 amino acid (aa 592 to 623) sequence with some α-helical character and acidic quality. In contrast, the *S. cerevisiae* C-terminal activation domain is ≈180 amino acids long and appears to be bipartite with one domain responsible for activation (aa 595 to 713) and the adjacent sequences (aa 713 to 780) have a supporting function for the activator. The tomato HSFs apparently have a third type activation motif located in the C-terminus which is composed of acidic sequences that contain a central tryptophan residue.

The activation of transcription by mammalian HSF, and the specific domains involved are not well understand, so we have used the heterologous GAL4 DNA binding domain (DBD) fusions to assess the activity of HSF sequences. We have concentrated on the C-terminal half of the mHSF1 protein, and these studies have demonstrated that mHSF1 has a strong transcriptional activating region in the C-terminus between amino acids 395 and 471. In the context of the GAL4 DBD, the HSF1 sequences are constitutive activators suggesting that deletion of N-terminal sequences results in loss of negative regulation. This activation region of mHSF1 is acidic and includes part of leucine zipper 4 (aa 395 to 406) which is conserved in metazoan HSFs. Deletion of only the leucine zipper 4 sequences from the activator results in significantly lower activation (20-fold) suggesting that hydrophobic interactions between individual activation domains in the trimer may be necessary for activator function.

A Model For The Regulation Of HSF1 Activation

When sufficient levels of HSPs have been produced, the heat shock response can be turned off, and indeed HS transcription attenuates after a period of several hours at the elevated temperature. This transcriptional down regulation requires the conversion of the trimeric HSF1 back to the latent non-DNA-binding monomer. The attenuation of the HSP70 transcriptional response is correlated with the release of bound HSF1. Utilizing genomic footprinting, the equilibrium dissociation rate of HSF1 from the HSE in vivo is shown to be ≈10-fold faster than occurs in vitro suggesting an active process that facilitates the release of active HSF1 (Abravaya et al, 1991a). The attenuation and release of HSF1 correlates with increased levels of HSP70. Evidence for the association of HSP70 with HSF has been obtained by analysis of the composition of complexes observed in gel shift experiments (Abravaya et al, 1992; Baler et al, 1992). The addition of anti-HSP70 antibodies causes an upward mobility shift in the migration of the HSF:HSE complexes (Figure 2.9, lane 3). This suggests that HSP70 is in a stable complex with HSF and that this complex can still bind DNA. Notably, the HSP70:HSF complex is dissociated upon addition at ATP (Figure 2.9, lanes 2 and 4), a cofactor known to mediate the release of bound substrates from HSP70 (Hartl et al, 1992; Hendrick and Hartl, 1993). The association between HSP70 and HSF is most readily observed during the attenuation phase of the heat shock response which suggests a role for HSP70 in disassembly of the HSF trimer. It is unlikely that HSP70 acts alone to accomplish this process as there are known co-chaperones which act in concert with HSP70 to facilitate protein folding (Hartl et al, 1992; Craig, 1993; Craig et al, 1993).

We propose a scenario for the activation and attenuation of mammalian HSF1 activity based on the evidence accumulated to date (Figure 2.10). (1) In the initial heat shock results in increased levels of unfolded substrates that require HSP70 and other chaperones to efficiently catalyze their correct refolding. This sequestration of HSP70 releases HSF1 from negative regulation, and the HSF monomer translocates to the nucleus.

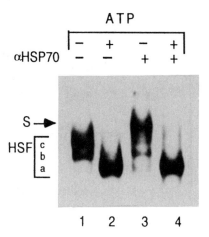

Figure 2.9 HSP70 is in an ATP dissociable complex with HSF1. Whole-cell extracts from heat-shocked HeLe cells were used in a gel retardation assay as described previously (Mosser et al, 1988). Prior to initiation of the binding reaction, some samples were preincubated with ATP and/or anti-HSP70 antibody. The HSF:HSE complexes are denoted (labeled a, b, and c). The S indicates the supershifted HSF:HSE complex formed when anti-HSP70 antibody is present in the binding reaction. Lanes: (1) control HSF binding reaction; (2) with ATP preincubation; (3) with anti-HSP70 antibody; (4) with both ATP and anti-HSP70 antibody. (Reprinted with permission of Cold Spring Harbor Press, from Abravaya et al, 1992)

(2) Upon entry to the nucleus, HSF1 trimerizes, and (3) binds to the HSE in the promoters of HS genes. (4) HS induced HSF1 is phosphorylated, and transcriptional activation by HSF1 results in expression of HSP70 and other inducible chaperones in the cytoplasm. (5) As heat induced protein damage is repaired, the released HSP70 protein transiently reassociates with HSF and facilitates the release of HSF from the HSE. (6) HSF1 remains complexed with HSP70, and HSF1 trimers are then converted to monomeric state. The maintenance of HSF1 in the latent state is most likely due to the continued transient association of HSP70. Perhaps in the unstressed cell the periodic unfolding of HSF1 is perceived as an unwanted event and HSP70 assists in the refolding process. There is supporting evidence for the role of HSP70 in HSF1 regulation since cell lines that overexpress HSP70 are delayed in the activation of HSF in response to heat (Mosser et al, 1993). This suggests that the increased pool of free HSP70 present in these cells requires more denatured or damaged proteins in order to permit HSF activation.

Pharmacological Manipulation Of The Heat Shock Response

Some recent studies on the activation of the heat shock response have focused on methods to uncouple and modify the activation of HSF and

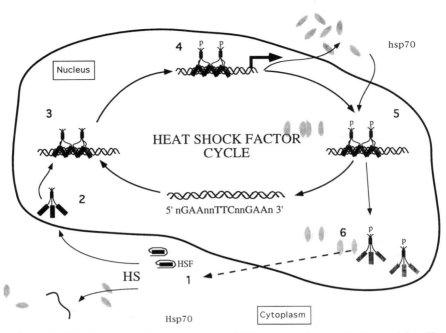

Figure 2.10 The heat shock factor cycle: a model for the regulation of HSF1 activity. The activation by HS of latent cytoplasmic HSF1 (step 1) is shown with the accompanying translocation to the nuclear compartment and oligomerization into an active trimer (step 2). The interaction of two HSF1 trimers with the HSP70 HSE (step 3); HSF1 phosphorylation and activation of HSP70 transcription (step 4) are also shown. After sufficient HSP70 has been synthesized, HSF1 dissociates from the HSE facilitated by the binding of HSP70 (step 5) to the HSF1:HSE complex. HSF1 remains associated with HSP70 and until it is converted back into a latent monomer in the cytoplasm (step 6).

thus affect HS gene expression. Studies with salicylate, a classical inducer of chromosome puffing, have demonstrated that it is possible to activate HSF1 trimerization and translocation to the nucleus with this compound; however, it does not activate HSP70 transcription efficiently (Jurivich et al, 1992). Salicylate is an inhibitor of arachidonic acid metabolism which has also been shown to activate HSF (Jurivich et al, 1994). Activation of HSF by arachidonic acid, a potent inflammatory cytokine, has been shown to occur synergistically with mild heat stress suggesting that temperatures which are physiologically approached during fever or inflammatory processes might activate the heat shock response. The activation of HSF1 has also been observed in cells treated with specific prostaglandins (PGA_2), additional products of arachidonic acid metabolism (Amici et al, 1992; Holbrook et al, 1992). These naturally occurring compounds have antiproliferative properties and strongly activated the heat shock response suggesting a role for HSP70 in growth arrest.

Other studies with the flavanoid compound quercetin have demonstrated that HSF DNA binding activity can be blocked prior to heat shock (Hosokawa et al, 1992). Further analysis has demonstrated that quercetin inhibits the heat induced phosphorylation of HSF1 and suggests that phosphorylation has a role in HSF1 binding to DNA (Kroeger, 1994). The results with quercetin, a known kinase inhibitor, suggest the existence of one or more kinases in the activation pathway for HSF1. It seems likely that the use of specific kinase and phosphatase inhibitors will aid in elucidating the pathway of HSF activation in response to stress. Thermotolerance, the ability to survive periods of lethal stress, was originally discovered in *Drosophila* and is now a major focus in the heat shock field, particularly as it pertains to cancer therapy (Li and Werb, 1982; Landry et al, 1989; Li et al, 1992; Lavoie et al, 1993; Parsell et al, 1993). The ability to specifically block the heat shock response could be enormously beneficial in hypothermic therapy where thermotolerance currently limits its effectiveness.

Conclusions

Heat shock represents an excellent model system to address a number of fundamental questions in cellular physiology. The response to stressful events is remarkably well conserved throughout evolution, and yet there has been diversification in the strategies used by organisms to respond to these threatening events. In yeast, perhaps due to the immediate threat of elevated temperature for a small unicellular organism, HSF is poised to respond already bound to the DNA. In *Drosophila* HSF is latent; however, there is ample evidence that the HSP70 promoter is primed with the presence of an engaged RNA polymerase II transcription complex. Finally, in mammalian systems, where presumably heat shock is not as rapid in its effects, the HSF1 protein is negatively regulated and cytoplasmic. There is currently no evidence that the mammalian HSP70 genes have a poised polymerase; however, there is basal transcription due to the other elements in the promoter, and this may contribute to the readiness of the cell to respond to stress.

The primary objectives of future studies will be the elucidation of the pathways that are utilized by cells to respond to specific events. Recent studies in yeast on the endoplastic reticulum (ER) chaperone GRP78/Bip have identified a ER localized kinase (ire1) that responds to unfolded substrates and results in the activation of a factor that induces GRP78 transcription (Mori et al, 1992; Kohno et al, 1993). The question of whether GRP78 is involved in the regulation of ire1 remains to be answered.

In contrast to signaling mechanisms in which a receptor has been identified that results in a cascade of phosphorylation events, the heat shock response appears to require less interplay between factors. The response centers around damage to proteins, and it seems likely that titration of HSP70 to these new substrates is responsible in part for the activation of HSF and the subsequent induction of HSP70 gene expression. The classical auto regulatory loop that is proposed to explain the regulation of HSF activity will likely become more complex as there are probably intermediate events which have not been uncovered.

The other question that needs to be addressed is how HSF leads to the enhanced transcription of HSP genes. Elucidation of the HSF activation domains is the first step toward a complete understanding of this process. Further studies will attempt to identify the components of the basal transcription complex that interact with each HSF. Over the last several years it has become apparent that activators such as VP16 of HSV activate transcription through their direct interaction with the basal transcription machinery. If HSF contacts a specific basal factor (e.g. TFIID, TFIIB) or RNA polymerase II directly, and how this accelerates transcription, remains to be established, but will be fruitful ground for further study.

References

Abravaya K, Myers MP, Murphy SP, Morimoto RI (1992): The human heat shock protein hsp70 interacts with HSF, the transcription factor that regulates heat shock gene transcriptions. *Genes & Dev* 6: 1153–1164

Abravaya K, Phillips B, Morimoto RI (1991a): Heat shock-induced interactions of heat shock transcription factor and the human hsp70 promoter examined by in vivo footprinting. *Mol Cell Biol* 11: 586–592

Abravaya K, Phillips B, Morimoto RI (1991b): Attenuation of the heat shock response in HeLa cells is mediated by the release of bound heat shock transcription factor and is modulated by changes in growth and in heat shock temperatures. *Genes & Dev* 5: 2117–2127

Agoff SN, Hou J, Linzer DI, Wu B (1993): Regulation of the human hsp70 promoter by p53. *Science* 259: 84–87

Amici C, Sistonen L, Santoro MG, Morimoto RI (1992): Anti-proliferative prostaglandins activate heat shock transcription factor. *Proc Natl Acad Sci USA* 89: 6227–6231

Amin J, Ananthan J, Voellmy R (1988): Key features of heat shock regulatory elements. *Mol Cell Biol* 8: 3761–3769

Anathan T, Goldberg AL, Voellmy R (1986): Abnormal proteins serve as eukaryotic stress signals and trigger the activation of heat shock genes. *Science* 232: 522–524

Aoki M, Abe K, Kawagoe JI, Sato S, Nakamura S, Kogure K (1993): Temporal profile of the induction of heat shock protein 70 and heat shock cognate protein 70 mRNAs after transient ischemia in gerbil brain. *Brain Res* 601: 185–192

Ashburner M (1970): Pattern of puffing activity in the salivary gland chromosomes of *Drosophila*. V. Response to environmental treatments. *Chromosoma* 31: 356–376

Baler R, Welch WJ, Voellmy R (1992): Heat shock gene regulation by nascent polypeptides and denatured proteins: hsp70 as a potential autoregulatory factor. *J Cell Biol* 117: 1151–1159

Banerji SS, Theordorakis NG, Morimoto RI (1984): Heat-shock-induced translational control of hsp70 and globin synthesis in chicken reticulocytes. *Mol Cell Biol* 4: 2437–2448

Becker PB, Rabindran SK, Wu C (1991): Heat shock-regulated transcription in vitro from a reconstituted chromatin template. *Proc Natl Acad Sci USA* 88: 4109–4113

Beckmann RP, Mizzen LE, Welch WJ (1990): Interaction of Hsp 70 with newly synthesized proteins: implications for protein folding and assembly. *Science* 248: 850–854

Benjamin IJ, Kroger B, Williams RS (1992): Induction of stress proteins in cultured myogenic cells: Molecular signals for the activation of heat shock transcription factor during ischemia. *J Clin Invest* 89: 1658–1689

Bienz M, Pelham HRB (1986): Heat shock regulatory elements function as an inducible enhancer in the Xenopus *hsp70* gene and when linked to a heterologous promoter. *Cell* 45: 753–760

Blackwell TK, Weintraub H (1990): Differences and similarities in DNA-binding preferences of myoD and E2A protein complexes revealed by binding site selection. *Science* 250: 1104–1110

Blake MJ, Gershon D, Fargnoli J, Holbrook NJ (1990a): Discordant expression of heat shock protein mRNAs in tissues of heat-stressed rats. *J Biol Chem* 265: 15275–15279

Blake MJ, Nowak TS, Holbrook NJ (1990b): In vivo hyperthermia induces expression of HSP70 mRNA in brain regions controlling the neuroendocrine response to stress. *Mol Brain Res* 8: 89–92

Blake MJ, Udelsman R, Feulner GJ, Norton DD, Holbrook NJ (1991): Stress-induced heat shock protein 70 expression in adrenal cortex: an adrenocorticotropic hormone-sensitive, age-dependent response. *Proc Natl Acad Sci USA* 88: 9873–9877

Bonner JJ, Ballou C, Fackenthal DL (1994): Interactions between DNA-bound trimers of the yeast heat shock factor. *Mol Cell Biol* 14: 501–508

Capdevila MD, Garcia-Bellido A (1974): Development and genetic analysis of bithorax phenocopies in *Drosophila*. *Nature* 250: 500–502

Chen Y, Barlev NA, Westergaard O, Jakobsen BK (1993): Identification of the C-terminal activator domain in yeast heat shock factor: independent control of transient and sustained transcriptional activity. *EMBO J* 12: 5007–5018

Choi HS, Lin Z, Li B, Liu A-C (1990): Age-dependent decrease in the heat-inducible DNA sequence-specific binding activity in human diploid fibroblasts. *J Biol Chem* 265: 18005–18011

Clos J, Rabindran S, Wisniewski J, Wu C (1993): Induction temperature of human heat shock factor is reprogrammed in a Drosophila cell environment. *Nature* 364: 252–255

Clos J, Westwood JT, Becker PB, Wilson S, Lambert K, Wu C (1990): Molecular cloning and expression of a hexameric Drosophila heat shock factor subject to negative regulation. *Cell* 63: 1085–1097

Corces V, Holmgren R, Freund R, Morimoto R, Meselson M (1980): Four heat shock proteins of Drosophila melanogaster coded within a 12-kilobase region in chromosome subdivision 67B. *Proc Natl Acad Sci USA* 77: 5390–5393

Corces V, Pellicer A, Axel R, Meselson M (1981): Integration, transcription, and control of a Drosophila heat shock gene in mouse cells. *Proc Natl Acad Sci USA* 78: 7038–7042

Cotto J (1994): personal communication

Craig EA (1993): Chaperones: Helpers along the pathway to protein folding. *Science* 260: 1902–1903

Craig EA, Gambill BD, Nelson RJ (1993): Heat shock proteins: molecular chaperones of protein biogenesis. *Microbiol Rev* 57: 402–414

Craig EA, McCarthy BJ, Wadsworth S (1979): Sequence organization of two recombinant plasmids containing genes for the major heat shock induced protein in *Drosophila melanogaster*. *Cell* 16: 575–583

Currie RW, White FP (1993): Heat shock and limitation of tissue necrosis during occlusion/reperfusion in rabbit hearts. *Circulation* 87: 963–971

DiDomenico BJ, Bugaisky GE, Lindquist S (1982): The Heat Shock Response is Regulated at both the Transcriptional and Posttranscriptional Levels. *Cell* 31: 593–603

Dorner AJ, Wasley LC, Kaufman RJ (1992): Overexpression of GRP78 mitigates stress induction of glucose regulated proteins and blocks secretion of selective proteins in Chinese hamster ovary cells. *EMBO J* 11: 1563–1571

Ferris DK, Harel-Bellan A, Morimoto RI, Welch WJ, Farrar WL (1988):Mitogen and lymphokine stimulation of heat shock proteins in T lymphocytes. *Proc Natl Acad Sci USA* 85: 3850–3854

Gallo GJ, Schuetz TJ, Kingston RE (1991): Regulation of heat shock factor in *Schizosaccharomyces pombe* more closely resembles regulation in mammals than in *Saccharomyces cerevisiae*. *Mol Cell Biol* 11: 281–288

Georgopoulos C, Welch WJ (1993): Role of major heat shock proteins as molecular chaperones. *Ann Rev Cell Biol* 9: 601–635

Gething M-J, Sambrook J (1992): Protein folding in the cell. *Nature* 355: 33–45

Goff SA, Goldberg AL (1985): Production of abnormal proteins in *E. coli* stimulates transcription of *lon* and other heat shock genes. *Cell* 41: 587–595

Goldschmidt R (1935): Gen und Ausseneigenschaft. 1. (Untersuchung an *Drosophila*). *Z Indukt Abstammungs Vererbungst* 69: 38–131

Greene JM, Kingston RE (1990): TATA-dependent and TATA-independent function of the basal and heat shock elements of a human hsp70 promoter. *Mol Cell Biol* 10(4): 1319–1328

Greene JM, Larin Z, Taylor IC, Prentice H, Gwinn KA, Kingston RE (1987): Multiple basal elements of a human hsp70 promoter function differently in human and rodent cell lines. *Mol Cell Biol* 7(10): 3646–3655

Hartl FU, Martin J, Neupert W (1992): Protein folding in the cell: the role of molecular chaperones Hsp70 and Hsp60. *Annu Rev Biophys Biomol Struct* 21: 292–322

Hendrick JP, Hartl F-U (1993): Molecular chaperone functions of heat-shock proteins. *Annu Rev Biochem* 62: 349–384

Heydari AR, Wu B, Takahashi R, Strong R, Richardson A (1993): Expression of heat shock protein 70 is altered by age and diet at the level of transcription. *Mol Cell Biol* 13: 2909–2918

Hightower LE (1991): Heat shock, stress proteins, chaperones, and proteotoxicity. *Cell* 66: 191–197

Holbrook NJ, Carlson SG, Choi AMK, Fargnoli J (1992): Induction of HSP70 gene expression by the antiproliferative prostaglandin PGA_2: a growth-dependent response mediated by activation of heat shock transcription factor. *Mol Cell Biol* 12: 1528–1534

Holbrook NJ, Udelsman R (1994): Heat shock protein gene expression in response to physiologic stress and aging. In: *The Biology of Heat Shock Proteins and Molecular Chaperones*. Morimoto RI, Tissieres A, Georgopoulos C, eds. Cold Spring Harbor, NY: Cold Spring Harbor Laboratory Press (in press)

Holmgren R, Corces V, Morimoto R, Blackman R, Meselson M (1981): Sequence homologies in the 5′ regions of four *Drosophila* heat-shock genes. *Proc Natl Acad Sci USA* 3775–3778

Holmgren R, Livak K, Morimoto R, Freund R, Meselson M (1979): Studies of cloned sequences from four Drosophila heat shock loci. *Cell* 18: 1359–1370

Hosokawa N, Hirayoshi K, Kudo H, Takechi H, Aoike A, Kawai K, Nagata K (1992): Inhibition of activation of heat shock factor in vivo and in vitro by flavanoids. *Mol Cell Biol* 12: 3490–3498

Hunt C, Morimoto RI (1985): Conserved features of eukaryotic hsp70 genes revealed by comparison with the nucleotide sequence of human hsp70. *Proc Natl Acad Sci USA* 82: 6455–6459

Jakobsen BK, Pelham HR (1988): Constitutive binding of yeast heat shock factor to DNA in vivo. *Mol Cell Biol* 8: 5040–5042

Jakobsen BK, Pelham HRB (1991): A conserved heptapeptide restrains the activity of the yeast heat shock transcription factor. *EMBO J* 10: 369–375

Jurivich D, Sistonen L, Sarge KD, Morimoto RI (1994): Arachidonate is a potent modulator of human heat shock gene transcription. *Proc Natl Acad Sci USA* 91: 2280–2284

Jurivich DA, Sistonen, L, Kroes, RA, Morimoto RI (1992): Effect of sodium salicylate on the human heat shock response. *Science* 255: 1243–1245

Kingston RET, Schuetz TJ, Larin Z (1987): Heat-inducible human factor that binds to a human hsp70 promoter. *Mol Cell Biol* 7: 1530–1534

Kline M (1994): unpublished observation

Kohno K, Normington K, Sambrook J, Gething MJ, Mori K (1993): The promoter region of the yeast KAR2 (BiP) gene contains a regulatory domain that responds to the presence of unfolded proteins in the endoplasmic reticulum. *Mol Cell Biol* 13: 877–890

Kroeger P (1994): unpublished observation

Kroeger P, Morimoto R (1994): Selection of new HSF1 and HSF2 DNA binding sites reveals differences in trimer cooperativity. *Mol. Cell Biol*: in press

Kroeger PE, Sarge KD, Morimoto RI (1993): Mouse heat shock transcription factors 1 and 2 prefer a trimeric binding site but interact differently with the HSP70 heat shock element. *Mol Cell Biol* 13: 3370–3383

Landry J, Chretien P, Lambert H, Hickey E, Weber A (1989): Heat shock resistance conferred by expression of the human HSP27 gene in rodent cells. *J Cell Biol* 109: 7–15

Larson JS, Schuetz TJ, Kingston RE (1988): Activation *in vitro* of sequence-specific DNA binding by a human regulatory factor. *Nature* 335: 372–375

Lavoie JN, Gingras-Breton, G, Tanguay RM, Landry J (1993): Induction of chinese hamster HSP27 gene expression in mouse cells confers resistance to heat shock. *J Biol Chem* 268: 3420–3429

Lee H, Kraus KW, Wolfner MF, Lis JT (1992): DNA sequence requirements for generating paused polymerase at the start of hsp70. *Genes Dev* 6: 284–295

Li GC, Li LG, Liu RY, Rehman M, Lee WM (1992): Heat shock protein hsp70 protects cells from thermal stress even after deletion of its ATP-binding domain. *Proc Natl Acad Sci USA* 89: 2036–2040

Li GC, Werb Z (1982): Correlation between synthesis of heat shock proteins and development of thermotolerance in Chinese fibroblast. *Proc Natl Acad Sci USA* 79: 3218–3222

Li WW, Sistonen L, Morimoto RI, Lee AS (1994): Stress induction of mammalian GRP78/Bip protein gene: in vivo genomic footprinting and the identification of p70CORE from human nuclear extract as a DNA binding component to the stress regulatory element. *Mol Cell Biol*: in press

Lindquist S (1980): Translational efficiency of heat induced messages in *Drosophila melanogaster* cells. *J Mol Biol* 137: 151–158

Lindquist S (1986): The Heat-Shock response. *Ann Rev Biochem* 55: 1151–1191

Lindquist S, Craig EA (1988): The heat shock proteins. *Annu Rev Genet* 22: 631–677

Lindquist-Mckenzie SL, Meselson M (1977): Translation in vitro of *Drosophila* heat shock messages. *J Mol Biol* 117: 279–283

Lindquist-Mckenzie SL, Henikoff S, Meselon M (1975): Localization of RNA from heat-induced polysomes at puff sites in *Drosophila melanogaster*. *Proc Natl Acad Sci USA* 72: 1117–1121

Lis J, Wu C (1993): Protein traffic on the heat shock promoter: parking, stalling, and trucking along. *Cell* 74: 1–4

Liu AY, Lin Z, Choi HS, Sorhage F, Li B (1989): Attenuated induction of heat shock gene expression in aging diploid fibroblasts. *J Biol Chem* 264: 12037–12045

Liu Y, Kato H, Nakata N, Kogure K (1992): Protection of rat hippocampus against ischemic neuronal damage by pretreatment with sublethal ischemia. *Brain Res* 586: 121–124

Livak KJ, Freund R, Schwebe M, Wensink PC, Meselson M (1978): Sequence organization and transcription at two heat shock loci in Drosophila. *Proc Natl Acad Sci USA* 75: 5613–5617

Lowe DG, Fulford WD, Moran LA (1983): Mouse and Drosophila genes encoding the major heat shock protein (Hsp70) are highly conserved. *Mol Cell Biol* 3: 1540–1543

Lu Q, Wallrath LL, Granok H, Elgin SC (1993): (CT)n (GA)n repeats and heat shock elements have distinct roles in chromatin structure and transcriptional activation of the Drosophila hsp26 gene. *Mole Cell Biol* 13: 2802–2814

Lum LSY, Sultzman LA, Kaufman RJ, Linzer DIH, Wu B (1990): A cloned human CCAAT-box-binding factor stimulates transcription from the human hsp70 promoter. *Mol Cell Biol* 10: 6709–6717

Marber MS, Latchman DS, Walker JM, Yellon DM (1993): Cardiac stress protein elevation 24 hours after brief ischemia or heat stress is associated with resistance to myocardial infarction. *Circulation* 88: 1264–1272

Mathur S, Sistonen L, Brown IB, Murphy SP, Sarge KD, Morimoto RI (1994): Deficient induction of human HSP70 gene transcription in Y79 retinoblastoma cells despite activation of HSF1. *Proc Natl Acad Sci USA*: in press

Milarski KL, Morimoto RI (1986): Expression of human HSP70 during the synthetic phase of the cell cycle. *Proc Natl Acad Sci USA* 83: 9517–9521

Mirault M-E, Southgate R, Delwart E (1982): Regulation of heat shock genes: a

DNA sequence upstream of Drosophila hsp70 genes is essential for their induction in monkey cells. *EMBO J* 1: 1279–1285

Moran L, Mirault ME, Tissieres A, Lis J, Schedl P, Artranis-Tsakonas S, Gehring WJ (1979): Physical map of two Drosophila melanogaster DNA segments containing sequences coding for the 70,000 dalton heat shock protein. *Cell* 17: 1–8

Morgan WD (1989): Transcription factor Sp1 binds to and activates a human HSP70 gene promoter. *Mol Cell Biol* 9: 4099–4104

Morgan WD, Williams GT, Morimoto RI, Greene J, Kingston RE, Tjian R (1987): Two transcriptional activators, CCAAT-box binding transcription factor and heat shock transcription factor, interact with a human HSP70 gene promoter. *Mol Cell Biol* 7: 1129–1138

Mori K, Sant A, Kohno K, Normington K, Gething MJ, Sambrook JF (1992): A 22 bp cis-acting element is necessary and sufficient for the induction of the yeast KAR2 (BiP) gene by unfolded proteins. *EMBO J* 11: 2583–2593

Morimoto RI (1991): Heat shock: the role of transient inducible responses in cell damage, transformation, and differentiation. *Cancer Cells* 3: 297–301

Morimoto RI (1993): Chaperoning the nascent polypeptide chain. *Curr Biol* 3: 101–102

Morimoto RI, Milarski KL (1990): Expression and function of vertebrate hsp70 genes. In: *Stress Proteins in Biology and Medicine*. Morimoto RI, Tissieres A, Georgopoulos C, eds. Cold Spring Harbor, NY: Cold Spring Harbor Laboratory Press

Morimoto RI, Abravaya K, Mosser D, Williams GT (1990): Transcriptional regulation of the human HSP70 gene: cis-acting elements and transacting factors involved in basal, adenovirus E1a, and stress-induced expression. In: *Stress Proteins*. Schlesinger M, Santoro MG, Garaci E, eds. Berlin: Springer-Verlag

Morimoto RI, Hunt C, Huang S-Y, Berg KL, Banerji SS (1986): Organization, nucleotide sequence, and transcription of the chicken HSP70 gene. *J Biol Chem* 261: 12692–12699

Morimoto RI, Jurivich DA, Kroeger PE, Mathur SK, Murphy SP, Nakai A, Sarge K, Abravaya K, Sistonen L (1994): The regulation of heat shock gene expression by a family of heat shock factors. In: *The Biology of Heat Shock Proteins and Molecular Chaperones*. Morimoto AI, Tissieres A, Georgopoulos C, eds. Cold Spring Harbor, NY: Cold Spring Harbor Laboratory Press

Mosser DD, Duchaine J, Massie B (1993): The DNA-binding activity of the human heat shock transcription factor is regulated in vivo by hsp70. *Mol Cell Biol* 13: 5427–5438

Mosser DD, Kotzbauer PT, Sarge KD, Morimoto RI (1990): In vitro activation of heat shock transcription factor DNA-binding by calcium and biochemical conditions that affect protein conformation. *Proc Natl Acad Sci USA* 87: 3748–3752

Mosser DD, Theodorakis NG, Morimoto RI (1988): Coordinate changes in heat shock element-binding activity and hsp70 gene transcription rates in human cells. *Mol Cell Biol* 8: 4736–4744

Murphy S, Phillips B (1994): unpublished observation

Nakai A, Morimoto RI (1993): Characterization of a novel chicken heat shock transcription factor, HSF3, suggests a new regulatory pathway. *Mol Cell Biol* 13: 1983–1997

Nakai A, Nagata K, Morimoto R (1994): unpublished observation

Nelson RJ, Ziegelhoffer T, Nicolet C, Werner-Washburne M, Craig EA (1992): The translation machinery and seventy kilodalton heat shock protein cooperate in protein synthesis. *Cell* 71: 97–105

Nieto-Sotelo J, Wiederrecht G, Okuda A, Parker CS (1990): The yeast heat shock transcription factor contains a transcriptional activation domain whose activity is repressed under nonshock conditions. *Cell* 62: 807–817

Nowak TS, Abe H (1994): The postischemic stress response in brain. In: *The Biology of Heat Shock Proteins and Molecular Chaperones*. Morimoto RI, Tissieres A, Georgopoulos C, eds. Cold Spring Harbor, NY: Cold Spring Harbor Laboratory Press (in press)

Parsell DA, Taulien J, Lindquist S (1993): The role of heat-shock proteins in thermotolerance. *Philoa Trans R Soc Lond Biol* 339: 279–285

Pederson DS, Fidrych T (1994): Heat shock factor can activate transcription while bound to nucleosomal DNA in *Saccharomyces cerevisiae*. *Mol Cell Biol* 14: 189–199

Pelham HRB (1982): A regulatory upstream promoter element in the Drosophila hsp 70 heat-shock gene. *Cell* 30: 517–528

Pelham HRB, Bienz M (1982): A synthetic heat-shock promoter element confers heat-inducibility on the herpes simplex virus thymidine kinase gene. *EMBO J* 1: 1473–1477

Perisic O, Xiao H, Lis JT (1989): Stable binding of Drosophila heat shock factor to head-to-head and tail-to-tail repeats of a conserved 5 bp recognition unit. *Cell* 59: 797–806

Peteranderl R, Nelson HCM (1992): Trimerization of the heat shock transcription factor by a triple-stranded α-helical coiled-coil. *Biochemistry* 31: 12272–12276

Phillips B, Morimoto RI (1991): Transcriptional regulation of human hsp70 genes: relationship between cell growth, differentiation, virus infection, and the stress response. In: *Heat Shock and Development*. Hightower LE, Nover L, eds. Heidelberg: Springer Verlag Press

Pleet H, Graham J, Smith JM, Smith DW (1981): Central nervous system and facial defects associated with maternal hyperthermia at four to 14 weeks gestation. *Pediatrics* 67: 785–789

Pollack R, Treisman R (1990): A sensitive method for the determination of protein-DNA binding specificities. *Nuc Acids Res* 18: 6197–6204

Pulsinelli, WA, Brierley JB, Plum F (1982): Temporal profile of neuronal damage in a model of transient forebrain ischemia. *Ann Neurol* 11: 491–498

Rabindran SK, Giorgi G, Clos J, Wu C (1991): Molecular cloning and expression of a human heat shock factor, HSF1. *Proc Natl Acad Sci USA* 88: 6906–6910

Rabindran SK, Haroun RI, Clos J, Wisniewski J, Wu C (1993): Regulation of heat shock factor trimer formation: role of a conserved leucine zipper. *Science* 259: 230–234

Ritossa FM (1962): A new puffing pattern induced by a temperature shock and DNP in *Drosophila*. *Experientia* 18: 571–573

Rothman JE (1989): Polypeptide chain binding proteins: catalysts of protein folding and related processes in cells. *Cell* 59: 591–601

Rougive AE, Lis JT (1988): The RNA polymerase II molecule at the 5' end of the uninduced hsp70 gene in *D. melanogaster* is transcriptionally engaged. *Cell* 54: 795–804

Rougive AE, Lis JT (1990): Postinitiation transcriptional control in Drosophila melanogaster. *Mol Cell Biol* 10: 6041–6045

Sarge KD, Murphy SP, Morimoto RI (1993): Activation of heat shock gene transcription by HSF1 involves oligomerization, acquisition of DNA binding activity, and nuclear localization and can occur in the absence of stress. *Mol Cell Biol* 13: 1392–1407

Sarge KD, Park-Sarge OY, Kirby D, Mayo K, Morimoto RI (1994): Regulated expression of heat shock factor 2 in mouse testis: potential role as a regulator of HSP gene expression during spermatogenesis. *Biol Reprod*: 50: 1334–1343

Sarge KD, Zimarino V, Holm K, Wu C, Morimoto RI (1991): Cloning and characterization of two mouse heat shock factors with distinct inducible and constitutive DNA-binding ability. *Genes & Dev* 5: 1902–1911

Scharf K-D, Rose S, Zott W, Schoff F, Nover L (1990): Three tomato genes code for heat stress transcription factors with a remarkable degree of homology to the DNA-binding domain of the yeast HSF. *EMBO J* 9: 4495–4501

Schuetz TJ, Gallo GJ, Sheldon L, Tempst P, Kingston RE (1991): Isolation of a cDNA for HSF2: evidence for two heat shock factor genes in humans. *Proc Natl Acad Sci USA* 88: 6910–6915

Silar P, Butle G, Thiele DJ (1991): Heat shock transcription factor activates transcription of the yeast metallothionein gene. *Mol Cell Biol* 11: 1232–1238

Sistonen L, Sarge KD, Morimoto R (1994): Human heat shock factors 1 and 2 are differentially activated and can synergistically induce hsp70 gene transcription. *Mol Cell Biol* 14: 2087–2099

Sistonen L, Sarge KD, Phillips B, Abravaya K, Morimoto R (1992): Activation of heat shock factor 2 during hemin-induced differentiation of human erythroleukemia cells. *Moll Cell Biol* 12(9): 4104–4111

Skroch P, Buchman C, Karin M (1993): Regulation of human and yeast metallothionein gene transcription by heavy metal ions. *Prog Clin Biol Res* 380: 113–128

Sorger PK (1990): Yeast heat shock factor contains separable transient and sustained response transcriptional activators. *Cell* 62: 793–805

Sorger PK, Nelson HCM (1989): Trimerization of a yeast transcriptional activator via a coiled-coil motif. *Cell* 59: 807–813

Sorger PK, Pelham HRB (1988): Yeast heat shock factor is an essential DNA-binding protein that exhibits temperature-dependent phosphorylation. *Cell* 54: 855–864

Sorger PK, Lewis MJ, Pelham HRB (1987): Heat shock factor is regulated differently in yeast and HeLa cells. *Nature* 329: 81–84

Spradling A, Pardue ML, Penman S (1977): Messenger RNA in heat-shocked *Drosophila* cells. *J Mol Biol* 109: 559–587

Spradling A, Penman S, Pardue ML (1975): Analysis of Drosophila mRNA by in situ hybridization: Sequences transcribed in normal and heat shock cultured cells. *Cell* 4: 395–404

Storti RV, Scott MP, Rich A, Pardue ML (1980): Translational control of protein synthesis in response to heat shock in D. melanogaster cells. *Cell* 22: 825–834

Taylor ICA, Workman JL, Schuetz TJ, Kingston RE (1991): Facilitated binding of GAL4 and heat shock factor to nucleosomal templates: differential function of DNA-binding domains. *Genes & Dev* 5: 1285–1298

Theodorakis NG, Zand DJ, Kotzbauer PT, Williams GT, Morimoto RI (1989): Hemin-induced transcriptional activation of the hsp70 gene during erythroid maturation in K562 cells is due to a heat shock factor-mediated stress response. *Mol Cell Biol* 9: 3166–3173

Tissieres A, Mitchell KH, Tracy VM (1974): Protein synthesis in salivary glands of *Drosophila melanogaster*: Relation to chromosome puffs. *J Mol Biol* 84: 389–398

Treuter E, Nover L, Ohme K, Scharf KD (1993): Promoter specificity and deletion analysis of three tomato heat stress transcription factors. *Mol Gen Genet* 240: 113–125

Tsukiyama T, Becker P, Wu C (1994): ATP-dependent nucleosome disruption at a heat-shock promoter mediated by the binding of GAGA transcription factor. *Nature* 367: 525–532

Udelsman R, Blake MJ, Stagg CA, Li D, Putney DJ, Holbrook NJ (1993): Vascular heat shock protein expression in response to stress. *J Clin Invest* 91: 465–473

Voellmy R, Ahmed A, Schiller P, Bromley P, Rungger D (1985): Isolation and functional analysis of a human 70,000 dalton heat shock protein gene segment. *Proc Natl Acad Sci USA* 82: 4949–4953

Voellmy R, Goldschmidt-Clermont, Southgate R, Tissieres A, Levis R, Coehring W (1981): A DNA segment isolated from chromosomal site 67B in Drosophila melanogaster contains four closely linked heat shock genes. *Cell* 23: 261–270

Vogel JP, Misra M, Rose MD (1990): Loss of BiP/GRP78 function blocks translocation of secretory proteins in yeast. *J Cell Biol* 110: 1885–1895

Watowich SS, Morimoto RI, Lamb RA (1991): Flux of the paramyxovirus hemagglutinin-neuraminidase glycoprotein through the endoplasmic reticulum activates transcription of the GRP78-BiP gene. *J Virol* 65: 3590–3597

Webster WS, Gerrain MA, Edwards MJ (1985): The introduction of microthalmia, encephalocele, and other heat defects following hyperthermia during the gastrulation process in the rat. *Teratology* 31: 73–82

Welch WJ, Feramisco JR (1984): Nuclear and nucleolar localization of the 72,000 dalton heat shock protein in heat-shocked cells. *J Biol Chem* 259: 4501–4513

Westwood JT, Clos J, Wu C (1991): Stress-induced oligomerization and chromosomal relocalization of heat-shock factor. *Nature* 353: 822–827

Westwood JT, Wu C (1993): Activation of *Drosophila* heat shock factor: conformational change associated with a monomer-to-trimer transition. *Mol Cell Biol* 13: 3481–3486

Wiederrecht G, Seto D, Parker CS (1988): Isolation of the gene encoding the S. cerevisiae heat shock transcription factor. *Cell* 54: 841–853

Williams GT, McClanahan TK, Morimoto RI (1989): E1a transactivation of the human HSP70 promoter is mediated through the basal transcriptional complex. *Mol Cell Biol* 9: 2574–2587

Williams GT, Morimoto RI (1990): Maximal stress-induced transcription from the human hsp70 promoter requires interactions with the basal promoter elements independent of rotational alignment. *Mol Cell Biol* 10: 3125–3136

Williams RS, Benjamin IJ (1993): Human HSP70 protects murine cells from injury during metabolic stress. *J Clin Invest* 92: 503–508

Wooden SK, Li LJ, Navarro D, Qadri I, Pereira L, Lee AS (1991): Transactivation of the grp78 promoter by malfolded proteins, glycosylation block, and calcium ionophore is mediated through a proximal region containing a CCAAT motif which interacts with CTF/NF-I. *Mol Cell Biol* 11: 5612–5623

Wu B, Hunt C, Morimoto RI (1985): Structure and expression of the human gene encoding major heat shock protein HSP70. *Mol Cell Biol* 5: 330–341

Wu B, Hurst H, Jones N, Morimoto RI (1986a): The E1a 13S product of adenovirus 5 activates transcription of the cellular human HSP70 gene. *Mol Cell Biol* 6: 2994–2999

Wu BJ, Kingston RE, Morimoto RI (1986b): Human HSP70 promoter contains at least two distinct regulatory domains. *Proc Natl Acad Sci USA* 83: 929–633

Wu C (1980): The 5′ ends of *Drosophila* heat shock genes in chromatin are hypersensitive to DNase I. *Nature* 286: 854–860

Wu C (1984): Two protein-binding sites in chromatin implicated in the activation of heat-shock genes. *Nature* 309: 229–234

Wu C, Wilson S, Walker B, David I, Paisley T, Zimarino V, Ueda H (1987): Purification and properties of *Drosophila* heat shock activator protein. *Science* 238: 1247–1253

Xiao H, Lis JT (1988): Germline transformation used to define key features of the heat shock response element. *Science* 239: 1139–1142

Xiao H, Perisic O, Lis JT (1991): Cooperative binding of Drosophila heat shock factor to arrays of a conserved 5 bp unit. *Cell* 64: 585–593

Zhong T, Arndt K (1993): The yeast SIS1 protein, a DnaJ homolog, is required for the initiation of translation. *Cell* 73: 1175–1186

Zimarino V, Wu C (1987): Induction of sequence-specific binding of Drosophila heat shock activator protein without protein synthesis. *Nature* 327: 727–730

3

The Role and Regulation of the Jun Proteins in Response to Phorbol Ester and UV Light

PETER ANGEL

Introduction

The genetic program of all biological systems including the cells of mammals is extensively determined by the conditions of the immediate environment. Mammalian cells are exposed to many environmental cues such as cytokines or growth factors, as well as extraorganismic influences, such as heat, high concentrations of heavy metal ions, chemical carcinogens such as alkylating agents, tumor promoters, and radiation. A major adverse effect of the latter harmful substances is damage to DNA. By analogy to the bacterial system where exposure to DNA-damaging agents induces the SOS response (Little and Mount, 1982; Walker, 1985), mammalian cells actively respond to those agents by activating DNA repair enzymes and initiating a transcriptional induction response known as the UV response (Karin and Herrlich, 1989; Ronai et al, 1990; Holbrook and Fornance, 1991; Herrlich et al, 1992).

In general, alterations in the transcription of a specific set of cellular genes in response to environmental cues is mediated by signal transduction pathways to the nucleus. These pathways influence specific regulatory DNA binding proteins, known as transcription factors, that directly regulate gene expression by binding to specific DNA sequences in the promoter regions (Figure 3.1) (Karin and Smeal, 1992). Much of our present knowledge about transcription factors comes from the discovery and study of the AP-1 factor family. AP-1 (and the transcription factor $NF_\kappa B$) has served to detect one of the decisive DNA binding motifs required for gene regulation by tumor promoters, such as PMA (Phorbol 12-myristate 13-acetate) and carcinogens, including UV irradiation and other DNA damaging agents (Curran and Franza, 1988; Vogt and Bos, 1990; Angel and Karin, 1991). One of its members, the heterodimer Fos-Jun, was found in the 1980's as a protein complex containing the viral

INDUCIBLE GENE EXPRESSION, VOLUME 1
P.A. Baeuerle, Editor
© 1995 Birkhäuser Boston

oncogene product Fos, without a clue to its function (Müller et al, 1982; Van Beveren et al, 1983; Van Straaten et al, 1983). The term AP-1 (activating protein-1) was coined for an activity that supports basal level transcription in vitro at the metallothionein IIa promoter (Lee et al, 1987a). AP-1 was recognized as the decisive control element of the human collagenase I promoter in vivo, and it was demonstrated that it could be activated by external stimulation with the tumor promoter PMA (Angel et al, 1987a, 1987b; Lee et al, 1987b) or UV irradiation (Stein et al, 1989) to enhance transcription of collagenase I or other AP-1-dependent genes.

In this review, by reversing the unidirectional signal transduction pathway from the cell membrane to the nucleus (Figure 3.1), I will first

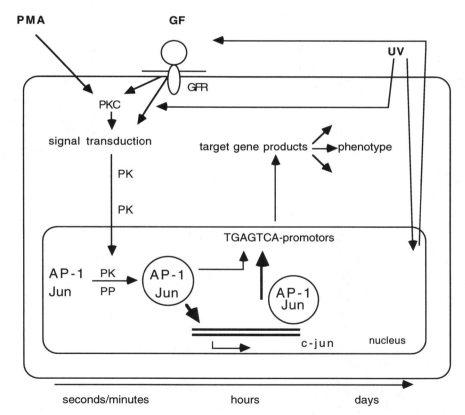

Figure 3.1 Transcription factors convert extracellular short term signals into long lasting cellular responses. A schematic illustration of signal transduction pathways regulating cJun/AP-1 in response to stimulation by growth factors (GF), phorbol esters (e.g. PMA) and carcinogens is shown. UV: UV irradiation. GFR: growth factor receptor. PKC: protein kinase C. PK: protein kinase; PP: protein phosphatase. Note that UV acts both on components of the inner cell membrane (within minutes) and by DNA damage in the nucleus inducing secretion of growth factors (II-1α, bFGF) which may act by an autocrine loop.

focus on the receiving end of these pathways, the Jun and Fos proteins, by discussing the structural properties and the various regulatory routes that regulate their activities. I will then summarize our current knowledge about the importance of these regulatory mechanisms for AP-1-dependent physiological and pathological processes regulated by tumor promoters and carcinogens, such as PMA or UV irradiation.

During the past few years the number of subunits of the AP-1 family has increased as additional members of the CREB/ATF protein family and previously identified proteins of unknown function that are capable of forming heterodimers with Jun (and possibly Fos) have been identified (Vogt and Bos, 1990; Busch and Sassone-Corsi, 1990; Angel and Karin, 1991). As will be described in the subsequent section, taking the current number of subunits and assuming that any member of the Jun, Fos or ATF/CREB families could form homo- or heterodimers (which is not strictly possible) we could predict more than 200 different heterodimers. However, the existence and function as well as the regulation of the majority of those dimers remains to be determined.

The Jun proteins may be the most extensively analyzed molecules in regard to structural and regulatory properties of transcription factors. For this reason, I will primarily focus on the Jun family in this review.

The Terminal Acceptor: The Members of the Nuclear Proto-Oncoprotein Family *jun*

Structural Characteristics of the Jun Proteins

According to its function in controlling gene expression the prototype of a transcription factor has to comprise at least two properties: a region of the protein that is responsible for binding to a specific DNA recognition sequence (DNA binding domain), and a second region that is required for transcriptional activation (transactivation domain) once the protein is bound to DNA.

The transactivation domain of the Jun proteins is located within the N-terminal half of the protein while the DNA binding domains of Jun is located at the C-terminus (Figure 3.2). In contrast, the transactivation domains of the members of the Fos and CREB/ATF proteins have not yet been determined precisely, but, in the case of Fos, transactivation seems to be influenced by amino acids at both the N-terminus and C-terminus of the protein. The DNA binding domain of Fos is located near the center of the protein (Vogt and Bos, 1990; Busch and Sassone-Corsi, 1990).

In vivo mutation analysis of the Jun proteins has identified three sub-

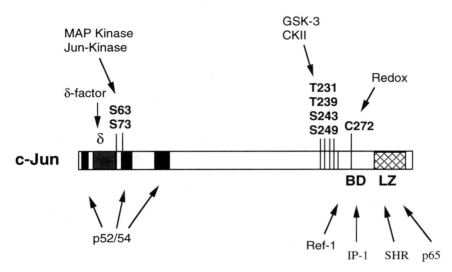

Figure 3.2 Scheme of the c-Jun protein structure and site of action of various agents. LZ: leucine zipper; BD: basic domain; solid boxes: activation domains. δ: δ-domain, only present in c-Jun but not in v-Jun. The phosphoserines and threonines and the redox site (Cys-272) are indicated. Factors that have been postulated to modulate Jun function are also shown. SHR: steroid hormone receptor. p65: the p65 subunit of $NF_\kappa B$. IP-1: inhibitor protein-1. See the text for details and the original references.

domains that together form the transactivation domain (Angel et al, 1989; Hirai et al, 1990). The sub-domains are characterized by an abundance of acidic amino acids (acidic-blob-type) which are essential for activity (Angel et al, 1989). In addition, in vitro, a fourth region near the DNA binding domain has been identified (Bohmann and Tjian, 1989). These regions are thought to be responsible for the link between the transcription factor bound to DNA and the RNA polymerase II-pre-initiation complex. Jun, however, does not contact this complex directly but seems to depend on the presence of an intermediary protein (p52/54) which has been identified by in vivo competition and immunoprecipita-tion analysis. This protein interacts with the transactivation domain of Jun, JunB (and possibly JunD), and a yet unknown component of the basal transcription machinery (Oehler and Angel, 1992). The transactiva-tion domain represents an independent biological module. Domain swapping experiments showed that the transactivation domain can be fused to a heterologous DNA binding domain to form a potent transcription factor of new promoter specificity (Angel et al, 1989).

In contrast to the transactivation domains, whose structural properties are only poorly understood, a great body of information on the DNA binding domains of Jun and Fos has been collected over the past few years (Vogt and Bos, 1990; Busch and Sassone-Corsi, 1990; Ransone et al, 1990).

Mutation analysis has revealed characteristic properties that are evolutionarily conserved between the Jun, Fos and CREB/ATF proteins, thus defining the protein family called bZip proteins (Landschulz et al, 1988). bZip stands for the amino acid sequences of the two independently acting sub-regions of the DNA binding domain. One, the basic domain, is rich in basic amino acids which are responsible for contacting the DNA. The other is the leucine-zipper region characterized by heptad repeats of leucine that are part of the well known 4-3 repeats forming a coiled-coil structure (O'Shea et al, 1989), and which are responsible for dimerization (which is a pre-requisite for DNA binding) (Kouzarides and Ziff, 1988; Sassone-Corsi et al, 1988; Gentz et al, 1989; Turner and Tjian, 1989; Neuberg et al, 1989b). In addition to the leucines, other hydrophobic and charged amino acid residues within the leucine region are responsible for specificity and stability of homo- or heterodimer formation between the various Jun, Fos or CREB/ATF proteins. The Fos proteins do not form stable homodimers but heterodimerize efficiently with the Jun proteins. The Jun proteins can form homodimers, although with reduced stability compared to Jun/Fos. While amino acid substitutions or deletions in the leucine zipper region greatly affect dimerization, mutations in the basic domain abolish DNA binding without affecting dimerization. Domain swapping experiments have shown that both domains are interchangeable among the different bZip proteins without loss of their physical properties (Neuberg et al, 1989a; Sellers and Struhl, 1989; Kouzarides and Ziff, 1989; Cohen and Curran, 1990).

In addition to the DNA binding and transactivation domains, transcription factors may also contain specific regions responsible for (1) interaction with other cellular proteins distinct from components of the RNA polymerase initiation complex (modulation domains), (2) nuclear translocation, and (3) regulation of protein stability. In the Jun (and Fos) proteins, regions have been identified that are involved in the association with other cellular proteins, such as steroid hormone receptors or the p65 subunit of NFkB (Jonat et al, 1990, Yang-Yen et al, 1990; Schüle et al, 1990a; Stein et al, 1993). While the nuclear localization signal in both Jun and Fos has been identified within the basic domain (Tratner and Verma, 1991; Chida and Vogt, 1992), specific regions involved in the rapid degradation of these proteins, possibly regulated by phosphorylation and ubiquitination (Papavasiliou et al, 1992; Bohmann, 1994) have not yet been precisely defined. Despite the very high degree of homology in the overall structural features described above, the different members of the Jun (and Fos) families exhibit significant differences which lead to subtle differences in DNA binding and transcriptional activation (Ryseck and Bravo, 1991; Hai and Curran, 1991; Chiu et al, 1989; Hirai et al,

1989; Deng and Karin, 1993) and which suggest specific functions in gene regulation for individual dimers.

In summary, the formation of specific homo- and heterodimers in a given cell depends on the relative abundance of each individual member of the bZip protein family. The mix of dimers will change with any change of a given subunit's abundance. Due to the unique properties of the specific domains of the individual bZip proteins, AP-1-dependent genes will be activated according to the prevalent AP-1 dimers present. The following section describes the different regulatory pathways to alter the level and activity of the Jun proteins in response to extracellular signals.

Transcriptional Regulation of the *jun* Genes

The *jun* (and *fos*) genes are members of a class of cellular genes, termed early response or immediate-early genes, which are characterized by a rapid and transient activation of transcription in response to changes of environmental conditions (Hirai et al, 1989; Ryseck et al, 1988; Quantin and Beathnach, 1988; Ryder et al, 1988, 1989; Angel et al, 1988). Transcription of c-*jun* and *junB*, but not *junD*, is rapidly (within 15 min) and highly enhanced in response to growth factors, cytokines, tumor promoters, carcinogens and expression of certain oncogenes. Subsequently, enhanced transcription drops back to basal level within two to three hours. Since this type of regulation of promoter activity is also observed in the absence of ongoing protein synthesis, it is generally accepted that, as a primary response to extracellular signals such as the phorbol ester PMA or UV irradiation, preexisting factors, whose activity gets altered by changes in posttranslational modification (described in detail in the subsequent section), are doing the job.

While the initial analysis of deletion mutants of the promoter regions of the *junB* and *junD* genes led to the identification of various essential cis-acting elements recognized by DNA binding proteins of mostly unknown identity (de Groot et al, 1991a, 1991b), regulation of c-*jun* promoter activity has been investigated in much more detail. Analysis of deletion mutants of the c-*jun* promoter identified two AP-1-like binding sites (Jun1, Jun2) which are involved in transcriptional regulation in response to UV irradiation, the phorbol ester PMA, or the E1A product of adenovirus (Angel et al, 1988; van Dam et al, 1990, 1993; Stein et al, 1992; Herr et al, 1994). The sequence of both sites differ from the consensus AP-1 site by the presence of an additional base pair. Based on these differences both sites are preferentially recognized by heterodimers composed of members of the Jun and ATF-2 protein families (van Dam et al, 1993; Herr et al, 1994).

For/Jun heterodimers which interact very efficiently with the consensus AP-1 site do not bind to the c-*jun* sites (Jun2) or only with very low affinity (Jun1). Most importantly, in vivo footprinting analysis revealed full occupation of both Jun1 and Jun2 in nonstimulated cells (Hagmeyer et al, 1993; Rozek and Pfeifer, 1993; Herr et al, 1994). This is in contrast to Jun/Fos-dependent target genes, e.g. the collagenase gene, where binding to the consensus AP-1 site is visible only at later time points after treatment of the cells, most likely due to enhanced synthesis of the Jun and Fos proteins (König et al, 1992). In fact, synthesis of Fos and Jun has been found to be absolutely required for enhanced collagenase expression in response to PMA (Schönthal et al, 1988). During transcriptional activation of c-*jun* at early time points after PMA or UV treatment, as well as during subsequent repression of the promoter, significant alterations in neither the DNA binding activity nor the composition of factors binding to Jun1 and Jun2 can be detected (Hagmeyer et al, 1993; Rozek and Pfeifer, 1993; Herr et al, 1994). Most likely, both activation and repression of the c-*jun* promoter in response to PMA and UV irradiation are mediated by the different types of posttranslational modification described below of promoter-bound c-Jun (and possibly ATF). The scenario described for the c-*jun* promoter closely resembles the situation that has been postulated for the c-*fos* promoter (Herrera et al, 1989), suggesting that rapid changes in the activity of prebound factors may be a hallmark of transcriptional regulation of immediate-early genes. It should be noted, however, that in addition to factors binding to Jun1 and Jun2, other DNA binding proteins including Sp1 and CTF, which have been described to modulate basal level activity of the c-*jun* promoter (Unlap et al, 1992; van Dam et al, 1993), and which are fully associated with the c-*jun* gene in both stimulated and unstimulated cells (Hagmeyer et al, 1993; Rozek and Pfeifer, 1993; Herr et al, 1994) may be important to stably assemble such types of preactivated protein complexes sitting on the c-*jun* promoter in unstimulated cells.

Regulation of Jun by Posttranslational Modifications

Kinases and Phosphatases Regulating Jun's DNA Binding Activity

The most common posttranslational modification known to modulate protein activity is phosphorylation (Hunter and Karin, 1992). Examination of the c-Jun protein from various cell types of human, mouse and chicken revealed that c-Jun is a phosphoprotein. Two-dimensional peptide maps and phosphoamino acid analysis have identified at least five serine and threonine residues in the c-Jun protein which, depending on extracellular signals, carry phosphates (Boyle, et al, 1991).

In nonstimulated cells, the c-Jun protein is phosphorylated in the C-terminal half. The corresponding amino acid residues are part of a common tryptic peptide, 227–252, located just upstream of the basic region of the DNA binding domain. Phosphopeptide analysis has identified these residues, either threonine-231 and/or serine-243 and serine-249 (Boyle et al, 1991). In vivo, casein kinase II (CKII) seems to be the major protein kinase responsible for the phosphorylation at positions 231 and 249 (Lin et al, 1992). In vitro phosphorylation studies showed that the threonine-239 and serine-243 may also serve as a phosphorylation acceptor site for phosphorylation by glycogen synthase kinase 3 (GSK-3; Boyle et al, 1991).

Upon treatment of cells with PMA or UV at doses that enhance DNA binding activity of Jun, the net phosphorylation of peptide 227-252 is decreased, suggesting that reduction in phosphorylation may enhance DNA binding. This assumption appears to be true, since in vitro phosphorylation of bacterially expressed Jun by GSK-3, acting on peptide 227-252, inhibits c-Jun DNA binding (Boyle et al, 1991). Furthermore, overexpression of GSK-3 and the analogous *Drosophila* protein kinase *shaggy* can reduce activity of AP-1-dependent promoters (de Groot et al, 1993). On the other hand, a c-Jun mutant missing all possible phosphorylation sites in the DNA binding domain is a much more potent transcriptional activator compared to wild-type c-Jun, most likely by preventing the constitutive, negatively acting down-modulation of DNA binding by phosphorylation (Hagmeyer et al, 1993). Microinjection of an excess of synthetic peptides representing CKII substrates into target cells results in an activation of AP-1-dependent genes, most likely by competitive inhibition of phosphorylation of the DNA binding domain of c-Jun (Lin et al, 1992).

The exact mechanism of TPA-induced DNA binding by reduction of phosphorylation is only poorly understood. Casein kinase II has been found to be constitutively active throughout the cell cycle, and treatment of cells with PMA (Carroll et al, 1988) or growth factors such as EGF (Ackermann and Osheroff, 1989) even enhance CKII activity. These findings argue against CKII being the decisive player in regulating c-Jun's DNA binding activity in response to extracellular signals. It is important to note, however, that CKII does not phosphorylate serine-243, which is a prerequisite for phosphorylation of threonine-231 and serine-249 by CKII (Lin et al, 1992). Therefore, the activity of CKII on c-Jun obviously depends on another kinase, possibly GSK-3 (since it can phosphorylate serine-243), or another, yet unidentified kinase. This yet unknown kinase may be the actual target for PMA or UV-dependent regulation of DNA binding of Jun. Alternatively, a specific phosphatase activated by PMA or UV may dephosphorylate the various amino acid residues in the DNA binding domain (or simply phosphorylation of serine-243). The existence of such a phosphatase, however, has yet to be confirmed.

Kinases and Phosphatases Affecting the Transactivation Domain of Jun

In contrast to the negative effect of hyperphosphorylation on DNA binding, enhanced phosphorylation at the N-terminus is required for the activation of the transactivation function of Jun. All stimuli that lead to increased transactivating potential of Jun, such as growth factors, PMA, or UV irradiation, cause hyperphosphorylation at two amino acid residues, serine-63 and serine-73 (Smeal et al, 1992; Devary et al, 1992; Radler-Pohl et al, 1993a). Both sites are also targeted following expression of various oncogenes including Ha-*ras* (Binetruy et al, 1991; Smeal et al, 1991, 1992). Depending on the stimulus and the cell type, phosphorylation at additional sites can be detected (Pulverer et al, 1991; Hagmeyer et al, 1993; Radler-Pohl et al, 1993a), whose locations have not yet been precisely identified.

The importance of the phosphorylation event for the biological function of c-Jun has been confirmed by analyzing Jun proteins carrying amino acid substitutions at positions 63 and 73. The basal activity of the transactivation domain of these mutants, either in the context of wild-type c-Jun protein or by fusing it to a heterologous DNA binding domain to activate transcription, is greatly impaired, and the positive action of PMA, UV or Ha-*ras* on the transactivation function of Jun is completely blocked (Pulverer et al, 1991; Smeal et al, 1991; Franklin et al, 1992; Devary et al, 1992; Radler-Pohl et al, 1993a). Phosphorylation of both serines 63 and 73 are also required for c-Jun's ability to cooperate with Ha-*ras* in the transformation of rat embryo fibroblasts (Smeal et al, 1992).

How is the PMA, UV or Ha-*ras*-induced hyperphosphorylation of c-Jun translated into enhanced transcription of Jun-dependent target genes? Since the transactivation domain, by definition, represents the region of the transcription factor, interacting directly or indirectly with components of the RNA polymerase II initiation complex, phosphorylation may affect those interactions. Recently, an intermediary factor, p52/54, has been described which specifically interacts with the transactivation domain of Jun and yet unknown components of the basal transcription machinery (Oehler and Angel, 1992). In vivo competition experiments revealed the necessity of serines 63 and 73 for c-Jun to interact efficiently with the intermediary factor (Oehler and Angel, 1993), suggesting that enhanced phosphorylation of c-Jun in response to PMA or UV may prolong the physical interaction between Jun and p52/54 leading to a more stable assembling of the preinitiation complex, and enhanced initiation of transcription. It is possible that p52/54 is also a phospho-protein regulated by TPA, or UV induced alterations in its phosphoryla-tion pattern. This phosphorylation may contribute to the regulation of p52/54-c-Jun interaction. Hyperphosphorylation of the transactivation domain of c-Jun, moreover, may also cause a release of a cell-type specific inhibitor interacting with the δ-domain of c-Jun (Baichwal and Tjian, 1990; Baichwal et al, 1991) to allow physical interaction with p52/54 or other proteins interacting with the transactivation domain.

The nature of the protein kinase that phosphorylates the stimulatory N-terminal sites serines 63 and 73 is still an open matter, but the family of ERK/mitogen activated protein (MAP) kinases is likely to harbour candidates for which c-Jun is a target. As pointed out by the given name, the activity of these kinase isoforms with a molecular weight of 40–46 kD is rapidly increased by MAP kinase kinases (MAPKK) in response to mitogens, such as NGF, EGF, and PDGF (Cobb et al, 1991; Pelech and Sanghere, 1992; Blenis, 1993). The regulatory phosphorylation sites in pp42-MAPK are Thr-183 and Tyr-185 (Payne et al, 1991). Hyperpho-sphorylation of pp42-MAPK is also observed in response to PMA and UV irradiation (Radler-Pohl et al, 1993a). In vitro, c-Jun is an efficient substrate for this kinase to be phosphorylated at serines 63 and 73 (Pulverer et al, 1991). In addition, in extracts of TPA treated cells, a Jun kinase copurifies with the pp42 and pp54 MAP kinases, suggesting that the action of these kinases is of physiological relevance for Jun phosphorylation in vivo (Pulverer et al, 1991, 1992). This assumption was further supported by the fact that dominant mutants of pp42 MAPK interfere, at least in part, with transcriptional activation of AP-1-dependent promoters in response to PMA and UV (Radler-Pohl and Sachsenmaier, 1994). In line with an essential role of MAP kinases in UV and PMA-induced signalling, Raf kinase, which was found to activate MAP kinases (Kyriakis et al, 1992), is also an essential component of UV-regulated signal transduction pathways (Devary et al, 1992, Radler-Pohl et al, 1993a). In addition, several studies have shown the role of Ras in Raf activation (Wood et al, 1992; Zhang et al, 1993).

Despite these different lines of evidence for an essential role of these kinases in Jun phosphorylation, recent data suggest that pp42 MAPK may not be the only Jun kinase that is commonly activated by growth factors, PMA, and UV irradiation. For example, UV irradiation is a much stronger inducer of c-*jun* transcription (Devary et al, 1991; Stein et al, 1992) and hyperphosphorylation of c-Jun protein compared to PMA (Radler-Pohl et al, 1993a). In contrast, however, UV irradiation results in only an incomplete activation of pp42 MAPK, while activation is complete following PMA stimulation of the cells (Radler-Pohl et al, 1993a). Most recently, two kinases with an apparent molecular weight of 46 kD and 55 kD have been identified that phosphorylate c-Jun at serines 63 and 73. These Jun N-terminal kinases (JNKs) were found to be affected most efficiently by UV (Hibi et al, 1993). Kinase activity is also enhanced in cells expressing Ha-*ras*. Although, the exact nature of JNKs is not yet resolved, both forms appear to be distinct from MAP kinases since they are neither phosphorylated at tyrosine (which is required for MAPK activity) nor recognized by anti-MAPK antibodies (Hibi et al, 1993).

Recently, an additional protein kinase has been partially purified by binding to a c-Jun affinity column, and has been shown to phosphorylate the amino terminus of Jun (Adler et al, 1992). However, the exact nature of this 67 kD kinase remains to be determined.

While a great body of information is now available on the activation of c-Jun activity by phosphorylation, only little is known about the enzyme(s) reverting the activation process. A putative candidate that counteracts protein kinase activity on Jun is phosphatase 2A (PP2A), which has been shown to remove phosphates from c-Jun synthesized in vitro (Black et al, 1991). In line with the model that enhanced phosphorylation of c-Jun is required for transcriptional activation of the c-*jun* promoter (Rozek and Pfeifer, 1993; Herr et al, 1994), inhibitors of PP2A, such as ocadaic acid, have been shown to enhance gradually c-*jun* transcription (Schönthal et al, 1991). The physiological requirement of PP2A in vivo for regulation of c-Jun activity remains to be confirmed. Clearly, much more work is required to sort out the importance and participation of individual kinases and phosphatases in signal transduction pathways initiated by different extracellular signals.

Other Modifications Affecting AP-1 Activity

In addition to phosphorylation, other posttranslational modifications have been identified which affect AP-1 activity. In vitro binding studies identified redox-dependent binding of Jun/Jun or Jun/Fos to DNA (Abate et al, 1990). This is of particular interest since many extracellular signals affecting AP-1, including PMA and UV, are known to induce intracellular free oxygen radical formation which, in turn, is expected to result in a shift of the redox state of cellular components (Cerutti, 1985; Cerutti and Trump, 1991). In fact, PMA-induced induction of c-*jun* or collagenase was found to be inhibited in the presence of oxygen radical scavengers such as N-acetylcysteine (Devary et al, 1992). In vitro, redox-regulated binding of Jun is stimulated by an ubiquitous 37 kD nuclear protein, Ref-1, which not only stimulates DNA binding of AP-1 but also of other transcription factors including Myb, NFkB and members of the ATF family (Xanthoudakis and Curran, 1992). However, in vitro binding analysis as well as in vitro transactivation studies clearly showed that simply mutating the cysteine residue at position 252 of c-Jun (to prevent oxidation) results in a complete loss of DNA binding in vitro and transcriptional activation of the collagenase I promoter in vivo by the Jun mutant protein (Oehler et al, 1993; Morgan et al, 1993). Redox-independent DNA binding and transcriptional activation of collagenase, however, is regained upon mutation of a phosphorylation site located in the DNA binding domain (Ser-243), suggesting that redox-independent activity of Jun depends both on the lack of phosphorylation of the DNA binding domain as well as the inability to oxidize the cysteine residue (Oehler et al, 1993; Morgan et al, 1993). Interestingly, these amino acids in the DNA binding domain are the only differences between c-Jun and its viral counterpart, v-Jun, leading to the hypothesis that v-Jun has acquired, at least in part, its oncogenic properties by escaping down-modulation of AP-1-dependent gene expression by phosphorylation and redox regulation (Vogt and Bos, 1990).

In addition to phosphorylation and redox regulation, the Jun protein has been found to undergo PMA-dependent ubiquitination, which appears to be responsible, at least in part, for regulating the half-life of the Jun protein (D. Bohmann, 1994). Jun was also found to be glycosylated (Jackson and Tjian, 1988). However, the regulation and function of this type of modification is completely unknown.

Interference Between Jun and Other Cellular and Viral Proteins Affecting Jun

Regulation of c-Jun activity is not restricted to direct modifications of Jun but can also be altered by interaction with other proteins. First of all, as described above, the choice of partner in the heterodimeric complex greatly affects the DNA binding activity of Jun: complex formation with members of the Fos protein family greatly enhance DNA binding; in contrast, heterodimer formation with JunB renders c-Jun incapable of activating transcription (Chiu et al, 1989; Deng and Karin, 1993; Vogt and Bos, 1990; Angel and Karin, 1991). Furthermore, dimerization with members of the CREB/ATF-2 protein family alters the DNA binding specificity from an AP-1 site to a sequence resembling the cAMP-responsive element (CRE) (Benbrook and Jones, 1990; Hai and Curran, 1991). Recently, the protein IP-1 has been described, which regulates DNA binding of AP-1 in a very rapid and phosphorylation-dependent manner (Auwerx and Sassone-Corsi, 1991). Treatment of cells with PMA inactivates IP-1 (resulting in efficient binding of AP-1 components), most likely by dephosphorylation. Although IP-1 appears to interact directly with the bZip region of Fos/Jun, the exact molecular mechanism of IP-1 action is still unknown.

The bZip region of c-Jun appears also to be the target for interaction with several members of the steroid hormone receptor family, such as the glucocorticoid receptor or the estrogen receptor. Except for one example of positive interference between AP-1 and the estrogen receptor on the regulation of the ovalbumin gene (Gaub et al, 1990), coexpression of Fos/Jun and activated members of the steroid hormone receptor superfamily results in mutual repression of AP-1 and hormone regulated genes (Schüle and Evans, 1991; Miner et al, 1991; Ponta et al, 1992). Repression occurs either by competitive binding to overlapping binding sites, for example in the promoter of the osteocalcin (Schüle et al, 1990b), and α-fetoprotein (Zhang et al, 1991) genes, and possibly the composite element of the proliferin gene (Diamond et al, 1990). On the other hand, Jun/Fos has been found to physically interact with steroid hormone receptors (Jonat et al, 1990; Yang-Yen et al, 1990). This fact may explain the ability of one factor to inhibit the target gene of the second transcription factor in the absence of an appropriate binding site. For example, PMA-induced collagenase I expression is completely repressed in the presence of glucocorticoids. In vivo footprinting analysis revealed that PMA-induced DNA binding of AP-1 is not affected suggesting that interaction of the receptor with Fos/Jun through the bZip region somehow disturbs the transactivation function of promoter-associated AP-1 by inhibiting contact formation between Fos/Jun and components of the RNA polymerase II preinitiation complex (König et al, 1992). Regardless of the exact mechanism of down-regulation, inhibition of PMA-induced expression of AP-1-regulated genes may provide an explanation for the anti-inflammatory and anti-tumor promoting effect of glucocorticoids, for example in the two stage mouse model of tumor formation induced by carcinogens and tumor promoters such as PMA (Belman and Troll, 1972; Scribner and Slaga, 1973; Allison, 1988).

c-Jun has also been shown to physically interact with MyoD; this interaction results in an inactivation at the transcriptional level and may contribute to Jun-mediated inhibition of myogenesis (Bengal et al, 1992; Li et al, 1992). Analyzing transcriptional regulation of the human papilloma virus type 18 promoter, a cross talk between AP-1 and the transcriptional repressor YY1 has been identified. Depending on the cell, either positive or negative interference between both factors takes place, possibly by physical interaction between YY1 and Jun (and possibly Fos) (Bauknecht et al, 1992; Bauknecht et al, 1994).

Most recently, a synergistic action of AP-1 and the transcription factor NFκB has been found (Stein et al, 1993). This is particularly interesting since the activity of both transcription factors is altered in response to an almost identical set of extracellular signals, such as cytokines (e.g. II-1, TNFα), PMA, or UV irradiation (Schreck and Baeuerle, 1991; Angel and Karin, 1991). While overexpression of Jun and/or Fos enhances the transcription of NF$_\kappa$B-dependent genes, overexpression of the p65 subunit of NF$_\kappa$B (Baeuerle, 1991), but not the p50 subunit, further enhances the transcription of AP-1-dependent promoters (e.g. collagenase I) without direct contact between p65 and the promoter (Stein et al, 1993). This phenomena is likely to be caused by direct interaction between Jun/Fos and p65. In Jun and Fos, the bZip regions have been identified to be required for interaction; in p65 the rel domain (Baeuerle, 1991) has been found to be essential (Stein et al, 1993). The exact mechanism of interaction remains to be elucidated. It is important to note, however, that Fos/Jun interacts only with the activated, nuclear form of p65 but does not associate with nonactive p65 molecules from untreated cells that are located in the cytoplasm complexed to the inhibitor I$_\kappa$B (Stein et al, 1993).

In contrast to the cellular proteins described above which interact directly with Jun and/or Fos, the E1A product of adenovirus modulates AP-1 activity without apparent direct interaction (Offringa et al, 1990). Most interestingly, E1A appears to be able to distinguish between different dimer combinations to either positively or negatively regulate activity. On one hand, dimers composed of c-Jun and members of the ATF-2 family are activated (van Dam et al, 1993), most likely by hyperphosphorylation of Jun (Hagmeyer et al, 1993) and possibly ATF-2 through an E1A-regulated kinase or phosphatase. This type of regulation appears to be responsible for enhanced transcription of the c-*jun* gene in adenovirus transformed cells. In contrast, the activity of Jun homodimers or Jun/Fos heterodimers is completely inhibited by E1A resulting in a complete loss of PMA-induced transcription of the collagenase I, stromelysin I or CD44 genes (Offringa et al, 1988, 1990; Hofmann et al, 1993) whose transcription completely depends on AP-1. In vivo footprinting analysis of the collagenase I gene has demonstrated that, in contrast to steroid hormone receptors, repression of transcription is mediated by interfering with Jun/Jun or Jun/Fos binding to DNA (Hagmeyer et al, 1993). The exact mechanism of inhibition is at present unknown. However, changes in phosphorylation or the redox state of Jun are clearly not involved in E1A-dependent inhibition of binding (Hagmeyer et al, 1993).

The Initial Target: Cell Membrane, Nucleus, or Both?

The major adverse effect of UV is damage to DNA caused by pyrimidine dimers, leading to somatic mutations. DNA damage has also been observed after PMA treatment, at least in certain cell types (Cerutti, 1985). Since the common program of alterations in gene expression is also elicited by other DNA-damaging agents, such as ionizing radiation, chemical carcinogens (e.g. mitomycin C, 4-nitroquinolineoxide), or hydrogen peroxide, DNA damage or by-products of DNA damage were hypothesized to be the primary signal in the cell that initiated such altered gene expression. This assumption appears to be confirmed by studying the expression of AP-1-dependent genes (collagenase I and MTIIa) in cells deficient in repair of UV-induced DNA lesions. In fibroblasts from patients with Xeroderma pigmentosum (XP), the UV dose required for maximal induction of collagenase is about 10% of what is required in wild-type cells (Schorpp et al, 1984; Angel et al, 1986; Stein et al, 1989). In addition, the production of the UV-induced secreted factor EPIF (Schorpp et al, 1984), containing interleukin 1α and bFGF (Krämer et al, 1993), initiates the UV response in nonirradiated cells and is also induced by low doses of UV in XP cells (Schorpp et al, 1984). Another line of evidence supporting the role of DNA damage as the initial signal of altered gene expression comes from the analysis of the action spectrum of UV-induced gene expression. Maximal levels are reached between 265 and 275 nm (Stein et al, 1989). Within this range nucleobase-containing compounds such as NAD, RNA, DNA, or other aromatic compounds are the most likely targets.

Since the DNA repair process takes hours, the XP system described above is not useful for determining the primary target of UV in the immediate early induction of c-*jun* transcription. On the other hand, the secretion of growth factors, such as II-1α or bFGF (and additional factors making up EPIF) in any measurable amount is a slow process and is, therefore, unlikely to account for the immediate early response such as the induction of c-*jun* and c-*fos*, as well as the alterations in the activity of the protein kinases and phosphatases regulating c-Jun activity. However, there is strong evidence that growth factor receptors or proteins associated with growth factor receptors are involved in the UV response. The earliest detectable cellular alterations in response to UV (within five minutes) is hyperphosphorylation of the EGF receptor (Sachsenmaier et al, 1994) and an activation of Src-family tyrosine kinases, followed by activation of Ha-ras, the cytoplasmic serine-threonine kinase Raf-1 and p42 MAP kinase (Devary et al, 1992; Radler-Pohl et al, 1993a). These components have been characterized as parts of signal transduction pathways initiated by growth factors (Pelech and Sanghere, 1992; Karin and Smeal, 1992; Blenis, 1993), suggesting that UV and growth factors regulate gene expression through common routes. The requirement for specific components of the signal transduction cascade has been demonstrated by using tyrosine kinase inhibitors or transdominant negative mutants of *src*, Ha-*ras*, Raf-1 or MAP-2 kinase (Devary et al, 1992; Radler-Pohl et al, 1993a, 1993b; Devary et al, 1993; Sachsenmaier et al, 1994). Activation of pp42 MAPK, as well as hyperphosphorylation of c-Jun and enhanced transcription of the c-*jun* gene or collagenase I promoter activity is blocked in the presence of Suramin (Sachsenmaier et al, 1994; Radler-Pohl et al, 1993b), a well known inhibitor of growth factor receptor activity (Betsholz et al, 1986; Coffey et al, 1987). However, Suramin does not affect signaling pathways that bypass receptors, elicited upon activation of v-Src, or in response to PMA treatment, (Radler-Pohl et al, 1993b; Sachsenmaier et al, 1994) which directly activates protein kinase C (Nishizuka, 1986), which in turn may activate Raf-1 kinase (Kölch et al, 1993).

The second line of evidence for an essential role of components at or near the plasma membrane is based on a phenomenon in which cells become what is known as refractory which means that treatment of cells with a specific inducer, such as growth factors, PMA or UV will not be effective when the cells are pretreated with the same agent. It is assumed that a cellular component present within cells in limited amounts is consumed during the first round of induction and is, therefore, not available upon restimulation of the cells. Thus, cells treated with PMA become refractory to a second PMA stimulation, but still respond to UV or EGF treatment (Büscher et al, 1988; Devary et al, 1991). Pretreatment of cells, however, with either EGF, bFGF or II-1α block, at least partially, subsequent UV induction (Sachsenmaier et al, 1994), suggesting the requirement of a component that is an essential part of signal transduction pathways initiated by UV or the various growth factors. In either case, the consumable component must be upstream of Raf-1 (which is essential for both UV and PMA action), since pretreatment of cells of PMA does not interfere with an additional round of induction following restimulation with UV (Büscher et al, 1988; Devary et al, 1991; Sachsenmaier et al, 1994). The consumable component may even be the growth factor receptors themselves, since pretreatment of the cells with one growth factor does not induce cross-refractoriness to a second different growth factor (Sachsenmaier et al, 1994).

In summary, these data strongly suggest that the UV signaling cascade activating Jun is initiated at or near the plasma membrane and feeds into common signal transduction pathways whose components are largely shared between growth factors, PMA and UV.

In the case of UV, the critical signal generated upon irradiation that initiates the immediate early events in the plasma membrane is at present unknown. Recently, the production of oxidative stress has been proposed to be the elicitor of the signaling cascade because N-acetylcysteine (NAC), a potent intracellular free oxygen radical scavenger, attenuates Src activation and induction of c-*jun* transcription (Devary et al, 1992). However, treatment of cells with PMA also produces oxidative stress (Cerutti, 1885; Schreck and Baeuerle, 1991), but does not induce identical patterns of phosphorylation of Jun or activation of Jun kinases, nor does it result in cross-refractoriness between PMA and UV. Clearly, the late UV responses, such as the induction of collagenase expression, appear not be induced through oxygen radicals, since wild-type and xeroderma pigmentosum cells do not differ in the repair of DNA lesions induced by reactive oxygen intermediates but exhibit an at least 10-fold difference in the UV dose required for collagenase induction. Possibly UV does not induce gene transcription by generating reactive oxygen stress but rather needs a fairly high constitutive level of reactive oxygen intermediates (which can be blocked by NAC) in order to function.

Is there any evidence for a contribution of DNA damage in the rapid initiation of the processes at or near the plasma membrane? A prerequisite of such reverse signal flow has to involve molecules activated by DNA damage that rapidly diffuse out of the nucleus into the cytoplasm to reach directly or indirectly (by activating cytoplasmic kinases) the cell membrane. To test this possibility, HeLa cells were enucleated by cytochalasin-B treatment. Such cytoplasts were still responsive to UV in respect to activation of Jun kinases (JNKs) and enhanced DNA binding of NFκB (Devary et al, 1993), arguing against the requirement of a nuclear signal in the immediate early response to UV irradiation. However, the cytoplast preparation used in this study still contained traces of mitochondrial DNA which may substitute, at least in part, for damaged genomic DNA.

Role of the Jun proteins in Physiology and Pathology

As described above, radiation and chemical carcinogens are characterized by their ability to damage DNA resulting in the formation of mutations in the genome, which is thought to be one of the initial steps leading to cell death or neoplastic transformation. Therefore, an obvious, naive concept for the function of an inducible transcription factor like AP-1 may be the induced production of DNA repair enzymes in order to rapidly block such harmful consequences. However, up to now, there is no clear example of a DNA repair gene whose transcription is efficiently induced by AP-1. In fact, overexpression of Fos has even been found to increase the rate of chromosomal aberrations and rearrangements (van den Berg et al, 1991). However, in this case, c-Fos is constitutively expressed rather than following the transient type of increase as found after PMA or UV treatment. Most recently, experimental evidence has been provided that supports a possible involvement of AP-1-regulated processes in the protection of cells against the toxic effects of UV. Inhibition of tyrosine kinases, which are immediately activated upon UV irradiation, potentiates cell killing by UV (Devary et al, 1992). These results, of course, do not rule out the involvement of other transcription factors distinct from AP-1, whose activity is controlled directly or indirectly by tyrosine phosphorylation. Nevertheless, at least three AP-1-regulated genes have been identified thus far whose gene products are involved in detoxification of DNA damaging agents. Glutathione transferase catalyses the conjunction of electrophilic compounds with glutathione, a potent oxygen radical scavenger. Overexpression of this enzyme protects cells from the influence of a number of genotoxic and cytotoxic agents (Nakagawa, 1990). The promoter region of the GT gene contains two imperfect AP-1 sites (Okuda et al, 1990; Friling et al, 1992) which are responsible for enhanced transcription of the GT gene in response to PMA (Sakai et al, 1992; Bergelson et al, 1994). An AP-1 binding site has also been described to be part of the antioxidant response element (ARE) of the quinone oxidoreductase (NQO) gene. Mutations in this region of the gene abolishes basal and inducible activity (Li and Jaiswal, 1992; Bergelson et al, 1994). This enzyme is induced by a number of carcinogens with quinone intermediates and protects against free radical toxicity (Li and Jaiswal, 1992). Metallothioneins are one of the first examples of genes that have been identified to be regulated by PMA and UV through AP-1 (Angel et al, 1986; 1987a). In respect to detoxification, these proteins bind very efficiently to heavy metal ions and are very efficient radical scavengers (Karin, 1985). Surprisingly, overexpression of MT protects cells against heavy metals but does not generate resistance against gamma-radiation, which is thought to exert its toxicity by oxygen radical formation. However, MT overexpressing cells are significantly more resistant against several other DNA damaging agents, such as N-methyl-N-nitrosourea, morphalan, chlorambucil and cisplatin (Kelley et al, 1988; Kaina et al, 1990). The molecular mechanism by which MT counteracts these cytotoxic agents is at present unknown. Enhanced c-*jun* and MT expression may, however, explain the rapid resistance to cisplatin of some ovarian cancer patients during chemotherapy (Bauknecht et al, 1993).

In summary, the present data suggest that the UV response allows enhanced survival of cells by inactivating genotoxic and cytotoxic agents prior to DNA damage rather than enhancing DNA repair mechanisms. In the future it will be interesting to determine whether the UV-induced secreted factor EPIF (Schorpp et al, 1984) or individual components of EPIF, such as II-1α and bFGF (Krämer et al, 1993), which have not been found to damage DNA to a significant extent, can induce this type of protection program in noninduced cells.

As suggested by the enhanced genomic instability in response to constitutively elevated c-Fos levels described above (van den Berg et al, 1991), it should be stressed that the alterations in AP-1 to induce the proposed beneficial events have to be tightly controlled. Any type of disregulation by by-passing regulatory mechanisms may, eventually, have fatal consequences. Clearly, members of the Jun protein family play a decisive role in controlling cell proliferation, since microinjection of Jun-specific antibodies interferes with cell cycle progression (Kovary and Bravo, 1991). However, it should be noted that the various Jun proteins have different functions in cell cycle control (Catellazzi et al, 1991): while c-Jun appears to be a positive regulator of cell proliferation, JunD seems to negatively regulate cell growth. Overexpression of JunD results in slower growth and an increase in the percentage of cells in G0/G1 while c-Jun expression produces larger S/G2 and M phase populations (Pfarr et al, 1994).

The requirement of appropriate control of AP-1 is further underlined by two findings. First, constitutive overexpression of c-Jun results in transformation of immortalized Rat-1a fibroblasts. In primary rat fibroblasts, Jun is not able to transform on its own but cooperates with *ras* (Schütte et al, 1989a; Alani et al, 1991). On the other hand, expression of transdominant negative mutants of Jun reverts the transformed phenotype of cells overexpressing *ras* (Lloyd et al, 1991). In line with the studies on cell proliferation, JunD is a negative regulator of c-Jun in *ras*-induced transformation (Pfarr et al, 1994). JunB, which is a negative regulator of c-Jun-dependent transactivation (Chiu et al, 1989) also counteracts cell transformation by c-Jun (Schütte et al, 1989b). The potency of c-Jun in cell transformation seems to be independent of Fos, but depends on an authentic, intact transactivation domain, which cannot be replaced by the potent transactivation domain of the yeast transactivator GCN4 (Oliviero et al, 1992).

The second finding is that a viral counterpart of c-Jun, but not JunB and JunD, has been isolated from a chicken retrovirus, ASV 17 (Maki et al, 1987). ASV 17 virus transforms chicken embryo fibroblasts (CEFs) in culture and induces fibrosarcomas in young chickens. The *jun* sequences excised from ASV17 and inserted into a retroviral expression vector allow efficient transformation of CEFs (Vogt and Bos, 1990). The transforming potential of v-Jun is encoded by the very few differences between v-Jun and c-Jun: a small deletion in the N-terminus (δ domain) resulting in the loss of association with a cell-type specific repressor (Bohmann and Tjian, 1989), and two point mutations leading to a loss of down-modulation by phosphorylation and redox (Vogt and Bos, 1990). In addition, the v-*jun* m-RNA is much more stable than c-*jun* due to the deletion of destabilizing sequences in the 3'-untranslated region (Vogt and Bos, 1990). Also, cell cycle dependent control of nuclear localization of v-Jun is lost (Chida and Vogt, 1992).

Although being able to efficiently transform CEFs, simply overexpressing v-Jun (or c-Jun) is not sufficient to induce tumor development in an animal model system. Transgenic mice overexpressing v-Jun or c-Jun in many tissues do not show an increased incidence of spontaneous tumors (Schuh et al, 1990; Grigoriadis et al, 1993). However, obligatory wounding of the dermis of v-Jun transgenic mice induces hyperplasia and the development of sarcomas at the site of wounding, suggesting that the cooperative action of v-Jun and cofactors that are activated during wounding or wound healing cause oncogenic transformation (Schuh et al, 1990).

As described in previous sections, the transactivation potential of Jun is enhanced by coexpression of specific oncogenes, such as *src*, Ha-*ras* or *raf*. In respect to tumor formation, it is important to note that a variety of human and animal tumors created by chemical or physical carcinogens contain an activated *ras* oncogene (Barbacid, 1986). According to the intracellular localization of the forementioned oncogenic products in the plasma membrane or cytoplasm, Jun has been hypothesized to be at the receiving end of signal transduction pathways (Herrlich and Ponta, 1989; Angel and Karin, 1991; Karin and Smeal, 1992). Because of the unidirectional nature of such pathways a hierarchical order of oncogene action has been established both on the level of transactivation of AP-1-regulated genes and cell transformation (Herrlich and Ponta, 1989; Angel and Karin, 1991). However, oncogene-induced cellular events have also been found in cell systems lacking functional AP-1 activity, which clearly demonstrates that other yet to be identified nuclear receptors for oncogene action must exist (Herrlich and Ponta, 1989; Angel and Karin, 1991).

Are the mutations in Jun, like the mutations found in v-Jun (possibly established by radiation or chemical mutagens), also involved in the generation and maintenance of human tumors? So far, only a few reports are available regarding alterations in c-*jun* expression in human tumors. High levels of c-*jun* transcripts have been detected in human renal cell cancer and human lung cancer cell lines, but the gene is also highly expressed in the corresponding normal tissue (Minna et al, 1989; Koo et al, 1992). With the potential synergistic and antagonistic interactions which can occur between members of the AP-1 family and between AP-1 and other transcription factors, as well as the posttranslational modifications (and mutants of c-Jun abolishing these regulatory modifications) which can alter AP-1 activity, measuring only changes in the level of c-*jun* transcripts appears not to be sufficient anyway. For example, in the mouse skin model system of chemically induced squamous cell cancer, expression of c-Jun (and c-Fos) is not altered at the mRNA level in either benign or malignant tumors compared to normal skin (Toftgard et al, 1985; Hashimoto et al, 1990). However, both benign and malignant tumors have increased expression of AP-1-regulated genes, such as urokinase and metallothionein (Hashimoto et al, 1990). Additionally, the expression of stromelysin is significantly upregulated in carcinomas compared to benign papillomas (Ostrowski et al, 1988) suggesting that enhanced AP-1 activity during skin tumor progression apparently occurs without changes in *jun* and *fos* transcription. Transgenic mice with an AP-1-dependent promoter linked to an appropriate reporter gene should, however, allow analysis in AP-1 activity at discrete stages of carcinogenesis. Recently isolated mice that lack a functional c-Fos protein (Johnson et al, 1992; Wang et al, 1992) may even be a more powerful system to confirm the role and requirement of specific dimers of AP-1 in such processes. These and other future studies should help elucidate the mechanisms by which Jun and Jun-related proteins function during the normal course of a cell's life and its pathogenesis.

Conclusions

Over the past decade AP-1 has been identified as a transcription factor and has become the paradigm of the field. The AP-1 family plays crucial roles in cell growth, proliferation, differentiation and apoptosis. It is the endpoint of several pathways of signal transduction, including one that triggers cancerous growth induced by either chemical or physical mutagens or by expression of certain oncogenes. Alterations in AP-1 activity are initiated by changes in posttranslational modification of preexisting molecules which appear to be required for the subsequent transcriptional control of the various members of the AP-1 family. Jun and Fos proteins therefore represent ideal molecules to study how posttranslational modifications (phosphorylation, ubiquitination, redox) regulate the activity of a protein. Studies of AP-1 have also allowed us to understand how short-term extracellular signals from the mico-environment of the cell are translated into long-lasting cellular responses, including the identification of the components of signal transduction pathways and the discovery of regulatory cross-talk between transcription factors. For example, AP-1 is modulated by viral gene products, and by steroid and retinoic acid receptors during the process of anti-inflammation.

Exemplified by the AP-1 family, the present review describes a development observed with several eucaryotic transcription factors, namely that a sequence-specific DNA binding activity, originally thought to be a single protein, turned out to be encoded by a family of structurally related proteins. For DNA binding dimerization is required. Since the various members of the protein family exhibit slight differences in function and regulation, combinatorial homo- and heterodimerization yield a great number of distinct transcription factors with subtle differences in DNA sequence specificity. In addition, combinatorial dimerization opens the possibility that specific heterodimers are addressed by different signalling pathways at the same time.

Despite the great body of information of AP-1 in cell culture systems, we are just at the beginning of understanding the individual role of the Jun and Fos proteins by using the powerful technique of homologous recombination in mice. Using these animals as well as cell lines derived from these animals, however, may have a major draw-back: in the complete animal, selection for viability may lead to compensation. For example, to create nonlethal Fos-minus mutations, one may force other members of the AP-1 family to replace Fos, which, under physiological conditions may not be of importance. Clearly, such mice have demonstrated the absolute requirement for Jun and Fos proteins for certain physiological processes, since inactivation of the appropriate gene loci results in the development of specific pathological phenotypes. However, the appropriate target genes responsible for these pathological phenotypes are still far from being identified. In addition, and in contrast to tissue culture cells, expression of AP-1 dependent genes in an animal system may be greatly influenced by tissue-specific factors interacting directly or indirectly with AP-1 on the promoter of AP-1-dependent target genes, by tissue-specific growth factors or cytokines, and by cell-cell or cell-matrix contacts.

In summary, although being the best studied transcription factor, AP-1 is far from getting boring. It still maintains a lot of its mystery, and further research may yield an even more complex picture of function and regulation of AP-1 than exists at present.

Acknowledgments

I am grateful to Dr. Larry Sherman for critical reading and Ingrid Kammerer for help with preparing the manuscript. The work in the author's laboratory is funded by the Deutsche Forschungsgemeinschaft (An 182/6-1) and the European Economic Community Biomedicine and Health Program.

References

Abate C, Patel L, Rauscher III FJ, Curran T (1990): Redox regulation of Fos and Jun DNA-binding activity in vitro. *Science* 249: 1157–1161

Ackermann P, Osheroff N (1989): Regulation of casein kinase II activity by epidermal growth factor in human A-432 carcinoma cells. *J Biol Chem* 264: 11958–11965

Adler V, Polotskaya A, Wagner F, Kraft AS (1992): Affinity-purified c-Jun amino-terminal protein kinase requires serine/threonine phosphorylation for activity. *J Biol Chem* 267: 17001–17005

Alani R, Brown P, Binétruy B, Dosaka H, Rosenberg RK, Angel P, Karin M, Birrer MJ (1991): The transactivating domain of the c-Jun proto-oncoprotein is required for cotransformation of rat embryo cells. *Mol Cell Biol* 11: 6286–6295

Allison AC (1988): *Immunopathogenic Mechanisms of Arthritis*. Goodacre J, Diek WC, eds. Boston: MIT Press

Angel P, Karin M (1991): The role of Jun, Fos and the AP-1 complex in cell-proliferation and transformation. *Biochem Biophys Acta* 1072: 129–157

Angel P, Baumann I, Stein B, Delius H, Rahmsdorf HJ, Herrlich P (1987b): 12-0-tetradecanoyl-phorbol-13-acetate induction of the human collagenase gene is mediated by an inducible enhancer element located in the 5′-flanking region. *Mol Cell Biol* 7: 2256–2266

Angel P, Hattori K, Smeal T, Karin M (1988): The jun proto-oncogene is positively autoregulated by its product, Jun/AP-1. *Cell* 55: 875–885

Angel P, Smeal T, Meek J, Karin M (1989): Jun and v-Jun contain multiple regions that participate in transcriptional activation in an interdependent manner. *New Biol* 1: 35–43

Angel P, Imagawa M, Chiu R, Stein B, Imbra RJ, Rahmsdorf HJ, Jonat C, Herrlich P, Karin M (1987a): Phorbol ester-inducible genes contain a common cis element recognized by a TPA-modulated trans-acting factor. *Cell* 49: 729–739

Angel P, Pöting A, Mallick U, Rahmsdorf HJ, Schorpp M, Herrlich P (1986): Induction of metallothionein and other mRNA species by carcinogens and tumor promoters in primary human skin fibroblasts. *Mol Cell Biol* 6: 1760–1766

Auwerx J, Sassone-Corsi P (1991): IP-1: a dominant inhibitor of Fos/Jun whose activity is modulated by phosphorylation. *Cell* 64: 983–993

Baeuerle PA (1991): The inducible transcription factor NF-κB: Regulation by distinct protein subunits. *Biochim Biophys Acta* 1072: 63–80

Baichwal VR, Tjian R (1990): Control of cJun activity by interaction of a cell-specific inhibitor. *Cell* 63: 815–825

Baichwal VR, Park A, Tjian R (1991): v-Src and EJ Ras alleviate repression of c-Jun by a cell-specific inhibitor. *Nature* 352: 165–168

Barbacid M (1986): Mutagenes, oncogenes and cancer. *TIG* 2: 188–192

Bauknecht T, Angel P, Royer HD, zur Hausen H (1992): Identification of a negative regulatory domain in the human papillomavirus type 18 promoter: interaction with the transcriptional repressor YY1. *EMBO J* 11: 4607–4617

Bauknecht T, Angel P, Kohler M, Kommoss F, Birmelin G, Pfleiderer A, Wagner A (1993): Gene structure and expression analysis of the epidermal growth factor receptor, transforming growth factor-alpha, myc, jun and metallothionein in human ovarian carcinomas. *Cancer* 71: 419–429

Belman S, Troll W (1972): The inhibition of croton oil-promoted mouse skin tumorigenesis by steroid hormones. *Cancer Res* 32: 450–454

Benbrook DM, Jones NC (1990): Heterodimer formation between CREB and JUN proteins. *Oncogene* 5: 295–302

Bengal E, Ransone L, Scharfmann R, Dwarki VJ, Tapscot SJ, Weintraub H, Verma IM (1992): Functional antagonism between c-Jun and MyoD proteins: a direct physical association. *Cell* 68: 507–519

Bergelson S, Pinkus R, Daniel V (1994): Induction of AP-1 (Fos/Jun) by chemical agents mediates activation of glutathione S-transferase and quinone reductase gene expression. *Oncogene* 9: 565–571

Betsholtz C, Johnsson A, Heldin C-H, Westermark B (1986): Efficient reversion of simian sarcoma virus-transformation and inhibition of growth factor-induced mitogenesis by suramin. *Proc Natl Acad Sci USA* 83: 6440–6444

Binétruy B, Smeal T, Karin M (1991): Ha-Ras augments c-Jun activity and stimulates phosphorylation of its activation domain. *Nature* 351: 122–127

Black EJ, Street AJ, Gillespie DAF (1991): Protein phosphatase 2A reverses phosphorylation of c-Jun specified by the delta domain in vitro: correlation with oncogenic activation and regulated transactivation activity. *Oncogene* 6: 1949–1958

Blenis J (1993): Signal transduction via the MAP kinases: Proceed at your own RSK. *Proc Natl Acad Sci USA* 90: 5889–5892

Bohmann D (1994): personal communication

Bohmann D, Tjian R (1989): Biochemical analysis of transcriptional activation by Jun: differential activity of c- and v-Jun. *Cell* 59: 709–717

Boyle WJ, Smeal T, Defize LHK, Angel P, Woodgett JR, Karin M, Hunter T (1991): Activation of protein kinase C decreases phosphorylation of c-Jun at sites that negatively regulate its DNA-binding activity. *Cell* 64: 573–584

Busch SJ, Sassone-Corsi P (1990): Dimers, leucine-zippers and DNA binding domains. *TIG* 6: 36–40

Büscher M, Rahmsdorf HJ, Litfin M, Karin M, Herrlich P (1988): Activation of the c-fos gene by UV and phorbol ester: different signal transduction pathways converge to the same enhancer element. *Oncogene* 3: 301–311

Carroll D, Santoro N, Marshak DR (1988): Regulating cell growth: casein kinase II-dependent phosphorylation of nuclear oncoproteins. *Cold Spring Harbor Symp Quant Biol* 53: 91–95

Catellazzi M, Spyrou G, La V, Dangy J, Piu F, Yaniv M, Brun G (1991): Over-expression of c-jun, junB, or junD affects cell growth differently. *Proc Natl Acad Sci USA* 88: 8890–8894

Cerutti PA (1985): Prooxidant states and tumor promotion. *Science* 227: 375–381

Cerutti PA, Trump BF (1991): Inflammation and oxidative stress in carcinogenesis. *Cancer Cells* 3: 1–7

Chida K, Vogt PK (1992): Nuclear translocation of viral Jun but not of cellular Jun is cell cycle dependent. *Proc Natl Acad Sci USA* 89: 4290–4294

Chiu R, Angel P, Karin M (1989): Jun-B differs in its biological properties from, and is a negative regulator of, cJun. *Cell* 59: 979–986

Cobb MH, Boulton TG, Robbins DJ (1991): Extracellular signal-regulated kinases-ERKs in progress. *Cell Reg* 2: 965–978

Coffey Jr, RJ, Leof EB, Shipley GD, Moses HL (1987): Suramin inhibition of growth factor receptor binding and mitogenicity in AKR-2B cells. *J Cell Physiol* 132: 143–148

Cohen DR, Curran T (1990): Analysis of dimerization and DNA binding functions in Fos and Jun by domain-swapping: involvement of residues outside the leucine zipper/basic region. *Oncogene* 5: 929–939

Curran T, Franza Jr, BR (1988): Fos and Jun: The AP-1 connection. *Cell* 55: 395–397

de Groot RP, Auwerx J, Karperien M, Staels B, Kruijer W (1991a): Activation of junB by PKC and PKA signal transduction through a novel cis-acting element. *Nucleic Acids Res* 19: 775–781

de Groot RP, Karperien M, Pals C, Kruijer W (1991b): Characterization of the mouse junD promoter-high basal level activity due to an octamer motif. *EMBO J* 10: 2523–2532

de Groot RP, Auwerx J, Bourouis M, Sassone-Corsi P (1993): Negative regulation of Jun/AP-1: conserved function of glycogen synthase kinase 3 and the Drosophila kinase shaggy. *Oncogene* 8: 841–847

Deng T, Karin M (1993): JunB differs from c-Jun in its DNA-binding and dimerization domains, and represses c-Jun by formation of inactive heterodimers. *Genes Dev* 7: 479–490

Devary Y, Gottlieb RA, Lau LF, Karin M (1991): Rapid and preferential activation of the c-jun gene during the mammalian UV response. *Mol Cell Biol* 11: 2804–2811

Devary Y, Gottlieb RA, Smeal T, Karin M (1992): The mammalian ultraviolet response is triggered by activation of Src tyrosine kinases. *Cell* 71: 1081–1091

Devary Y, Rosette C, DiDonato JA, Karin M (1993): NF-κB activation by ultraviolet light not dependent on a nuclear signal. *Science* 261: 1442–1445

Diamond MI, Miner JN, Yoshinaga SK, Yamamoto KR (1990): Transcription factor interactions: Selectors of positive or negative regulation from a single DNA element. *Science* 249: 1266–1272

Franklin CC, Sanchez V, Wagner F, Woodgett JR, Kraft AS (1992): Phorbol ester-induced amino-terminal phosphorylation of human JUN but not JUNB regulates transcriptional activation. *Proc Natl Acad Sci USA* 89: 7247–7251

Friling RS, Bergelson S, Daniel V (1992): Two adjacent AP-1-like binding sites form the electrophile-responsive element of the murine glutathione S-transferase Ya subunit gene. *Proc Natl Acad Sci USA* 89: 668–672

Gaub M-P, Bellard M, Scheuer I, Chambon P, Sassone-Corsi P (1990): Activation of the ovalbumin gene by the estrogen receptor involves the Fos-Jun complex. *Cell* 63: 1267–1276

Gentz R, Rauscher III FJ, Abate C, Curran T (1989): Parallel association of Fos and Jun leucine zippers juxtaposes DNA binding domains. *Science* 243: 1695–1699

Grigoriadis AE, Schellander K, Wang Z-Q, Wagner EF (1993): Osteoblasts are target cells for transformation in c-fos transgenic mice. *J Cell Biol* 122: 685–701

Hagmeyer BM, König H, Herr I, Offringa R, Zantema A, van der Eb AJ, Herrlich P, Angel P (1993): Adenovirus E1A negatively and positively modulates transcription of AP-1 dependent genes by dimer-specific regulation of the DNA binding and transactivation activities of Jun. *EMBO J* 12: 3559–3572

Hai T, Curran T (1991): Cross-family dimerization of transcription factors Fos/Jun and ATF/CREB alters DNA binding specificity. *Proc Natl Acad Sci USA* 88: 3720–3724

Hashimoto Y, Tajima O, Hashiba H, Nose K, Kuroki T (1990): Elevated expression of secondary, but not early, responding genes to phorbol ester tumor promoters in papillomas and carcinomas of mouse skin. *Mol Carcinog* 3: 302–308

Herr I, van Dam H, Angel P (1994): Binding of promoter-associated AP-1 is not altered during induction and subsequent repression of the c-jun promoter by TPA and UV irradiation. *Carcinogenesis* 15: 1105–1113

Herrera R, Ro HS, Robinson GS, Xanthopoulos KG, Spiegelman (1989): A direct role for C/EBP and the AP-1-binding site in gene expression linked to adipocyte differentiation. *Mol Cell Biol* 9: 5331–5339

Herrlich P, Ponta H (1989): "Nuclear" oncogenes convert extracellular stimuli into changes in the genetic program. *TIG* 5: 112–116

Herrlich P, Ponta H, Rahmsdorf HJ (1992): DNA damage-induced gene expression: signal transduction and relation to growth factor signaling. *Rev of Physiol Biochem Pharmacol* 119: 187–223

Hibi M, Lin A, Smeal T, Minden A, Karin M (1993): Identification of an oncoprotein- and UV-responsive protein kinase that binds and potentiates the c-Jun activation domain. *Genes & Dev* 7: 2135–2148

Hirai S-I, Ryseck R-P, Mechta F, Bravo R, Yaniv M (1989): Characterization of junD: a new member of the jun proto-oncogene family. *EMBO J* 8: 1433–1439

Hirai S-I, Bourachot B, Yaniv M (1990): Both Jun and Fos contribute to transcription activation by the heterodimer. *Oncogene* 5: 39–46

Hofmann M, Rudy W, Günthert U, Zimmer SG, Zawadzki V, Zöller M, Lichtner RB, Herrlich P, Ponta H (1993): A link between RAS and metastatic behavior of tumor cells: ras induces CD44 promoter activity and leads to low-level expression of metastasis-specific variants of CD44 in CREF cells. *Cancer Res* 53: 1516–1521

Holbrook NJ, Fornace Jr, AJ (1991): Response to adversity: molecular control of gene activation following genotoxic stress. *New Biol* 3: 825–833

Hunter T, Karin M (1992): Control of transcription factor activity by protein phosphorylation. *Cell* 70: 375–388

Jackson SP, Tjian R (1988): O-glycosylation of eukaryotic transcription factors: implications for mechanisms of transcriptional regulation. *Cell* 55: 125–133

Johnson RS, Spiegelman BM, Papaioannou V (1992): Pleiotropic effects of a null mutation in the c-fos proto-oncogene. *Cell* 71: 577–586

Jonat C, Rahmsdorf HJ, Park K-K, Cato ACB, Gebel S, Ponta H, Herrlich P (1990): Anti-tumor promotion and antiinflammation: Down-modulation of AP-1 (Fos/Jun) activity by glucocorticoid hormone. *Cell* 62: 1189–1204

Kaina B, Lohrer H, Karin M, Herrlich P (1990): Overexpressed human metallothionein IIA gene protects Chinese hamster ovary cells from killing by alkylating agents. *Proc Natl Acad Sci USA* 87: 2710–2714

Karin M (1985): Metallothioneins: proteins in search of function. *Cell* 41: 9–10

Karin M, Herrlich P (1989): Cis- and trans-acting genetic elements responsible for induction of specific genes by tumor promoters, serum factors, and stress. In: *Genes and Signal Transduction in Multistage Carcinogenesis*, Colburn NH ed. New York-Basel: Marcel Dekker

Karin M, Smeal T (1992): Control of transcription factors by signal transduction pathways: The beginning of the end. *TIBS* 17: 418–422

Kelley SL, Basu A, Teicher BA, Hacker MP, Hamer DH, Lazo JS (1988): Over-expression of metallothionein confers resistance to anticancer drugs. *Science* 241: 1813–1815

Kölch W, Heidecker G, Kochs G, Hummel R, Vahidi H, Mischak H, Finkenzeller G, Marmè D, Rapp UR (1993). Protein kinase Cα activates RAF-1 by direct phosphorylation. *Nature* 364: 249–252

König H, Ponta H, Rahmsdorf HJ, Herrlich P (1992): Interference between pathway-specific transcription factors: glucocorticoids antagonize phorbol ester-induced AP-1 activity without altering AP-1 site occupation in vivo. *EMBO J* 11: 2241–2246

Koo AS, Chiu R, Soong J, deKernion JB, Belldegrun A (1992): The expression of c-jun and junB mRNA in renal cell cancer and in vitro regulation by transforming growth factor beta 1 and tumor necrosis factor alpha 1. *J Urol* 148: 1314–1318

Kouzarides JT, Ziff E (1988): Role of the leucine zipper in the fos-jun interaction. *Nature* 336: 646–651

Kouzarides T, Ziff E (1989): Leucine zippers of fos, jun and GCN4 dictate dimerization specificity and thereby control DNA binding. *Nature* 340: 568–571

Kovary K, Bravo R (1991): The Jun and Fos protein families are both required for cell cycle progression in fibroblasts. *Mol Cell Biol* 11: 4466–4472

Krämer M, Sachsenmaier C, Herrlich P, Rahmsdorf HJ (1993): UV-irradiation-induced interleukin-1 and basic fibroblast growth factor synthesis and release mediate part of the UV response. *J Biol Chem* 268: 6734–6741

Kyriakis JM, App H, Zhang X, Banerjee P, Brautigan DL, Rapp UR, Avruch J (1992): Raf-1 activates MAP kinase-kinase. *Nature* 358: 417–421

Landschulz WH, Johnson PF, McKnight SL (1988): The leucine zipper: a hypothetical structure common to a new class of DNA binding proteins. *Science* 240: 1759–1764

Lee W, Haslinger A, Karin M, Tjian R (1987a): Activation of transcription by two factors that bind promoter and enhancer sequences of the human metallothionein gene and SV40. *Nature* 325: 368–372

Lee W, Mitchell P, Tjian R (1987b): Purified transcription factor AP-1 interacts with TPA-inducible enhancer elements. *Cell* 49: 741–752

Li L, Chambard JC, Karin M, Olson EC (1992): Fos and Jun repress transcriptional activation by myogenin and MyoD: the amino terminus of Jun can mediate repression. *Genes Dev* 6: 676–689

Li Y, Jaiswal AK (1992): Regulation of human NAD(P)H:quinone oxireductase gene. *J Biol Chem* 267: 15097–15104

Lin A, Frost J, Deng T, Smeal T, Al-Alawi N, Kikkawa U, Hunter T, Brenner D, Karin M (1992): Casein kinase II is a negative regulator of c-Jun DNA binding and AP-1 activity. *Cell* 70: 777–789

Little JW, Mount DW (1982): The SOS regulatory system of *Escherichia coli. Cell* 29: 11–22

Lloyd A, Yancheva N, Wasylyk B (1991): Transformation suppressor activity of a Jun transcription factor lacking its activation domain. *Nature* 352: 635–638

Maki Y, Bos TJ, Davis C, Starbuck M, Vogt PK (1987): Avian sarcoma virus 17 carries the jun oncogene. *Proc Natl Acad Sci USA* 84: 2848–2852

Miner JN, Diamond MI, Yamamoto KR (1991): Joints in the regulatory lattice: composite regulation by steroid receptor AP-1 complexes. *Cell Growth Diff* 2: 525–530

Minna JD, Schütte J, Viallet J, Thomas F, Kaye FJ, Takahashi T, Nau M, Whang-Peng J, Birrer M, Gazdar AF (1989): Transcription factors and recessive oncogenes in the pathogenesis of human lung cancer. *Int J Cancer Suppl* 4: 32–34

Morgan IM, Asano M, Havarstein LS, Ishikawa H, Hiiragi T, Ito Y, Vogt PK (1993): Amino acid substitutions modulate the effect of Jun on transformation, transcriptional activation and DNA replication. *Oncogene* 8: 1135–1140

Müller R, Slamon DJ, Tremblay JM, Cline MJ, Verma IM (1982): Differential expression of cellular oncogenes during pre- and postnatal development of the mouse. *Nature* 299: 640–644

Nakagawa K, Saijo N, Tsuchida S, Sakai M, Tsunokawa Y, Yokata J, Muramatsu M, Sato K, Terada M, Tew KD (1990): Glutathione-S-transferase pi as a determinant of drug resistance in transfectant cell lines. *J Biol Chem* 265: 4296–4301

Neuberg M, Adamkiewicz J, Hunter JB, Müller R (1989a): A Fos protein containing the Jun leucine zipper forms a homodimer which binds to the AP1 binding site. *Nature* 341: 243–245

Neuberg, M, Schuermann M, Hunter JB, Müller R (1989b): Two functionally different regions in Fos are required for the sequence-specific DNA interaction of the Fos/Jun protein complex. *Nature* 338: 589–590

Oehler T, Angel P (1993): unpublished observation

Oehler T, Angel P (1992): A common intermediary factor (p52/54) recognizing "acidic-blob"-type domains is required for transcriptional activation by the Jun proteins. *Mol Cell Biol* 12: 5508–5515

Oehler T, Pintzas A, Stumm S, Darling A, Gillespie D, Angel P (1993): Mutation of a phosphorylation site in the DNA binding domain is required for redox-independent transactivation of AP1-dependent genes by v-Jun. *Oncogene* 8: 1141–1147

Offringa R, Gebel S, van Dam H, Timmers M, Smits A, Zwart R, Stein B, Bos JL, van der Eb A, Herrlich P (1990): A novel function of the transforming domain of E1a: repression of AP-1 activity. *Cell* 62: 527–538

Offringa R, Smits AMM, Houweling A, Bos JL, van der Eb AJ (1988): Similar effects of adenovirus E1A and glucocorticoid hormones on the expression of the metalloprotease stromelysin. *Nucleic Acids Res* 16: 10973–10984

Okuda A, Imagawa M, Sakai M, Muramatsu M (1990): Functional cooperativity between two TPA responsive elements in undifferentiated F9 embryonic stem cells. *EMBO J* 9: 1131–1135

Oliviero S, Robinson GS, Struhl K, Spiegelman BM (1992): Yeast GCN4 as a probe for oncogenesis by AP-1 transcription factors: transcriptional activation through AP-1 sites is not sufficient for cellular transformation. *Genes Dev* 6: 1799–1809

O'Shea E, Rutkowski R, Kim PS (1989): Evidence that the leucine zipper is a coiled coil. *Science* 243: 538–542

Ostrowski LE, Finch J, Krieg P, Matrisian L, Patskan G, O'Connell JF, Phillips J, Slaga TJ, Breathnach R, Bowden GT (1988): Expression pattern of a gene for a secreted metalloproteinase during late stages of tumor progression. *Molec Carcinogenesis* 1: 13–19

Papavassiliou AG, Chavrier C, Bohmann D (1992): Phosphorylation state and DNA-binding activity of cJun dependent on the intracellular concentration of binding sites. *Proc Natl Acad Sci USA* 89: 11562–11565

Payne DM, Rossomando AJ, Martino P, Erickson AK, Her J-H, Shabanowitz J,

Hunt DF, Weber MJ, Sturgill TW (1991): Identification of the regulatory phosphorylation sites in pp42/mitogen-activated protein kinase (MAP kinase). *EMBO J* 10: 885–892

Pelech SL, Sanghere JS (1992): MAP kinases: Charting the regulatory pathways. *Science* 257: 1355–1356

Pfarr CM, Mechta F, Spyrou G, Lallemand D, Carillo S, Yaniv M (1994): Mouse JunD negatively regulates fibroblast growth and antagonizes transformation by ras. *Cell* 76: 747–760

Ponta H, Cato ACB, Herrlich P (1992): Interference of pathway specific transcription factors. *Biochim Biophys Acta* 1129: 255–261

Pulverer BJ, Kyriakis JM, Avruch J, Nikolakaki E, Woodgett JR (1991): Phosphorylation of c-jun mediated by MAP kinases. *Nature* 353: 670–674

Pulverer BJ, Hughes K, Franklin CC, Kraft AS, Leevers SJ, Woodgett JR (1992): Co-purification of mitogen-activated protein kinases with phorbol ester-induced c-Jun kinase activity in U937 leukaemic cells. *Oncogene* 7: 407–415

Quantin B, Breathnach R (1988): Epidermal growth factor stimulates transcription of the c-jun proto-oncogene in rat fibroblasts. *Nature* 334: 538–539

Radler-Pohl A, Sachsenmaier C (1994): unpublished observation

Radler-Pohl A, Sachsenmaier C, Gebel S, Auer H-P, Bruder JT, Rapp U, Angel P, Rahmsdorf HJ, Herrlich P (1993a): UV-induced activation of AP-1 involves obligatory extranuclear steps including Raf-1 kinase. *EMBO J* 12: 1005–1012

Radler-Pohl A, Gebel S, Sachsenmaier C, König H, Krämer M, Oehler T, Streile M, Ponta H, Rapp U, Rahmsdorf H, Cato ACB, Angel P, Herrlich P (1993b): The activation and activity control of AP-1 (Fos/Jun). In: *Annals of the New York Academy of Sciences*, vol 684, M. Sluyser, G. Ab, A.O. Brinkman, R.A. Blankenstein, pp. 127–148. Meeting on "Zinc Finger Proteins in Oncogenesis: DNA binding and gene regulation"

Ransone LJ, Visvader J, Wamsley P, Verma IM (1990): Trans-dominant negative mutants of Fos and Jun. *Proc Natl Acad Sci USA* 87: 3806–3810

Ronai ZA, Lambert ME, Weinstein IB (1990): Inducible cellular responses to ultraviolet light irradiation and other mediators of DNA damage in mammalian cells. *Cell Biol Toxicol* 6: 105–126

Rozek D, Pfeifer GP (1993): In vivo protein-DNA interactions at the c-jun promoter: preformed complexes mediate the UV response. *Mol Cell Biol* 13: 5490–5499

Ryder K, Lanahan A, Perez-Albuerne E, Nathans D (1989): Jun-D: a third member of the Jun gene family. *Proc Natl Acad Sci USA* 86: 1500–1503

Ryder K, Lau LF, Nathans D (1988): A gene activated by growth factors is related to the oncogene v-jun. *Proc Natl Acad Sci USA* 85: 1487–1491

Ryseck RP, Bravo R (1991): cJun, JunB and JunD differ in their binding affinities to AP-1 and CRE consensus sequences: effect of Fos proteins. *Oncogene* 6: 533–542

Ryseck R-P, Hirai SI, Yaniv M, Bravo R (1988): Transcriptional activation of c-jun during the G_0/G_1 transition in mouse fibroblasts. *Nature* 334: 535–537

Sachsenmaier C, Radler-Pohl A, Zinck R, Nordheim A, Herrlich P, Rahmsdorf HJ (1994): Involvement of growth factor receptors in the mammalian UVC response. *Cell* in press

Sakai M, Muramatsu M, Nishi S (1992): Suppression of glutathione transferase P expression by glucocorticoids. *Biochem Biophys Res Comm* 187: 976–983

Sassone-Corsi P, Ransone LJ, Lamph WW, Verma IM (1988): Direct interaction between fos and jun nuclear oncoproteins: role of the "leucine zipper" domain. *Nature* 336: 692–695

Schönthal A, Herrlich P, Rahmsdorf HJ, Ponta H (1988): Requirement for fos gene expression in the transcriptional activation of collagenase by other oncogenes and phorbol esters. *Cell* 54: 325–334

Schönthal A, Alberts AS, Fost JA, Feramisco JR (1991): Differential regulation of jun family gene expression by the tumor promoter okadaic acid. *New Biol* 3: 977–986

Schorpp M, Mallick U, Rahmsdorf, HJ, Herrlich P (1984): UV-induced extracellular factor from human fibroblasts communicates the UV response to nonirradiated cells. *Cell* 37: 861–868

Schreck R, Baeuerle PA (1991): A role for oxygen radicals as second messengers. *Trends Cell Biol* 1: 39–42

Schuh AC, Keating SJ, Monteclaro FS, Vogt PK, Breitman ML (1990): Obligatory wounding requirement for tumorigenesis in v-jun transgenic mice. *Nature* 346: 756–760

Schüle R, Rangarajan P, Kliewer S, Ransone LJ, Bolado J, Yang N, Verma IM, Evans RM (1990a): Functional antagonism between oncoprotein c-Jun and the glucocorticoid receptor. *Cell* 62: 1217–1226

Schüle R, Umesono K, Mangelsdorf DJ, Bolado J, Pike JW, Evans RM (1990b): Jun-Fos and receptors for vitamins A and D recognize a common response element in the human osteocalcin gene. *Cell* 61: 497–504

Schüle R, Evans RM (1991): Cross-coupling of signal tranduction pathways: zinc finger meets leucine zipper. *TIG* 7: 377–381

Schütte J, Minna JD, Birrer MJ (1989a): Deregulated expression of human c-jun transforms primary rat embryo cells in cooperation with an activated c-Ha-ras gene and transforms Rat-1a cells as a single gene. *Proc Natl Acad Sci USA* 86: 2257–2261

Schütte J, Viallet J, Nau M, Segal S, Fedorko J, Minna J (1989b): Jun-B inhibits and c-fos stimulates the transforming and trans-activating activities of c-jun. *Cell* 59: 987–997

Scribner JD, Slaga TJ (1973): Multiple effects of dexamethasone on protein synthesis and hyperplasia caused by a tumor promoter. *Cancer Res* 33: 542–546

Sellers JW, Struhl K (1989): Changing Fos oncoprotein to a Jun-independent DNA-binding protein with GCN4 dimerization specificity by swapping 'leucine zipper'. *Nature* 341: 74–76

Smeal T, Binétruy B, Mercola DA, Birrer M, Karin M (1991): Oncogenic and transcriptional cooperation and Ha-ras requires phosphorylation of c-Jun on serines 63 and 73. *Nature* 354: 494–496

Smeal T, Binétruy B, Mercola D, Grover-Bardwick A, Heidecker G, Rapp, UR, Karin M (1992): Oncoprotein mediated signalling cascade stimulates cJun activity by phosphorylation of serines 63 and 73. *Mol Cell Biol* 12: 3507–3513

Stein B, Angel P, van Dam H, Ponta H, Herrlich P, van der Eb A, Rahmsdorf HJ (1992): Ultraviolet-radiation induced c-jun gene transcription: two AP-1 like binding sites mediate the response. *Photochem Photobiol* 55: 409–415

Stein B, Baldwin Jr AS, Ballard DW, Greene WC, Angel P, Herrlich P (1993): Cross-coupling of the NF-κB p65 and Fos/Jun transcription factors produces potentiated biological function. *EMBO J* 12: 3879–3891

Stein B, Rahmsdorf HJ, Steffen A, Litfin M, Herrlich P (1989): UV-induced DNA damage is an intermediate step in UV-induced expression of human immuno-deficiency virus type 1, collagenase, c-fos, and metallothionein. *Mol Cell Biol* 9: 5169–5181

Toftgard R, Roop DR, Yuspa SH (1985): Protooncogene expression during two-stage carcinogenesis in mouse skin. *Carcinogenesis* 6: 655–657

Tratner I, Verma IM (1991): Identification of a nuclear targeting sequence in the Fos protein. *Oncogene* 6: 2049–2053

Turner R, Tjian R (1989): Leucine repeats and an adjacent DNA binding domain mediate the formation of functional cFos-cJun heterodimers. *Science* 243: 1689–1694

Unlap T, Franklin CC, Wagner F, Kraft AS (1992): Upstream regions of the c-jun promoter regulate phorbol ester-induced transcription in U937 leukemic cells. *Nucleic Acids Res* 20: 897–902

van Beveren C, van Straaten F, Curran T, Müller R, Verma IM (1983): Analysis of FBJ-MuSV provirus and c-fos (mouse) gene reveals that viral and cellular fos gene products have different carboxy termini. *Cell* 32: 1241–1255

van Dam H, Duyndam M, Rottier R, Bosch A, de Vries-Smits L, Herrlich P, Zantema A, Angel P, van der Eb AJ (1993): Heterodimer formation of cJun and ATF-2 is responsible for induction of c-jun by the 243 amino acid adenovirus E1A protein. *EMBO J* 12: 479–487

van Dam H, Offringa R, Meijer I, Stein B, Smits AM, Herrlich P, Bos JL, van der Eb AJ (1990): Differential effects of the adenovirus E1A oncogene on members of the AP-1 transcription factor family. *Mol Cell Biol* 10: 5857–5864

van den Berg S, Kaina B, Rahmsdorf HJ, Ponta H, Herrlich P (1991): Involvement of Fos in spontaneous and ultraviolet light induced genetic changes. *Molec Carcinogenesis* 4: 460–466

van Straaten F, Müller R, Curran T, van Beveren C, Verma IM (1983): Complete nucleotide sequence of a human c-onc gene: deduced amino acid sequence of the human c-fos protein. *Proc Natl Acad Sci USA* 80: 3183–3187

Vogt PK, Bos TJ (1990): Jun: Oncogene and transcription factor. *Adv Cancer Res* 55: 1–35

Walker GC (1985): Inducible DNA repair systems. *Ann Rev Biochem* 54: 425–457

Wang Z-Q, Ovitt C, Grigoriadis AE, Möhle-Steinlein U, Rüther, U, Wagner EF (1992): Bone and haematopoietic defects in mice lacking c-fos. *Nature* 360: 741

Wood KW, Sarnecki C, Roberts TM, Blenis J (1992): Ras mediates nerve growth factor receptor modulation of three signal-transducing protein kinases: MAP-kinase, Raf-1, and RSK. *Cell* 68: 1041–1050

Xanthoudakis S, Curran T (1992): Identification and characterization of Ref-1, a nuclear protein that facilities AP-1 DNA-binding activity. *EMBO J* 11: 653–665

Yang-Yen H-F, Chambard J-C, Sun Y-L, Smeal T, Schmidt TJ, Drouin J, Karin M (1990): Transcriptional interference between c-Jun and the glucocorticoid receptor: mutual inhibition of DNA binding due to direct protein-protein interaction. *Cell* 62: 1205–1215

Zhang X-K, Dong J-M, Chiu J-F (1991): Regulation of α-fetoprotein gene expression by antagonism between AP-1 and the glucocorticoid receptor at their over-lapping bind site. *J Biol Chem* 266: 8248–8254

Zhang X, Settlerman J, Kyriakis JM, Suzuki E, Elledge J, Marshall M, Bruder J, Rapp UR, Avruch J (1993): Normal and oncogenic p21^{ras} proteins binds to the amino terminal regulatory domain of c-Raf-1. *Nature* 364: 308–313

4

NF-κB: A Mediator of Pathogen and Stress Responses

ULRICH SIEBENLIST, KEITH BROWN, AND GUIDO FRANZOSO

Introduction

The transcription factor NF-κB is a central regulator of defensive responses which are mounted by cells against many potentially threatening environmental challenges. Bacteria, viruses, parasites, injury, radiation, oxidative stress, numerous chemical agents and many cytokines released in response to such challenges are all well-studied and potent activators of this transcription factor in a number of different cell types. Activated NF-κB then induces the expression of many genes whose encoded functions play critical roles for the defense of the organism. The induced proteins have a wide range of activities, including anti-bacterial or anti-viral functions, antigen recognition, cellular migration and adhesion as well as hematopoietic cell differentiation and proliferation. Aside from regulating cellular genes, several viruses, including the human immunodeficiency virus, have diverted this factor for their own purposes. Since many cytokines are regulated by NF-κB, this transcription factor appears critical to a coordinated defense response. In an evolutionary sense, the association between defensive responses and NF-κB dates at least as far back as insects. Although NF-κB is present in many cells, its role appears to be most prominent in cells with obvious immunologic defensive functions, like monocytes/macrophages, B cells, T cells and endothelial cells, cells in which NF-κB can be readily activated by many stimuli.

Given NF-κB's activation by many mitogenic stimuli in certain immune cells, it may not be surprising to find recurrent genetic changes in genes encoding NF-κB activity or its regulators in some tumors of hematopoietic origin. This suggests a potential involvement of NF-κB in proliferation. A developmental role for this transcription factor may be

INDUCIBLE GENE EXPRESSION, VOLUME 1
P.A. Baeuerle, Editor
© 1995 Birkhäuser Boston

indicated also, most obviously by the Drosophila NF-κB-related protein dorsal, the essential morphogen for all ventral structures.

NF-κB is well suited for rapidly transmitting signals into the nucleus. It is already present in an inactive form in the cytoplasm of cells prior to stimulation, kept there by the inhibitory protein IκB-α. Upon appropriate stimulation, the inhibitor is inactivated within minutes; it is rapidly phosphorylated and proteolytically degraded, allowing the NF-κB transcription factor to then translocate to the nucleus and induce the transcription of many genes. It does so by binding to κB sites located within enhancers or promoters of these genes (the consensus κB sequence is 5'-GGGPuNN-PyPyCC-3') where it functionally interacts with other transcription factors to regulate expression. Thus, NF-κB appears to be critical for many rapid signal-dependent genetic responses in numerous cell types, in particular in response to those signals connected with a pathologic condition.

NF-κB activity is defined by many different dimeric complexes, all composed of members of the Rel/NF-κB family of polypeptides. This family consists of p50, p52 (p50B), RelA (p65), RelB, Rel (c-Rel), chicken v-Rel and the Drosophila proteins dorsal and Dif. Depending on cell and stimulation conditions, several of these dimeric complexes may be present and can be activated, although typically a dimer of p50 and p65 (RelA) predominates. Although most of the NF-κB dimers which can be generated by various combinations of Rel/NF-κB polypeptides appear to have similar activities, they also possess unique properties and differ in expression pattern. The diversification into several functionally distinct but similar complexes may explain why such a large array of genes can take advantage of this transcription factor system.

Prior to cloning of the genes encoding NF-κB activity and the subsequent development of specific reagents, the various NF-κB complexes could not be distinguished; therefore, what was described in the literature as NF-κB and thought to consist of a single complex actually consists of various different species, depending on cell and stimulation conditions. To be consistent with previous reports, we will use the term NF-κB or Rel/NF-κB to collectively denote all κB-binding activity due to this family of proteins, and we will refer to specific dimers by naming their subunits.

In this review we will concentrate on recent developments in the field. A number of excellent reviews have been published previously covering various aspects of NF-κB (Baeuerle, 1991; Blank et al, 1992; Bose, 1992; Bours et al, 1992b; Gilmore, 1992; Israel, 1992, Nolan and Baltimore, 1992; Schreck et al, 1992a; Beg and Baldwin, 1993; Collins, 1993; Gilmore and Morin, 1993; Grilli et al, 1993; Grimm and Baeuerle, 1993; Hay, 1993; Liou and Baltimore, 1993; Kaltschmidt et al, 1993; Muller et al, 1993; Wasserman, 1993; Baeuerle and Henkel, 1994; Lenardo and Siebenlist, 1994).

Molecular Structure

The family of Rel/NF-κB proteins

The NF-κB dimers are composed of members of the Rel/NF-κB family of proteins. All family members share a Rel/NF-κB homology domain (RHD) of about 300 amino acids in length, while the remaining parts of these proteins show little similarity. The RHDs of the vertebrate family members (p50, p52, RelA, RelB and Rel) exhibit between 42% and 61% identity and the Drosophila proteins dorsal and Dif are only slightly more diverged (Bours et al, 1992a; 1992b; Ryseck et al, 1992; Ip et al, 1993). New names for the individual members of the Rel/NF-κB and IκB families as well as previous or alternative names are listed in the Table (adapted from a consensus reached in October 1993 at a meeting entitled "NF-κB, Rel and Dorsal: Structure and Function," held at the Howard Hughes Medical Institute in Bethesda, MD). In accord with this proposed nomenclature, we will use the names p50, p52 (or their precursors p105, p100 respectively), RelA, Rel, v-Rel and RelB throughout this review.

The conserved RHD determines DNA binding, dimerization, nuclear translocation and interaction with the inhibitory IκB proteins. Deletions and site-directed mutagenesis have located the DNA-binding region in p50 to the N-terminal part of this domain (Logeat et al, 1991; Bressler et al, 1993; Coleman et al, 1993). In particular, a short stretch of amino acids at the beginning of the domain appears critical for binding (the RXXRXRXXC motif) and is likely to directly contact DNA (Kumar et al, 1992; Bressler et al, 1993; Toledano et al, 1993). The cysteine residue

Table 1. Table 1: Rel/NKκB and IκB proteins

Proteins	Other names
p50 or p105 (NF-κB1)	p110, KBF1, EBP-1
p52 or p100 (NF-κB2)	p50B or p97, p49 or p100, p55 or p98, Lyt10, H2FT1
Rel	c-Rel
v-Rel	
RelA	p65
RelB	I-Rel
dorsal	
Dif, Cif	dorsal-related immunity factor, cecropia immunoresponsive factor
IκB-α	MAD-3, pp40, RL/IF-1, ECI-6
IκB-β	
IκB-γ	p105/pdI, C-terminal portion of p105
Bcl-3	
cactus	

within this motif must be in a reduced state since its oxidation interfered with DNA-binding (Toledano and Leonard, 1991; Kumar et al, 1992; Matthews et al, 1992, 1993a; Toledano et al, 1993). It has been speculated that NF-κB activity may be redox-regulated at this cysteine (Toledano and Leonard, 1991), and experiments in which the exogenously expressed thioredoxin enhanced NF-κB binding further support this notion (Matthews et al, 1992; Hayashi et al, 1993). Nonetheless, there is no direct evidence that such regulation is physiological; on the contrary, cells exposed to oxidative stress actually activate NF-κB (see below). A second region in p50, located approximately 100 amino acids C-terminal to the first region, also contributes significantly to binding (Bressler et al, 1993). Neither region fits previously determined DNA-binding motifs present in other transcription factors, suggesting that this family of proteins encodes a novel DNA binding motif. A possible beta-turn-beta structure has recently been implicated (Liu et al, 1994), although ultimately this needs to be resolved by X-ray crystallography.

The C-terminal half of the RHD harbors the dimerization functions (Logeat et al, 1991; Bressler et al, 1993; Doerre et al, 1993; Ganchi et al, 1993). The structure of this region is also unknown. Dimerization with different partners may involve distinct amino acids. Two specific mutations in the dimerization domain severely interfere with homodimerization but not heterodimerization with p50 (Ganchi et al, 1993). The extreme C-terminal end of the RHD contains a nuclear localization sequence (NLS) which has been reported as important also for interaction with the inhibitory IκB proteins (see below) (Blank et al, 1991; Beg et al, 1992; Ganchi et al, 1992; Henkel et al, 1992; Matthews et al, 1993b; Zabel et al, 1993).

Two classes of Rel/NF-κB proteins

The Rel/NF-κB family can be divided into two groups; one comprises the p50 and p52 (p50B, p49) proteins, which are generated by proteolytic processing from their precursor forms p105 and p100 (p97, lyt10) respectively, (these proteins are also referred to as NF-κB1 and NF-κB2 respectively) (Bours et al, 1990; Ghosh et al, 1990; Kieran et al, 1990; Meyer et al, 1991; Neri et al, 1991; Schmid et al, 1991; Bours et al, 1992a; Mercurio et al, 1992), and the other group consists of the Rel (c-Rel), v-Rel, RelA (p65) and RelB (I-Rel) proteins (Stephens et al, 1983; Wilhelmsen et al, 1984; Brownell et al, 1989; Grumont and Gerondakis 1989; Nolan et al, 1991; Ruben et al, 1991; Ballard et al, 1992; Ruben et al, 1992; Ryseck et al, 1992), as well as the Drosophila proteins dorsal and

Dif (Steward, 1987; Ip et al, 1993) (see Table for nomenclature). The latter group of proteins contains activation domains which lie outside the RHD and which potently transactivate reporter constructs upon transfection of certain cells, while the p50 and p52 proteins, representing the former group, are not known to harbor such activation domains (see below).

The p50/p105 and p52/p100 proteins are the most highly related family members (Bours et al 1992a). Processing of the precursor p105 or p100 proteins into their mature forms may be somewhat upregulated during stimulation with extracellular signals (Mellits et al, 1993; Mercurio et al, 1993), but is otherwise a slow, constitutive process (Fan and Maniatis, 1991; Brown and Siebenlist, 1994). Processing of p105 was shown to be ATP-dependent (Fan and Maniatis, 1991). A terminal cleavage for both precursors occurs in a glycine-rich region located directly adjacent to the RHD. This region is likely to function as a flexible hinge in the precursor and may also provide ready access to cleavage by endoproteases. While the N-terminal halves of the precursors give rise to the mature proteins, the C-terminal halves appeared to be degraded during processing (Fan and Maniatis, 1991; Rice et al, 1992).

RelA (p65), Rel, RelB and the Drosophila protein dorsal (and most likely Dif) contain activation domains in their C-terminal halves (Bull et al, 1990; Kamens et al, 1990; Ip et al, 1991; Richardson and Gilmore, 1991; Schmitz and Baeuerle, 1991; Ballard et al, 1992; Dobrzanski et al, 1993). RelB also contains a second cooperating activation domain located in its unique N-terminal extension, a short region preceding the RHD which may encode a leucine-zipper-like motif (Dobrzanski et al, 1993). According to one report, RelB (termed I-Rel) acts as a non-transactivating inhibitor of NF-κB (Ruben et al, 1992), but ample evidence now indicates that RelB functions to potently induce transcription (Bours et al, 1992a; Ryseck et al, 1992; Dobrzanski et al, 1993; Bours et al, 1994). Rel contains two distinct regions which could participate in transactivation (Ishikawa et al, 1993; Sarkar and Gilmore, 1993). The more C-terminally postioned of these two domains of Rel as well as the potent transactivation domain present in RelA and the C-terminal domain of RelB may all belong to the class of acidic transactivators (Bull et al, 1990; Kamens et al, 1990; Schmitz and Baeuerle 1991; Dobrzanski et al, 1993). v-Rel lacks this particular transactivating domain (Kamens et al, 1990; Ishikawa et al, 1993; Sarkar and Gilmore, 1993), and this difference from Rel may be critical to the oncogenic potential of the viral form (see below). The residual transactivating function of v-Rel is apparent primarily in undifferentiated cells (Walker et al, 1992; Ishikawa et al, 1993; Inuzuka et al, 1994; Hrdlickova et al,

1994a), while Rel can transactivate in a wide range of cells (Kamens et al, 1990; Inoue et al, 1991; Ishikawa et al, 1993).

Transactivation is likely to be mediated by direct physical interaction with the basal transcription apparatus. RelA, dorsal, Rel and v-Rel have all been shown to associate with the TATA binding protein (TBP), a component of TFIID, although this has not been resolved in the case of v-Rel (Kerr et al, 1993; Xu et al, 1993). It is also uncertain which domain of Rel is responsible, with one report implicating only the N-terminal part of the RHD (Kerr et al, 1993), while another report implicates the two transactivation domains as critical for the interaction (Xu et al, 1993). Rel, v-Rel and RelA also have been found to contact TFIIB (Kerr et al, 1993; Xu et al, 1993), a basal transcription factor whose recruitment into the preinitiation complex may be rate-limiting.

The family of IκB proteins

The IκB family encompasses IκB-α, the precursor proteins p105 and p100, IκB-γ, Bcl-3 and the Drosophila protein cactus. They share a partially conserved domain which harbors between six and eight ankyrin motifs, each 33 amino acids in length (Blank et al, 1992, Nolan and Baltimore, 1992). That such motifs are important for NF-κB function was first recognized with the cloning of the p105 precursor protein (Bours et al, 1990; Kieran et al, 1990), where their presence inhibits DNA-binding of the N-terminal Rel/NF-κB homology domain (Bours et al, 1990; Ghosh et al, 1990; Kieran et al, 1990). The IκB proteins interfere with nuclear translocation and DNA binding of Rel/NF-κB complexes, with the notable exception of Bcl-3 (see below).

The IκB proteins belong to a larger family of proteins with more distantly related ankyrin-domains (Schmitz et al, 1991; Blank et al, 1992; Hatada et al, 1992; Michaely and Bennett, 1992; Nolan and Baltimore, 1992). There is no known biologic function common to all ankyrin-motif proteins although such may yet be discovered. Most likely, the ankyrin motifs simply define backbone structures for protein-protein interaction domains. They may form amphipathic α-helices which are bundled together (Gay and Ntwasa, 1993). The more diverged sequences in these domains, located in the putative loops between helices, may then determine binding to unique targets. In the case of IκB-α, Bcl 3 and p105 the whole ankyrin domain has been shown to be necessary for inhibitory activity, although some mutations could be tolerated; in the case of IκB-α and p105 a short negatively charged segment has been found to be needed in addition for full inhibition (Blank et al, 1991; Hatada et al, 1992; Inoue et al, 1992b; Wulczyn et al, 1992; Bours et al, 1993; Franzoso et al, 1993; Hatada et al, 1993).

IκB-α and the ankyrin domain of the p105 precursor (which is identical to that of the IκB-γ protein) interact with and shield the NLS located at the end of the RHD domain (Beg et al, 1992; Mellits et al, 1993; Zabel et al, 1993). IκB-α binds as a monomer, suggesting that it can mask the NLSs of both subunits of NF-κB (Hatada et al, 1993). The C-termini of Rel and dorsal may in addition assist in cytoplasmic retention (Hannink and Temin, 1989; Capobianco et al, 1990; Isoda et al, 1992; Norris and Manley, 1992; Diehl et al, 1993). In the case of RelA, the C-terminus has been reported to help in IκB-α-mediated inhibition of DNA-binding also (Ganchi et al, 1992). IκB-α tightly binds to and functionally inhibits all dimeric complexes containing any of the transactivating subunits (RelA, Rel, RelB). On the other hand, endogenous homodimers of p50 or p52 are not efficiently retained in the cytoplasm by IκB-α (Franzoso et al, 1992; Kang et al, 1992), although they bind IκB-α (Beg et al, 1992; Ganchi et al, 1992; Franzoso et al, 1993).

The strongly transactivating complexes containing either RelA, Rel or RelB are inhibited by IκB-α from binding DNA and, in addition, are dissociated from DNA if prebound (Baeuerle and Baltimore 1988; Zabel and Baeuerle, 1990; Haskill et al, 1991; Beg et al, 1992; Davis et al, 1992; Inoue et al, 1992b; Tewari et al, 1992). p50 and p52 homodimers, however, are essentially unaffected in DNA-binding (Beg et al, 1992; Kerr et al, 1992; Franzoso et al, 1993; Nolan et al, 1993). It is not known precisely how DNA binding of dimers containing RelA, Rel or RelB is interfered with. It has been reported that IκB-α may bind exclusively to the N-terminal DNA-binding region of Rel (Kerr et al, 1991), also that it binds to this domain and to the NLS (Diehl et al, 1993; Kumar and Gelinas, 1993); alternatively, it binds to the dimerization domain and the NLS of RelA (Ganchi et al, 1992, 1993). In the latter case, DNA-binding would be interfered with only indirectly. This model may more easily explain how IκB-α could dissociate even stably bound complexes from DNA, since direct access to the DNA-contacting portion would not be required.

Two distinct IκB-like protein fractions have been detected during purification, termed IκB-α and IκB-β (Zabel and Baeuerle, 1990; Link et al, 1992). IκB-α function appears to be encoded by the cloned human MAD-3 (Haskill et al, 1991), chicken pp40 (Davis et al, 1992), rat RL/IF-1 (Tewari et al, 1992) and porcine ECI-6 (de Martin et al, 1993) genes (Zabel et al, 1993). The identity of IκB-β remains unresolved although it behaves like a unique protein as judged by various parameters, including size, immunological properties and inactivation by phosphatases (Zabel and Baeuerle, 1990; Link et al, 1992; Zabel et al, 1993). IκB-γ contains the C-terminal half of the p105 precursor molecule, synthesized from a separate mRNA, which so far has been detected only in some mouse B cells (Inoue et al, 1992a; Liou et al, 1992). Its physiological relevance remains to be demonstrated.

The p105 and p100 precursor proteins function as IκB-like proteins (Blank et al, 1991; Henkel et al, 1992; Rice et al, 1992; Mercurio et al, 1993; Naumann et al, 1993; Scheinmann et al, 1993; Beraud et al, 1994). They dimerize with the transactivating subunits Rel, RelA and RelB and, through their ankyrin domains, inhibit these proteins from translocating to the nucleus, even in the absence of IκB-α (Henkel et al, 1992; Rice et al, 1992; Mercurio et al, 1993; Naumann et al, 1993). Since the precursor proteins have a relatively long half-life before they are processed, they may function as physiological inhibitors of NF-κB activity, and indeed such IκB-α-independent complexes can be found in cell cytoplasms (Rice et al, 1992). The precursor may be processed more rapidly in direct response to at least some signals (Mercurio et al, 1993). Therefore, precursor complexes could provide a pool of activatable NF-κB complexes in addition to those associated with IκB-α, although this remains to be demonstrated. The precursor-associated cytoplasmic complexes appear to primarily serve as a reservoir to replenish the signal-responsive IκB-α complexes.

Bcl-3 was first discovered by cloning of a translocation break point in the immunoglobulin locus in a subset of chronic lymphocytic leukemias (Ohno et al, 1990). In contrast to IκB-α, Bcl-3 prefers to interact with homodimers of p50 and p52 (Franzoso et al, 1992; Hatada et al, 1992; Wulczyn et al, 1992; Bours et al, 1993; Franzoso et al, 1993; Naumann et al, 1993; Nolan et al, 1993). Also, Bcl-3 does not necessarily interfere with the nuclear translocation; on the contrary, Bcl-3 is often found in cell nuclei (Bours et al, 1993; Franzoso et al, 1993; Nolan et al, 1993), although not in all cells (Naumann et al, 1993).

Regulation And Function Of NF-κB Dimers

Almost all theoretically possible homo- and heterodimers of the Rel/NF-κB family of proteins have been documented. Dimerization is a requirement for DNA binding (Logeat et al, 1991; Bressler et al, 1993). Several different members of the Rel/NF-κB family of proteins are usually coexpressed in the same cells, albeit to different extents, and they may compete for dimerizing partners. Different NF-κB dimers display different binding affinities with respect to certain κB sites (Urban and Baeuerle,

1990; Neri et al, 1991; Bours et al, 1992a; Kunsch et al, 1992; Perkins et al, 1992; Franzoso et al, 1993). This suggests some overlapping and some distinct physiological gene targets for the various complexes.

NF-κB dimers containing Rel, RelA or RelB

The p50/RelA (p50/p65) complex is present in almost all cells and is usually the most abundant dimeric complex. Homodimers of RelA, Rel or RelA/Rel heterodimers are usually much rarer, but may nevertheless play significant roles in the context of specific promoters (Hansen et al, 1992; Nakayama et al, 1992; Bakalkin et al, 1993; Costello et al, 1993; Ganchi et al, 1993; Kunsch and Rosen, 1993). Homodimerization of RelB may not readily occur (Ryseck et al, 1992; Dobrzanski et al, 1993), and heterodimers of this protein with RelA or Rel have not been noted either. RelA, Rel and RelB are usually found primarily in dimers with p50 or p52, indicating a possible preference for these combinations.

NF-κB dimers differ in their kinetics of activation. The ubiquitous p50/RelA dimer is always rapidly translocated to the nucleus in response to extracellular activating signals, while other complexes, such as p50/Rel, are usually delayed by several hours before reaching peak levels in the nucleus (Molitor et al, 1990; Doerre et al, 1993). Rel complexes have been proposed to function as later-acting competitive downregulators of genes induced by RelA dimers at early times after stimulation (Ballard et al, 1992; Doerre et al, 1993; La Rosa et al, 1994). However, the transfection data on which this conclusion is based may also simply reflect a relatively lower (but significant) transactivation potential of Rel in these cells. In other cells, including embryonal cells, Rel potently transactivated many κB-dependent reporter constructs (Inoue et al, 1991; Richardson and Gilmore, 1991; Ishikawa et al, 1993; Inuzuka et al, 1994).

Rel-containing complexes have been detected in many cell lines, but they appear to be most prevalent in hematopoietic cells, particularly in B cells, although the expression of Rel can be induced in many cells (Brownell et al, 1987, 1989; Feuillard et al, 1994). RelB complexes appear to be even more restricted in tissue since their expression was confined primarily to interdigitating dendritic cells in thymus and in spleen, although the type of cells that express RelB in spleen have not been clearly identified (Carrasco et al, 1993). RelB may be essential for antigen-presentation and T-cell activation and selection. In another study, RelB complexes have also been reported in at least some B cells (Lernbecher et al, 1993). RelB was also inducible in fibroblast cell lines when stimulated with serum (Ryseck et al, 1992). Together these studies indicate that while Rel and RelB are restricted in their expression in tissues, they may nevertheless have significant roles to play in many other tissues where their expression is normally low, but where these proteins may be induced in response to signals (Bull et al, 1989; Grumont and Gerondakis 1990; Ryseck et al, 1992).

v-Rel is the transforming gene carried by the avian retrovirus REV-T which causes fatal tumors of hematopoietic origin in young chicks. In vitro, chicken embryo fibroblasts, splenocytes and bone marrow cells can also be transformed (Rice and Gilden 1988; Boehmelt et al, 1992; Bose, 1992; Morrison et al, 1992). In addition to various amino acid differences with the cellular avian Rel protein, v-Rel also lacks the more C-terminally located transactivation domain. Various divergent theories have been put forth as to the mechanism by which v-Rel transforms cells (see Gilmore, 1992; Boehmelt et al, 1992; Bose, 1992; Walker et al, 1992). Recently a consensus appears to have been reached. While the cellular Rel protein can weakly transform cells, several differences in v-Rel relative to Rel are responsible for the much greater transforming ability of v-Rel; also, v-Rel appears to transform cells by inducing the transcription of specific target genes, as opposed to acting as a competitive inhibitor of NF-κB complexes, as previously proposed (Ballard et al, 1990, 1992; Inoue et al, 1991; Richardson and Gilmore, 1991; McDonnell et al, 1992). High expression of avian Rel can weakly transform at least some cells (Hrdlickova et al, 1994b; Kralova et al, 1994). C-terminal deletions of Rel as well as particular RHD mutations in Rel which match sequences present in v-Rel all enhance the tumorigenic potential of Rel. The C-terminal deletions eliminated the second transactivation domain as well as a putative cytoplasmic retention function (Hrdlickova et al, 1994b; Kralova et al, 1994; Nehyba et al, 1994). The amino acid differences between v-Rel and Rel located within a region which encompasses the C-terminal part of the RHD may change the interaction with the IκB-α inhibitor, since IκB-α was reported to be less efficient in inhibiting DNA binding by Rel proteins which carried these internal mutations (Diehl et al, 1993). Consequently, v-Rel may partially escape into the nucleus. The remaining transactivation domain of v-Rel is necessary for transformation, suggesting that transcriptional stimulation of at least some target genes is required for tumor formation (Boehmelt et al, 1992; Sarkar and Gilmore 1993; Hrdlickova et al, 1994a, 1994b; Nehyba et al, 1994). Consistent with the transforming potential of Rel in avian cells, disruptions at the Rel gene locus have been noted in a few human tumors although it remains to be shown how these changes relate to Rel function (Lu et al, 1991).

Rel may play an important role in apoptosis which may be mediated in part by its C-terminal transactivation domain, the domain that is deleted in v-Rel. High levels of Rel have been observed in various cells under-going apoptosis and autophagocytosis in developing chick embryos; in addition, avian bone marrow cells (but not fibroblasts) infected with Rel-expressing vectors undergo programmed cell death (Abbadie et al, 1993). In contrast to Rel, v-Rel may actually protect against cell death since v-Rel-transformed bursal lymphocytes were resistant to various inducers to apoptosis including radiation (Neiman et al, 1991).

Due to the coexistence of the structurally very similar p50 and p52 proteins in many cells, two similar sets of heterodimeric complexes are generated. Both proteins readily heterodimerize with RelA, Rel or RelB and the resulting heterodimers all can transactivate with no obvious significant differences depending on which of the two proteins is present as a partner (Bours et al, 1992b, Franzoso et al, 1994). Differences between these complexes may manifest themselves in the context of specific promoters (Perkins et al, 1992) or when p50 or p52 still exist in their precursor phase (p105 and p100 respectively) (Mercurio et al, 1993; Beraud et al, 1994).

Homodimers of p50 and p52

Homodimers of p50 appear to be ubiquitous and often localize to the nucleus, even in the absence of stimulation (Franzoso et al, 1993), presumably due to inefficient cytoplasmic retention by IκB proteins. p52 homodimers are less often observed as a result of a generally lower level of expression compared to that of p50. Many transfection studies in several different cells indicate that p50 homodimers (as well as p52 homodimers) are unable, by themselves, to significantly transactivate a variety of κB-dependent reporter constructs, and this is consistent with the lack of an identifiable transactivation domain on p50 (or p52) (Schmid et al, 1991; Schmitz and Baeuerle, 1991; Ballard et al, 1992; Bours et al, 1992a; Franzoso et al, 1992; Kunsch et al, 1992; Mercurio et al, 1992; Ryseck et al, 1992; Bours et al, 1993; Franzoso et al, 1993). However, p50 homodimers have also been reported to have transactiva-tion potential based primarily on in vitro transcription data (Fujita et al, 1992; Kretzschmar et al, 1992), but also on some additional experiments (Moore et al, 1993; Fujita et al, 1993). Consistent with a nontransactiva-tion function, however, p50 homodimers usually behave as transcriptional inhibitors in vivo, counteracting potent transactivation by p50/RelA heterodimers by direct competition for κB sites (Schmitz and

Baeuerle et al, 1991; Franzoso et al, 1992, 1993). This inhibition is particularly noticeable with κB sites that display a preference for p50 homodimers, such as that site present within the IL-2 receptor-α gene, a site with which these homodimers associate in a very stable manner (Franzoso et al, 1993). Since p50 homodimers can be found in nuclei of resting primary T cells, for example, their role may be to help protect some genes against inadvertent induction by low levels of the potently transactivating NF-κB dimers (Franzoso et al, 1993).

In vivo data further support an inhibitory role for p50 homodimers. The expression of IL-2 in resting, nontranformed mouse T-cell clones is under negative control by p50 homodimers. Only a complete stimulation protocol with peptide and antigen presenting cells (APC) results in expression of IL-2 and this correlates with the specific removal of p50 homodimers from DNA (Kang et al, 1992). p50 homodimers also appear to inhibit expression of MHC class I genes. Highly metastatic cell variants, expressing few class I genes, feature high levels of these homodimers, while the reverse is true with less tumorigenic cell variants (Plaksin et al, 1993). It is of course conceivable that p50 homodimers, although apparently unable to transactivate by themselves, can do so indirectly by cooperating with other transcription factors in the context of a particular promoter.

The p50 and p52 homodimers are regulated in their activities by the IκB family member Bcl-3, which preferentially targets these homodimers. Recent evidence suggests that unlike IκB-α, Bcl-3 activates transcription through κB sites rather than inhibiting it. Two mechanisms for activation have been proposed: an indirect one, in which Bcl-3 antagonizes inhibitory p50 homodimers (Franzoso et al, 1992, 1993), and a direct mechanism in which Bcl-3 acts as an accessory factor, converting non-transactivating p52 homodimers into transactivating ones (Bours et al, 1993). A conversion of p50 homodimers into a transactivating complex has also been proposed (Fujita et al, 1993). Bcl-3 inhibited DNA binding of p50 homodimers and also dissociated already bound homodimers (Hatada et al, 1992; Franzoso et al, 1993; Nolan et al, 1993). By removing tightly bound inhibitory p50 homodimers from DNA, Bcl-3 can free such sites for binding by potently transactivating heterodimers, like p50/RelA (Franzoso et al, 1992, 1993). Such a situation may exist during mitogenic stimulation of primary T cells when prebound p50 homodimers can block NF-κB heterodimers from engaging certain κB sites, unless Bcl-3 is present (Franzoso et al, 1993). Preliminary evidence suggests that normal antigenic signalling of non-transformed T cells induces Bcl-3 (Lenardo and Siebenlist, 1994). Thus, Bcl-3 could be the protein which removes p50 homodimers from the IL-2 promoter to allow expression of this cytokine. This form of regulation is very different from that of IκB-α in that it is positive and happens in the nucleus.

Bcl-3 can also directly transactivate through targeting of p52 homodimers (Bours et al, 1993), p52 homodimers are infrequently observed, with the exception of a few highly differentiated cells, such as myelomas (Bours et al, 1993; Chang et al, 1994; Franzoso and Siebenlist, 1994), and Bcl-3 is constitutively expressed in such more highly differentiated cells as well (Bhatia et al, 1991; Bours et al, 1993). Bcl-3 tightly associates with both homodimers, but in distinction from p50 homodimers, p52 homodimers are not as efficiently dissociated from their cognate binding sites. Rather, Bcl-3 and p52 homodimers form ternary complexes, at least transiently, with the κB sites. This enables these two proteins to induce transcription through the κB site, owing to transactivation domains residing on Bcl-3. Bcl-3 harbors two such domains, located on the N- and C-terminal parts of the protein, outside of the ankyrin domain (Bours et al, 1993). In our work, significant transactivation by Bcl-3 and p50 homodimers has not been observed, regardless of the p50 construct used for transfections, particularly when compared to the transactivation seen with p52 (Bours et al, 1993; Franzoso and Siebenlist, 1994). It has been reported, however, that Bcl-3 and p50 homodimers together could transactivate, albeit weakly (Fujita et al, 1993). It is conceivable that cell- or signal-dependent modifications of p50 or Bcl-3 (such as phosphorylation) determine whether these molecules can significantly transactivate. Bcl-3 is a highly phosphorylated protein in vivo and dephosphorylation in vitro interferes with the ability of Bcl-3 to dissociate p50 homodimers from DNA (Fujita et al, 1993; Nolan et al, 1993).

High levels of p52 homodimers are seen also in a number of human B- and T-cell tumors, in particular in cutaneous lymphomas (Neri et al, 1991; Fracchiolia et al, 1993), as a result of gene translocation. In all cases the translocation also disrupts the ankyrin domain, leading to p52-like proteins with variably sized C-terminal extensions which are partially processed into mature p52 proteins; both forms have been observed in nuclei, in contrast to the p100 precursor (Chang et al, 1994; Franzoso and Siebenlist, 1994). It is possible that homodimers of the truncated (but not yet fully processed) p100 proteins have some transactivation potential. It is also conceivable that the truncated and processed forms transactivate in conjunction with Bcl-3. Bcl-3 itself is overexpressed as a result of rare translocations (Ohno et al, 1990). Overexpression of Bcl-3 may also result in inappropriate transactivation of specific κB-dependent target genes, according to the mechanisms outlined above.

Stimuli And Intracellular Signalling Paths For NF-κB Activation

Inflammation and cytokines

The potent proinflammatory cytokines TNF-α, TNF-β and IL-1 activate NF-κB is a master regulator of defensive reactions (Osborn et al, 1989; Messer et al, 1990; Hohmann et al, 1990a, 1990b). These cytokines are secreted by many primary defense cells that sense pathogenic agents, and, in consequence, these cytokines are usually associated with inflammation. TNF-α, one of the most potent and best studied inducers of NF-κB activity, signals through the 55 kd TNF-I receptor. Although the immediate receptor proximal events are unknown, a phosphatidylcholine specific phospholipase C may be activated to generate 1,2-diacylglycerol (DAG) in response to ligand (Dressler et al, 1992; Schutze et al, 1992). DAG in turn may initiate a signalling cascade which involves, in order, the activation of acidic sphingomyelinases located in endosomal and lysosomal compartments, the subsequent generation of ceramide from sphingomyelin (Schutze et al, 1992), and the ceramide-dependent activation of a serine/threonine kinase (Joseph et al, 1993; Mathias et al, 1991). Alternatively, neutral sphingomyelinases located in the plasma membrane may be involved, independent of DAG (Yang et al, 1993). In support of a sphingomyelinase pathway for TNF-α, NF-κB has been activated in permeabilized cells by exogenously added phospholipase C, DAG analogs, purified acidic sphingomyelinase or ceramide (Schutze et al, 1992). Also, addition of sphingomyelinase or cell-permeable ceramide analogs to intact cells has induced NF-κB activity (Yang et al, 1993), although the effect of several of these agents remains somewhat controversial (Dbaibo et al, 1993).

Mitogen activated protein (MAP) kinase, a downstream effector of Raf function, has been tyrosine-phosphorylated and activated in response to TNF (Saklatvala et al, 1993). It is possible that the Raf pathway may be activated by signalling through ceramide, but no direct connection has been established to date. In support of such a connection, dominant negative Ras and Raf mutants have been reported to block TNF-α-mediated activation of NF-κB (Devary et al, 1993). In fact, Raf has been implicated as the kinase which may directly activate NF-κB via phosphorylation of IκB-α to effect its functional inactivation (see below). Indirect support for this comes from experiments in which constitutively active forms of Raf or Ras activated NF-κB or in which dominant negative mutants of Raf inhibited signalling not only by TNF-α, but also by UV or serum (Bruder et al, 1993; Devary et al, 1993; Finco and

Baldwin, 1993; Li and Sedivy, 1993). More direct evidence for Raf as the proximal mediator of NF-κB activation has been supplied by a yeast two-hybrid experiment which indicates a direct physical interaction between Raf and IκB-α (Li and Sedivy, 1993). Furthermore, IκB-α has been phosphorylated by Raf in vitro, although this by itself does not establish that IκB-α is a physiological target (Li and Sedivy, 1993). Mitochondria could be a downstream target of ceramide since inhibitors of mitochondrial electron transport functions impaired TNF-induced activation of NF-κB (Schulze-Osthoff et al, 1992), and since elimination of mitochondria had similar effects (Schulze-Osthoff et al, 1993). Mitochondria-generated reactive oxygen intermediates may be critical, since anti-oxidants inhibit NF-κB activation by many signals (see below). Another report implicates protein kinase C (PKC) zeta in TNF-α signalling to NF-κB, possibly as part of the sphingomyelin-initiated pathway (Diaz-Meco et al, 1993). Although TNF-α could cause the production of DAG (which activates PKC), the activation of NF-κB by TNF-α appears to be independent of classical PKC. For example, inhibitors of PKC, which block PMA-induced activation of NF-κB, nevertheless fail to block TNF-α-induced activation (Meichle et al, 1990).

IL-1 may induce the production of ceramide as well, and therefore, the IL-1 pathway and the TNF-α pathways may converge, as evidenced also by the largely overlapping biological activities of the two cytokines (Mathias et al, 1993). Herbimycin A, an inhibitor of tyrosine phosphorylation, interferes with IL-1α-induced NF-αB activation in T and B cells, suggesting a role for tyrosine kinases possibly during early phases of signalling by this cytokine (Iwasaki et al, 1992). Other cytokines which can activate NF-κB in at least some cells include interleukin-2 (IL-2), leukemia inhibitory factor (LIF), and possibly interferon-γ and PDGF (Olashaw et al, 1992; Grilli et al, 1993; Ohmori and Hamilton, 1993; Baeuerle and Henkel, 1994). The CD40-ligand may also activate NF-κB in B cells (Lalmanach-Girard et al, 1993). Critical components of these and other select signalling paths leading to NF-κB activation are summarized in Figure 4.1.

Physical and oxidative stress

UV, γ-irradiation, X-rays, photofrin plus red light, hypoxia, hydrogen peroxide and minimally oxidized lipids have all been shown to cause an activation of NF-κB, although the degree of this activation is variable (Andalibi et al, 1993; Brach et al, 1993; Parhami et al, 1993; Ryter and Gomer, 1993; Baeuerle and Henkel, 1994; Koong et al, 1994). Radiation

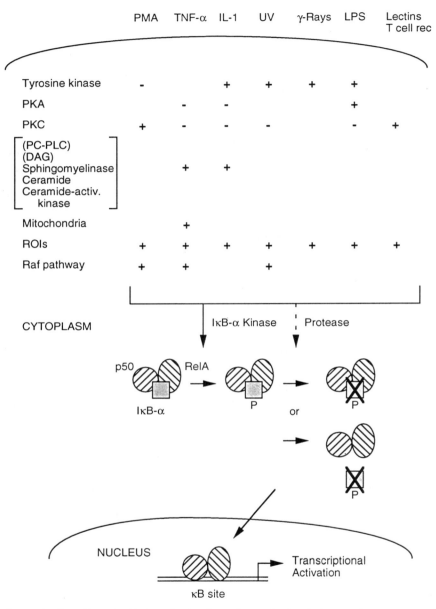

Figure 4.1 Signalling of NF-κB activation by various cell stimuli. Presumed components of signalling pathways are indicated as are the postulated mechanisms of signal-dependent inactivation of IκB-α. NF-κB is represented by a p50/RelA dimer. See text for details and references. Further references (Bomsztyk et al, 1991; Jamieson et al, 1991; Feuillard et al, 1991; Iwasaki et al, 1992; Deisher et al, 1993; Gross et al, 1993; Ray and Kennard, 1993; Uckun et al, 1993). The generation of ROIs by IL-1 may be cell-type dependent (Schreck et al, 1991; Stylianou et al, 1992). The dashed arrow indicates that a signal-dependent activation of the IκB-α protease has not been demonstrated.

damage may in part be caused by activation of NF-κB through subsequent induced expression of many defense genes. Ionizing radiation and UV are thought to mediate their effects through the rapid generation of reactive oxygen intermediates (ROIs) (Devary et al, 1993; Schieven et al, 1993). It has been proposed that many and possibly all inducers of NF-κB activity may generate reactive oxygen intermediates since levels for ROIs have been found to increase in response to various other signals as well, including TNF-α, IL-1, PMA and LPS, although the mechanism for this is not understood (Schreck et al, 1992a, 1992d, Meyer et al, 1993b, Geng et al, 1993; Schieven et al, 1993). It is possible that mitochondria are involved in these signal-induced increases, as suggested at least by studies with TNF-α (Schulze-Osthoff et al, 1992, 1993). More direct support for a role of reactive oxygen intermediates as common messengers comes from studies with many different antioxidants, which all appear to at least partially block activation of NF-κB in various cells stimulated in a variety of ways (Schreck et al, 1992a, 1992c, 1992d; Meyer et al, 1993b). Inhibitory antioxidants with diverse structures include N-acetyl-L-cysteine (NAC is a precursor of glutathione), vitamin E derivatives, dithiocarbamates and various other metal chelators. Pyrolidinedithiocarbamate (PDTC) has been repeatedly demonstrated to inhibit the TNF-α and PMA-induced activation of NF-κB in Jurkat T cells by apparently preventing the inactivation of the IκB-α inhibitor (Beg et al, 1993; Henkel et al, 1993; Sun et al, 1993). Activation of NF-κB is suppressed by NAC (Devary et al, 1993). Although a role for ROIs as a common denominator of all signals is very appealing, a direct functional role for ROIs in signalling to NF-κB remains to be shown. Among various ROIs added to cells only peroxides effectively activated NF-κB in at least certain HeLa and Jurkat cell lines (Schreck et al, 1991, 1992a; Meyer et al, 1993a, 1993b). While hydrogen peroxide by itself is usually only weakly activating, depending on the cell, it is reported to synergize strongly with the phosphatase inhibitors okadaic acid and calyculin A in activating NF-κB in primary lymphocytes (Menon et al, 1993). In cell lines these inhibitors of phosphatase 1 and 2A can activate NF-κB by themselves although the mechanism for this is not known (Thevenin et al, 1990; Menon et al, 1993).

Tyrosine kinases appear to be involved in signalling activation of NF-κB with both ionizing radiation and UV (Devary et al, 1993; Schieven et al, 1993). Such kinases are not generally implicated in signalling paths leading to NF-κB activation, making it less likely that they function downstream of the ROI; this assumes, of course, an obligatory role for ROIs as a common denominator for activation of NF-κB. While UV and other physical stress signals can damage DNA, the NF-κB response to

UV has now been demonstrated to be independent of such damage as it can occur in enucleated cells (Devary et al, 1993).

Activation of NF-κB by recognition of pathogens

Bacteria (e.g. Mycobacterium tuberculosis and Shigella flexneri) or various distinct bacterial cell wall products (lipopolysaccharides (LPS), muramyl peptides and G(Anh)MTetra) can activate NF-κB in a number of cells, including monocyte/macrophages, endothelial cells and B cells (Schreck et al, 1992b; Dyer et al, 1993; Baeuerle and Henkel, 1994; Dokter et al, 1994; Zhang et al, 1994). Bacteria may also activate NF-κB in T and B cells via antigen receptor-mediated recognition. Also, various bacterial toxins have been shown to activate NF-κB, including staphylococcus entertoxins A and B (SEA and SEB), toxic shock syndrome toxin-1 (TSST-1) and possibly cholera toxin; again, activation can occur in macrophages as well as in antigen-recognizing cells (Muroi and Suzuki, 1993; Parhami et al, 1993; Trede et al, 1993). LPS in particular has been widely employed as a stimulator and reportedly acts through tyrosine kinases and possibly also through cAMP-dependent protein kinase (PKA) (Geng et al, 1993; Muroi and Suzuki, 1993).

Stimulation of B or T cells through their respective antigen receptors activates NF-κB, as demonstrated by antigens in the context of appropriate antigen-presenting cells, or by stimulation with other agonists like anti-CD3 antibodies, lectins (e.g. PHA) and anti-IgM antibodies (Grilli et al, 1993). In T cells most antigen-receptor-mediated responses, including the activation of NF-κB, appear to depend, at least in part, on the action of the calcium-activated phosphatase calcineurin; a constitutively activated form of calcineurin can replace the calcium signal required for efficient activation of NF-κB in concert with protein kinase C (PKC) agonists (Frantz et al, 1994). Consequently, cyclosporin A and FK506, which inhibit calcineurin, can also inhibit activation of NF-κB in T cells (Schmidt et al, 1990; Frantz et al, 1994). Antigen-receptor stimulated lymphocytes probably require NF-κB to induce expression of the many cytokines that are secreted by such cells to coordinate the immune response. In addition, however, NF-κB may play a role in proliferation of the cells themselves; many mitogenic stimulants acting through other cell surface receptors, for example anti-CD2 and anti-CD28, also activate this factor in T cells (Bressler et al, 1991; Verweij et al, 1991; Grilli et al, 1993). NF-κB may be directly involved in growth control and/or may act indirectly through induced expression of autocrine/paracrine growth factors (e.g. IL-2) and receptors (e.g. IL-2 receptor-α). The association of NF-κB with growth control may not only be confined to lymphocytes since NF-κB is activated also during the transition of fibroblasts from the G0 to the G1 phase subsequent to serum stimulation (Baldwin et al, 1991). Finally, partial liver hepatectomy, a strong mitogenic signal that causes a rapid regenerative response in liver, activates NF-κB as well (Tewari et al, 1992).

Activation of NF-κB in virus-infected cells

A significant number of viruses induce NF-κB activity in cells upon infection. In some cases this may result from a defensive response of such cells to induce an anti-viral state, as for example in the case of infection with Newcastle disease virus or Sendai virus, viruses which cause the induction of interferon-β in fibroblasts, possibly by double-stranded RNA intermediates (Ten et al, 1993; Du et al, 1993). Other viruses, however, appear to deliberately activate NF-κB and/or cells in general, presumably because these viruses derive some benefit from such activation. Activation may be by virions or through synthesis of viral products after infection. These viruses may need to activate cells in order to allow their integration or replication. Viruses/viral proteins which appear to activate NF-κB by design include the human T-cell leukemia virus-I (HTLV-I) Tax protein, the hepatitis B virus (HBV) proteins Hbx and MHBs[t], the Epstein-Barr virus (EBV) proteins EBNA-2 and LMP, the cytomegalovirus (CMV), the herpes simplex virus-1 (HSV-1), HSV-6, adenovirus 5 and possibly the human immunodeficiency virus-1 (HIV-1) (Nielsch et al, 1991; Grilli et al, 1993; Baeuerle and Henkel, 1994).

HIV infection of monocytic cells reportedly activates NF-κB after several days (Bacherlerie et al, 1991; Paya et al, 1992; Roulston et al, 1993, 1993). This may help to express this virus whose transcription depends on cis-acting κB elements in the HIV LTR (Nabel and Baltimore, 1987; Ross et al, 1991). The HIV encoded protease has been proposed to be involved in this activation through processing of the p105 precursor protein (Riviere et al, 1991). However, these observations have not been confirmed, nor would they necessarily explain nuclear translocation of NF-κB. Activation of NF-κB in HIV-infected cultures may not have been due to the virus itself. In apparent contradiction to virus-induced activation, the HIV Nef product has been reported as an inhibitor of NF-κB (Niederman et al, 1992). HIV-1 may depend on environmental co-factors to stimulate propagation, as resting populations of primary cells generally do not integrate or replicate the virus (Pantaleo et al, 1993b). Inflammation may promote viral spread

(Embretson et al, 1993; Pantaleo et al, 1993a), possibly due to inflammatory products which activate NF-κB, such as TNF-α, bacterial toxins and neutrophil-generated H_2O_2.

T cells can be transformed to continued growth by infection with the HTLV I virus, a prerequisite for adult T-cell leukemias (Smith and Greene, 1991). In particular the HTLV-I Tax product has the ability to transform cells (Nerenberg et al, 1987; Grassman et al, 1989; Kitajima et al, 1993) by activating a number of cellular transcription factors, among them NF-κB. Tax-mediated activation of NF-κB, in turn, induces expression of many mitogen-response proteins (Kelly et al, 1992), including the IL-2 growth factor and IL-2 receptor-α (Hoyos et al, 1989; Smith and Greene, 1991). Tax has been reported to activate NF-κB indirectly, through Tax-induced transcription of NF-κB-encoding genes (Arima et al, 1991), or directly either by an unspecified posttranslational event by an unspecified posttranslational event (Lindholm et al, 1992; Schreck et al, 1992b) or by a mechanism which depends on the apparent physical interaction of Tax with p50/p105 (Hirai et al, 1992; Suzuki et al, 1993; Watanabe et al, 1993). Recently we have discovered two ways in which Tax may activate NF-κB. Tax induces increased turnover of the IκB-α protein, which may interfere with efficient inhibition, allowing some NF-κB complexes to escape into the nucleus (Kanno et al, 1994a). We also have demonstrated an effect of Tax on cytoplasmic pools of NF-κB which are independent of IκB-α: NF-κB dimers can complex with and be inhibited by p100 precursor proteins. Tax antagonizes the p100-mediated cytoplasmic inhibition, probably through a direct binding to the p100 protein (Kanno et al, 1994b). A preferential interaction of Tax with p100 has recently been described elsewhere (Beraud et al, 1994). While the physiological importance of the Tax-mediated release of NF-κB complexes from IκB-α-independent cytoplasmic stores remains to be shown, such a mechanism, together with induced turnover of IκB-α, can account for the strong constitutive levels of nuclear NF-κB observed.

Constitutive NF-κB activity

Apart from viral-induced constitutive NF-κB activity, mature B cells (but not preB cells) also show such activity, albeit at lower levels (Sen and Baltimore, 1986a, 1986b). Similar to what is seen in Tax-expressing cells (see above), these B cells also exhibit an increased turnover of IκB-α, relative to that seen in preB cells, for example (Miyamoto et al, 1994). IκB-α is continuously degraded at an increased rate but it is also resynthesized at a faster rate, presumably due to induced transcription by NF-κB itself (see below). Under these conditions, IκB-α may not be able to inhibit all complexes, especially p50/Rel complexes which were found to predominate in these B cells; p50/RelA dimers largely remained in the cytoplasm but could still be activated in response to various signals (Liou and Baltimore 1993; Miyamoto et al, 1994). It is possible that B cells are continually signalled by autocrine- or paracrine-acting cytokines like IL-1 and TFN-α, cytokines whose expression is positively controlled by NF-κB itself (see below).

Constitutive NF-κB activity may serve a developmental role in B cells, possibly by controlling expression of the immunoglobulin kappa light chain through its κB element in the intronic enhancer. NF-κB may induce sterile transcripts as well as locus demethylation as preparation for rearrangement of the κ light chain (Lichtenstein et al, 1994). Further-more, v-abl, which transforms cells at the preB stage, has been reported to block NF-κB activity as well as κ light chain transcription and rearrange-ment (Klug et al, 1994; Chen et al, 1994). Constitutive NF-κB activity may occur in other developing cells as well, since early developing thymocytes have been found to contain nuclear NF-κB, possibly due to an environ-ment rich in cytokines (Zuniga-Pflucker et al, 1993). A definitive connec-tion between NF-κB and development exists in insects where dorsal acts as the essential morphogen which determines dorsoventral polarity in the developing Drosophila embryos (Govind and Steward, 1991; Ip and Levine, 1992, St. Johnston and Nüsslein-Volhard, 1992). Finally, NTera-2 embryonal carcinoma cells contain little or no NF-κB proteins but can be induced with the differentiating agent retinoic acid to express these proteins and their activities (Segars et al, 1993).

IκB-α, The Target Of NF-κB-Activating Signals

Activation of NF-κB by a number of extracellular signals appears to cause functional inactivation and proteolytic degradation of the inhibitory IκB-α protein. To date there is no evidence that rapid signal-induced transloca-tion of NF-κB can occur independent of IκB-α inactivation, even though other cytoplasmic pools of NF-κB exist, for example the demonstrated precursor-associated pools discussed above. However, these IκB-α-inde-pendent pools may not be directly signal-responsive. NF-κB-activating signals must therefore converge on an effector molecule acting upstream of IκB-α, for example an IκB-α kinase, possibly connected with the action of ROIs (see above). Alternatively, IκB-α itself may be the common target of several different and possibly independent pathways.

IκB-α is nearly completely degraded proteolytically within minutes after stimulation of many different cells with numerous extracellular agents (Beg et al, 1993; Brown et al, 1993; Sun et al, 1993; Cordle et al, 1993; de Martin et al, 1993; Henkel et al, 1993; Mellits et al, 1993; Rice and Ernst 1993; Scott et al, 1993; Chiao et al, 1994; Read et al, 1994). Also, a posttranslational phosphorylation of IκB-α accompanies the degradation (Beg et al, 1993; Brown et al, 1993; Cordle et al, 1993; Sun et al, 1994). The modified form of IκB-α is detected only transiently shortly after stimulation of cells, prior to complete degradation. These observations suggest that phosphorylation may tag IκB-α for rapid degradation, although this remains to be demonstrated directly. The appearance of nuclear NF-κB closely correlated with the disappearance of IκB-α (Brown et al, 1993; Sun et al, 1993).

It is possible also that phosphorylation of IκB-α releases the inhibitor from NF-κB, which is then degraded rapidly because it is unstable in its free, uncomplexed form (Beg et al, 1993). In support of this view, several kinases have been reported to activate NF-κB in vitro simply by phosphorylation of IκB-α (Shirakawa and Mizel, 1989; Ghosh and Baltimore 1990). In this model proteolytic degradation would not be essential for activation. On the other hand, we have recently obtained evidence in support of an essential role for degradation in activating NF-κB. A slower-migrating, phosphorylated species of IκB-α which appears following stimulation remained associated with NF-κB, as demonstrated by co-immunoprecipitation with anti-RelA antibodies (Lin et al, 1994). This favors an essential involvement of proteases in activating NF-κB, presumably acting on the NF-κB-IκB-α complex in situ. Inhibition of NF-κB activation by chymotrypsin-like inhibitors which block IκB-α degradation also supports the importance of proteolysis (Henkel et al, 1993; Mellits et al, 1993; Chiao et al, 1994), but this interpretation may be complicated by the fact that these protease inhibitors also appear to block the signal-dependent modification of IκB-α (Lin et al, 1994). Assuming that activation proceeds via obligatory phosphorylation and degradation of IκB-α, the former may be sufficient to induce the latter, but a separate signal-dependent induction of protease activity cannot be ruled out. Figure 4.1 summarizes these observations.

Pathologic conditions such as toxic/sepsis, graft vs. host reactions, acute inflammatory conditions, acute phase responses, radiation damage and atherosclerosis all correlate with activated NF-κB (see below) and may be alleviated by blockers of NF-κB. Small synthetic molecules could be considered as therapeutic agents, potentially targeting the transcription factor itself or, alternatively, components of the signalling pathway, for example the IκB-α kinase, or the protease(s).

While all the intracellular components which are involved in transducing an NF-κB-activating signal have not been definitively identified (see discussion above and Figure 4.1), genetic analysis in Drosophila has identified the proteins tube and pelle as essential for activation of dorsal by positional cues. Though nothing is known about the function of tube, pelle is a kinase which may be a direct regulator of cactus, the Drosophila homolog of IκB-α (Shelton and Wasserman, 1993). The Drosophila signalling pathway may be conserved through evolution, since the toll receptor through which dorsal is activated contains structural similarity in its intracytoplasmic tail to the mammalian IL-1 receptor (Wasserman, 1993).

NF-κB-Induced Genes

Induction of genes encoding IκB-α and NF-κB components

Activation of NF-κB by numerous signals results in induction of IκB-α mRNA and protein. This occurs soon after IκB-α is initially degraded to allow nuclear translocation of NF-κB (Brown et al, 1993; Scott et al, 1993; Sun et al, 1993; Rice and Ernst, 1993; Chiao et al, 1994; Read et al, 1994). The induction of IκB-α is mediated by NF-κB subunits which induce endogenous IκB-α (Brown et al, 1993; Scott et al, 1993; Sun et al, 1993; Chiao et al, 1994). As predicted, the IκB-α promoter contains functionally important κB binding sites (de Martin et al, 1993; Le Bail et al, 1993; Chiao et al, 1994). Therefore, NF-κB potently induces its own inhibitor, presumably to try to restore the inhibited state (Brown et al, 1993). This feedback inhibition may be critical to limit activation and thus potential tissue damage due to inflammatory functions of NF-κB induced defense genes. A transient response is assured once the initiating event fades. newly synthesized IκB-α may actually transiently enter nuclei to remove already activated NF-κB, since in its absence NF-κB appears to persist in the nucleus, even without any further stimulation (Brown et al, 1993; Brown and Siebenlist, 1994). Also exogenously expressed IκB-α proteins and endogenous chicken pp40 proteins have been detected in cell nuclei (Cressman and Taub, 1993; Zabel et al, 1993; Davis et al, 1990) and IκB-α is known to be able to remove already bound NF-κB from its binding sites (Zabel et al, 1990). IκB-α proteins which are not free but bound to NF-κB, however, may not enter nuclei, possibly because of mutual inhibition.

The genes for the precursor proteins p105 and p100 are induced after cellular stimulation which also activates NF-κB (Gunter et al, 1989; Bours et al, 1990, 1992a), as are the genes for Rel and RelB (Bull et al,

1989; Ryseck et al, 1992). Induction is not as rapid as that of IκB-α, but these genes nevertheless appear to be regulated by NF-κB, as demonstrated in the case of p105 and Rel, whose genes contain NF-κB-responsive promoters with functional κB elements (Ten et al, 1992; Hannink and Temin, 1990; Capobianco and Gilmore, 1991); the genes encoding p100 (Sun et al, 1994) and RelB are likely to be controlled by NF-κB also. Induced expression of these genes is likely to replenish NF-κB activity and may be required for maintenance of nuclear activity during longer periods of stimulation, as reported for HL60 cells (Hohmann et al, 1991). The precursor proteins (prior to processing) may also function as IκB proteins to limit and inhibit NF-κB activation, at least initially. In contrast to these genes, the expression of the RelA-encoding gene appears to be largely unaffected by cellular stimulation, and there are no κB elements in the RelA promoter (Ueberla et al, 1993). The difference between the induction of Rel and RelA may explain the observed increase in amounts of Rel-containing dimers versus RelA-containing dimers in nuclei of Jurkat T cells depending on time of stimulation (Molitor et al, 1990; Doerre et al, 1993). Cells with constitutive NF-κB, such as B cells or HTLV 1 transformed T cells, also preferentially contain Rel in their nuclei (discussed above). Assuming distinct target genes for different dimeric NF-κB complexes, a change in dimers during cellular stimulation may control kinetic differences in induction of such genes.

Induction of cytokines

NF-κB is involved in the expression of many genes but appears not to be the sole determinant of gene expression, but rather functions in concert with one or several other transcription factors, some of which may also be regulated in activity. Nonetheless, NF-κB often appears to be the dominant signal-dependent factor and can be a powerful transactivator. As will be discussed, NF-κB at times functions by direct physical interaction with several other transcription factors. NF-κB induces many of the effectors of immune, inflammatory or acute phase responses. In particular, genes encoding cytokines/growth factors/chemokines, biological messengers which control and coordinate defensive responses, are regulated by NF-κB. Some of these messengers can use NF-κB for amplification via a positive autoregulatory loop. The pro-inflammatory cytokines TNF and IL-1 activate NF-κB and are themselves induced by NF-κB (Messer et al, 1990; Hiscott et al, 1993). The dependence of the TNF-α gene on NF-κB may vary depending on the cell type; NF-κB appears critical for the expression by monocytes/macrophages (Goldfeld et al, 1993; Ziegler-Heitbrock et al, 1993). The NF-κB-mediated amplification of the potentially toxic and widely-acting TNF-α cytokine (and other cytokines) may be the basis of septic shock and acute inflammatory conditions. It is in these pathologic conditions that inhibitors of NF-κB should be considered as therapeutic agents.

Other critical cytokines induced by NF-κB include the acute phase regulator IL-6 and various chemokines which summon cells to sites of inflammation such as IL-8, IP-10, Gro, and possibly also MIP1-α, MCP-1/JE and Rantes (Anisowicz et al, 1991; Grove and Plumb, 1993; Joshi-Barve et al, 1993; Danoff et al, 1994; Shattuck et al, 1994). NF-κB induces IL-6 and IL-8 in synergy with members of the C/EBP family of transcription factors through adjoining promoter binding sites (Kunsch and Rosen, 1993, Matsusaka et al, 1993; Stein et al, 1993b; Stein and Baldwin, 1993). C/EBP proteins are transcription factors containing basic leucine zipper (bZIP) DNA binding/dimerization motifs. The bZIP motifs of several C/EBP proteins have been reported to physically bind to several RHDs (Le Clair et al, 1992; Matsusaka et al, 1993; Stein et al, 1993b). In the IL-8 promoter, NF-κB binding at the κB site allowed C/EBP to cooperatively engage a relatively weak neighboring C/EBP binding site, resulting in synergistic transactivation (Stein and Baldwin, 1993). RelA homodimers may be the preferred and functional NF-κB complex for the IL-8 gene (Kunsch and Rosen, 1993, Stein and Baldwin, 1993). Another gene in which a unique NF-κB may be functional is the urokinase gene, where a RelA/c-Rel complex has been implicated (Hansen et al, 1992, 1994).

Administration of steroids can block induction of IL-6 which is dependent on functional synergy between NF-κB and C/EBP-β (NF-IL6). Steroids may carry out their anti-inflammatory functions via direct interaction of NF-κB with liganded steroid receptor proteins, specifically with dexamethasone-activated glucocorticoid receptors (Ray and Prefontaine, 1994). This inhibition involves direct physical association of RelA (p65) with the ligand-bound receptor. Conversely, exogenously expressed RelA can inhibit dexamethasone-induced activation of the mouse mammary tumor virus (Ray and Prefontaine, 1994). These results suggest that the general anti-inflammatory activities of steroids could be due to the physical association between steroid receptors and NF-κB.

The cytokine IFN-β gene is potently induced by viruses, in part through the activation of NF-κB (Thanos and Maniatis, 1992; Du et al, 1993). Induced expression of IFN represents an intracellular anti-viral defense response and may be initiated by double-stranded RNA (dsRNA) (Visvanathan and Goodbourn, 1989; Thanos and Maniatis

1992; Du et al, 1993). NF-κB cooperates with ATF-2-containing complexes to induce IFN-β expression; in addition, NF-κB cooperates with IRF-1 and HMG I/Y proteins (Miyamoto et al, 1988; Harada et al, 1989; Du and Maniatis, 1992; Reis et al, 1992; Thanos and Maniatis, 1992; Du et al, 1993). NF-κB physically interacts with ATF-2, a bZip motif transcription factor and may in this way bring the latter factor into close proximity to the transcriptional initiation complex, generating a DNA loop in the process (Thanos and Maniatis, 1992; De et al, 1993). Functional synergy between these proteins and presumably also formation of a DNA loop is critically dependent on the HMG I/Y proteins, proteins which may bend DNA. Binding sites for HMG I/Y flank the ATF-2 site, and another is located within the NF-κB binding site itself. HMG I/Y also physically interacts with NF-κB and with it cooperatively binds DNA, engaging AT base pairs in the minor groove; these contacts lie in the middle of rare κB sites. Since NF-κB bends DNA upon binding (Schreck et al, 1990), HMG I/Y may help this process. Together these factors appear to form a large stable protein-DNA complex at the promoter upon virus induction. Induction of IFN-β by other stimuli, may depend more critically on a functional interaction between NF-κB and IRF-1 (Fujita et al, 1989; Abdollahi et al, 1991).

The interaction between NF-κB and ATF or C/EBP factors may be similar to the observed interaction between NF-κB and c-Jun and c-Fos (Stein et al, 1993b), since all these partners of NF-κB are bZIP transcription factors, but are otherwise unrelated. The bZIP domains of c-Jun and c-Fos have been demonstrated to interact with the RHD of RelA (p65) (Stein et al, 1993a). Interactions between DNA binding/dimerization domains (such as bZIP and RHD) may be a common theme by which transcription factors physically and functionally cooperate, enhancing DNA binding and transactivation. The functional synergy of NF-κB with Jun and/or Fos may occur with only one or the other of their cognate binding sites, i.e. only one of the factors is required to contact DNA (Stein et al, 1993a). It remains to be shown which genes are regulated by synergistic interactions of NF-κB and AP-1. Other cytokine genes under the influence of NF-κB include IL-2, M-CSF, GM-CSF and G-CSF, proenkephalin, and possibly erythropoietin and TGF-β2 (Grilli et al, 1993; Lee-Huang et al, 1993; Baeuerle and Henkel, 1994).

Induction of immunoreceptors

Migration of immune cells into inflamed tissue is mediated by adhesion to the blood vessel endothelium and subsequent extravasation. This process requires expression of the cell surface adhesion proteins endothelial, leukocyte adhesion molecule 1 (E-selectin or ELAM-1) and vascular cell adhesion molecule 1 (VCAM-1), both of which appear to be induced by an NF-κB-dependent pathway (Iademarco et al, 1992; Neish et al, 1992; Kaszubska et al, 1993; Shu et al, 1993). The intercellular cell adhesion molecule 1 (ICAM-1) may also be regulated by NF-κB and acts, together with VCAM-1, to facilitate monocyte adherence to endothelial cells (Voraberger et al, 1991). Atheroscelorotic lesions, which begin with monocytes sticking to blood vessel walls may be initiated by the inappropriate expression of cytokines and adhesion receptors on endothelial cells, possibly in response to activation of NF-κB by oxidative stress signals, such as oxidized lipoproteins (Andalibi et al, 1993; Collins, 1993; Liao et al, 1993; Parhami et al, 1993). The physical interaction of NF-κB with ATF factors (discussed above in the case of the IFN-β gene) may be essential for the induction of the ELAM-1 gene as well (Kaszubska et al, 1993). This cell adhesion protein is induced by cytokines on endothelial cells where it acts to facilitate the binding and extravasation of neutrophils and a subset of leukocytes from the blood into sites of inflammation (Collins, 1993).

NF-κB may be also be involved in other adhesion processes since antisense RelA oligonucleotides caused embryonal stem cells and other cells to detach from the substratum (Narayanan et al, 1993; Sokoloski et al, 1993). PMA-induced adhesion of HL60 cells could be inhibited by competitive binding of NF-κB to κB oligonucleotides in vivo (Eck et al, 1993).

MHC class I and possibly also class II genes are induced by NF-κB. In the MHC class I promoter NF-κB and IRF-1 cooperate functionally through binding to adjoining DNA recognition sites. This explains the observed synergy between the cytokines TNF-α (through NF-κB) and interferon-γ (through IRF-1) in inducing MHC class I expression (Johnson and Pober, 1994; Ten et al, 1993), possibly by physical association of these transcription factors (Drew and Ozato, 1994).

Further immunoreceptor genes whose expression is at least partly induced by NF-κB include those encoding the T-cell receptor β chain, β2-microglobulin, MHC class II invariant chain Ii, tissue factor 1, the IL-2 receptor α chain and possibly also CD7 (Grilli et al, 1993; Baeuerle and Henkel, 1994). NF-κB may also interact with a proximally bound serum response factor complex to control the IL-2 receptor-α gene (Kuang et al, 1993).

NF-κB may functionally interact with basic helix-loop-helix (bHLH) transcription factors (bHLH) to induce expression of the immunoglobulin κ light chain, as indicated by the close proximity of their respective binding sites in the Ig κ enhancer (Staudt and Lenardo, 1991; Grilli et al,

1993). Cooperation with bHLH factors may be suspected also because of the demonstrated physical interaction of the Drosophila protein dorsal with several bHLH proteins (Jiang and Levine, 1993). When the κ enhancer is introduced into Drosophila embryos striped patterns of expression result; such expression is dependent on the interaction of dorsal and Drosophila bHLH proteins which presumably recognized the related mammalian NF-κB and bHLH factor binding sites present on this enhancer (Gonzalez-Crespo and Levine, 1994).

Other select genes induced by NF-κB

Several acute phase response proteins are induced by NF-κB. These include angiotensinogen, serum amyloid A precursor, complement factor B, complement factor C4 and possibly the urokinase-type plasminogen activator (Grilli et al, 1993; Baeuerle and Henkel, 1994). In addition, the nitric oxide (NO) synthetase gene, whose expression is induced during acute phase responses, is regulated by NF-κB (Lowenstein et al, 1993; Xie et al, 1994). NO synthetase, angiotensinogen and serum amyloid A are all examples in which NF-κB and C/EBP proteins cooperate (Ron et al, 1990, 1991; Betts et al, 1993), as discussed for the IL-6 and IL-8 genes above. Synergistic activation by these two transcription factors may explain the observed global synergy between the cytokines IL-1, a strong activator of NF-κB and IL-6, a strong activator of C/EBP, in regulating acute phase responses, T-cell activation and immunoglobulin secretion.

In addition to the many cytokine and receptor genes which participate in cell proliferation, NF-κB is involved in the induced expression of several genes whose encoded products may directly function in cell cycle progression, such as the c-myc oncogene/transcription factor and the transcription factors IRF-1 and IRF-2 (Duyao et al, 1990; Baldwin et al, 1991; Duyao et al, 1992; Kessler et al, 1992; Harada et al, 1994). Finally, the A20 zinc-finger containing transcription factor, which appears to protect cells from TNF-α-induced cytotoxicity, is also induced by NF-κB through two κB sites (Krikos et al, 1992).

Induction of virus expression

A number of viruses contain κB elements in their promoters/enhancers and utilize the cellular NF-κB transcription factor in their regulation. CMV activates and is transcriptionally stimulated by NF-κB (Sambucetti et al, 1989; Boldogh et al, 1993; Kowalik et al, 1993). Expression of HIV-1 is determined by two cooperating tandem κB sites located in its enhancer (Nabel and Baltimore, 1987, Pierce et al, 1988). This has been shown functionally for propagation of the HIV-related simian immunodeficiency virus (SIV) in monocytes/macrophages (Bellas et al, 1993), and it is likely to be the case also for HIV in such cells, as well as in primary T cells and at least some T-cell lines (Ross et al, 1991). The ubiquitous and apparently constitutively-acting Sp1 transcription factor has been shown to synergize with NF-κB to induce transcription of the HIV-1 LTR (Perkins et al, 1993). The spatial arrangement of the two respective adjoining binding sites has been found to be critical to this synergy, suggesting a possible direct interaction between these factors. Given constitutive SP-1 activity, NF-κB is the only transcription factor known that activates HIV-1 in response to signals. In contrast to HIV-1, HIV-2 possesses only one κB element; here, NF-κB may need to functionally interact with several other regulated factors which have been shown to be important for expression (Leiden et al, 1992; Hannibal et al, 1993). Other viruses responsive to NF-κB activation include the adenovirus, HSV-1 and potentially the human neurotropic virus (JCV) and SV40 (Grilli et al, 1993; Ranganathan and Khalili 1993; Baeuerle and Henkel, 1994). NF-κB could be considered as a therapeutic target to suppress the multiplication of viruses such as HIV-1. Since blockers of NF-κB may need to be administered for long periods, such treatments may lead to complications due to the many functions of NF-κB. However, approaches which target the action of NF-κB more specifically, for example the relatively unique interaction between NF-κB and SP1 on the HIV LTR, could yield useful therapeutics.

Defensive responses in insects

That the regulation of defense genes by NF-κB factors has been conserved through evolution is suggested by the finding that insects regulate their responses to bacterial infections through an NF-κB transcription factor. In the case of Drosophila this factor has been cloned, and is termed Dif (dorsal-related immunity factor); it may function as a homodimer (Hultmark, 1993, 1994; Ip et al, 1993). Unlike dorsal, Dif is not expressed during early embryogenesis but rather during later stages of development. Nuclear Dif activity is inducible from (presumably cactus-inhibited) cytoplasmic stores in cells of the fat body and in hemolymph. Ancient acute phase responses may thus be the original source of what has evolved into the family of factors which now includes the Rel, NF-κB, dorsal and Dif proteins. A role in embryogenesis (dorsal) and in vertebrate immune functions may have developed later (Ip et al, 1993; Hultmark, 1994).

Conclusions

Since the cloning in 1990 of the first gene shown to encode NF-κB activity (p50/p105), there has been a virtual explosion of information about this family of transcription factors. This wealth of data has raised a number of important questions which remain unanswered and which need to be addressed in the future. Unresolved issues include a) the three-dimensional structure of the DNA binding and dimerization domains encoded in the RHD; b) the three-dimensional structure of ankyrin domains and their mode of interaction with the RHD; c) the specific physiological roles of the various dimeric complexes; d) the molecular details and the physiological roles of the interactions between NF-κB dimers and other transcription factors, on and off DNA; e) the role of NF-κB in cell cycle progression; f) the role of NF-κB in apoptotic cell death; g) the role of NF-κB in vertebrate development; h) the role of NF-κB in response to injury; i) the signal transduction pathways which lead to activation of NF-κB, including viral transactivators; j) the identification of the kinase(s) and protease(s) which mediate the inactivation of IκB-α; k) the physiological roles of Bcl-3 and the prescursors p105 and p100; l) the modes of action by which various NF-κB/Rel proteins or some IκB proteins can contribute to tumorigenesis; m) the identification of anti-inflammatory therapeutic agents which act by inhibiting NF-κB activity; most likely these will be small synthetic molecules which inhibit NF-κB dimers or which inhibit signalling molecules essential for activation. Some of the questions related to the physiological role of NF-κB proteins will be addressed via analysis of transgenic animals, in particular via targeted disruptions of the various NF-κB/Rel/IκB genes. Research to date has established NF-κB as a model system for dissecting critical components of immune activation; in addition, NF-κB serves as a model for signalling from the membrane to the nucleus and for regulation of nuclear import. Given its central role in regulating responses to pathogens and stress, NF-κB will continue to be an intensively studied transcription factor.

Acknowledgments

We thank all members of our laboratory for their scientific contribution, and we are grateful to Dr. Anthony S. Fauci for his support. We apologize for not including all relevant research efforts nor citing all relevant publications due to necessary limits on the size of this review and the very large number of publications. We thank M. Rust for her skilled assistance in the preparation of this review.

References

Abbadie C, Kabrun N, Bouali F, Smardova, J, Stehelin D, Bandenbunder B, Enrietto PJ (1993): High levels of c-rel expression are associated with programmed cell death in the developing avian embryo and in bone marrow cells in vitro. *Cell* 75: 899–912

Abdollahi A, Lord KA, Hoffman-Liebermann B, Liebermann D (1991): Interferon regulatory factor 1 is a myeloid differentiation primary response gene induced by interleukin 6 and leukemia inhibitory factor: role in growth inhibition. *Cell Growth Differ* 2: 401–407

Andalibi A, Liao F, Imes S, Fogelman AM, Lusis AJ (1993): Oxidized lipoproteins influence gene expression by causing oxidative stress and activating the transcription factor NF-κB. *Biochem Soc Trans* 21: 651–655

Anisowicz A, Messineo M, Lee SW, Sager R (1991): An NF-κB-like transcription factor mediates IL-1/TNF-α induction of gro in human fibroblasts. *J immunol* 147: 520–527

Arima N, Molitor JA, Smith MR, Kim JH (1991): Human T-cell leukemia virus type I Tax induces expression of the Rel-related family of κB enhancer-binding proteins: evidence for a pretranslational component of regulation. *J Virol* 65: 6892–6899

Bachelerie F, Alcami J, Arenzana-Seisdedos F, Virelizier J-L (1991): HIV enhancer activity perpetuated by NF-κB induction on infection of monocytes. *Nature* 350: 709–712

Baeuerle PA (1991): The inducible transcription activator NF-κB: regulation by distinct protein subunits. *Biochem Biophys Acta* 1072: 63–80

Baeuerle PA, Baltimore D (1988): IκB: a specific inhibitor of the NF-κB transcription factor. *Science* 242: 540–546

Baeuerle PA, Henkel T (1994): Function and activation of NF-κB in the immune system. *Annu Rev Immunol* 12: 141–179

Bakalkin GYA, Yakovleva T, Terenius L (1993: NF-κB-like factors in the murine brain. Developmentally-regulated and tissue-specific expression. *Mol Brain Res* 20: 137–146

Baldwin AJ, Azizkhan JC, Jensen DE, Beg AA, Coodly LR (1991): Induction of NF-κB DNA-binding activity during the G0 to G1 transition in mouse fibroblasts. *Mol Cell Biol* 11: 4943–4951

Ballard DW, Dixon EP, Peffer NJ, Bogerd H, Doerre S, Stein B, Greene WC (1992): The 65-kDa subunit of human NF-κB functions as a potent transcriptional activator and a target for v-Rel-mediated repression. *Proc Natl Acad Sci USA* 89: 1875–1879

Ballard DW, Walker WH, Doerre S, Sista P, Molitor JA, Dixon EP, Peffer NJ, Hannink M, Greene WC (1990): The V-REL oncogene encodes a κB enhancer binding protein that inhibits NF-κB function. *Cell* 63: 803–814

Beg AA, Baldwin AS (1993): The IκB proteins: multifunctional regulators of Rel/NF-κB Transcription factors. *Genes Dev* 7: 2064–2070

Beg AA, Finco TS, Nantermet PV Baldwin AS (1993): Tumor necrosis factor and interleukin-1 lead to phosphorylation and loss of IκB α: a mechanism for NF-κB activation. *Mol Cell Biol* 13: 3301–3310

Beg AA, Ruben SM, Scheinman RI, Haskill S, Rosen CA, Baldwin AS (1992): IκB interacts with the nuclear localization sequences of the subunits of NF-κB: a mechanisms for cytoplasmic retention. *Genes Dev* 6: 1899–1913

Bellas RE, Hopkins N, Li Y (1993): The NF-κB binding site is necessary for efficient replication of simian immunodeficiency virus of macaques in primary macrophages but not in T cells in vitro. *J Virol* 67: 2908–2913

Beraud C, Sun SC, Ganchi P, Ballard DW, Green WC (1994): Human T-cell leukemia virus type I tax associates with and is negatively regulated by the NF-κB2 p100 gene product: implications for viral latency. *Mol Cell Biol* 14: 1374–1382

Betts JC, Cheshire JK, Akira S, Kishimoto T, Woo P (1993): The role of NF-κB and NF-IL-6 transactivating factors in the synergistic activation of human serum amyloid A gene expression by interleukin-1 and interleukin-6. *J Biol Chem* 268: 25624–25631

Bhatia K, Huppi K, McKeithan T, Siwarski D (1991): Mouse bcl-3: cDNA structure, mapping and stage-dependent expression in B lymphocytes. *Oncogene* 6: 1569–1573

Blank V, Kourilsky P, Israël A (1991): Cytoplasmic retention, DNA binding and processing of the NF-κB p50 precursor are controlled by a small region in its C-terminus. *EMBO J* 10: 4159–4167

Blank V, Kourilsky P, Israël A (1992): NF-κB and related proteins: Rel/dorsal homologies meet ankyrin-like repeats. *Trends Biochem Sci* 17: 135–140

Boehmelt G, Walker A, Kabrun N, Melitzer G, Beug H, Zenke M (1992): Hormone-regulated v-rel estrogen receptor fusion protein: reversible induction of cell transformation and cellular gene expression. *EMBO J* 11: 4641–4652

Boldogh I, Fons MP, Albrecht T (1993): Increased levels of sequence-specific DNA-binding proteins in human cytomegalovirus-infected cells. *Biochem Biophys Res Commun* 197: 1505–1510

Bomsztyk K, Rooney JW, Iwasaki T, Rachi NA, Dower SK, Sibley C (1991): Evidence that interleukin-1 and phorbolesters activate NF-κB by different pathways: of protein kinase C. *Cell Regul* 2: 329–335

Bose HJ (1992): The Rel family: models for transcriptional regulation and oncogenic transformation. *Biochim Biophys Acta* 1114: 1–17

Bours V, Azarenko V, Dejardin E, Siebenlist U (1994): Human RelB (I-Rel) functions as a κB site-dependent transactivating member of the family of Rel-related proteins. *Oncogene*: in press

Bours V, Burd PR, Brown K, Villalobos J, Park S, Ryseck R, Bravo R, Kelly K, Siebenlist U (1992a): A novel mitogen-inducible gene product related the p50-p105-NF-κB participates in transactivation through a κB site. *Mol Cell Biol* 12: 685–695

Bours V, Franzoso G, Brown K, Park S, Azarenko V, Tomita-Yamaguchi M, Kelly K, Siebenlist U (1992b): Lymphocyte activation and the family of NF-κB transcription factor complexes. *Curr Topics Microbiol Immunol* 182: 411–420

Bours V, Franzoso G, Azarenko V, Park S, Kanno T, Brown K, Siebenlist U (1993): The oncoprotein Bcl-3 directly transactivates through κB motifs via association with DNA-binding p50B homodimers. *Cell* 72: 729–739

Bours V, Villalobos J, Burd PR, Kelly K, Siebenlist U (1990): Cloning of a mitogen-inducible gene encoding a κB DNA-binding protein with homology to the rel oncogene and to cell-cycle motifs. *Nature* 348: 76–80

Brach MA, Gruss HJ, Kaisho T, Asano Y (1993): Ionizing radiation induces expression of interleukin 6 by human fibroblasts involving activation of nuclear factor-kappa B. *J Biol Chem* 268: 8466–8472

Bressler P, Brown K, Timmer W, Bours V, Siebenlist U, Fauci AS (1993): Mutational analysis of the p50 subunit of NF-κB and inhibition of NF-κB activity by trans-dominant p50 mutants. *J Virol* 67: 288–293

Bressler P, Pantaleo G, Demaria A, Fauci AS (1991): Anti-CD2 receptor antibodies activate the HIV long terminal repeat in T lymphocytes. *J Immunol* 147: 2290–2294

Brown K, Siebenlist U (1994): unpublished observation

Brown K, Park S, Kanno T, Franzoso G, Siebenlist U (1993): Mutual regulation of the transcriptional activator NF-κB and its inhibitor, I kappa B-α. *Proc Natl Acad Sci USA* 90: 2532–2536

Brownell E, Mathieson B, Young Ha, Keller J, Ihle JN, Rice NR (1987): Detection of c-rel-related transcripts in mouse hematopoietic tissues, fractionated lymphocyte populations, and cell lines. *Mol Cell Biol* 7: 1304–1309

Brownell E, Mittereder N, Rice NR (1989): A human rel protooncogene cDNA containing an Alu fragment as a potential coding exon. *Oncogene* 4: 935–942

Bruder JT, Heidecker G, Tan T-H, Weske JC, Derse D, Rapp UR (1993): Oncogene activation of HIV-LTR-driven expression via the NF-κB binding sites. *Nucl Acids Res* 21: 5229–5234

Bull P, Hunter T, Verma IM (1989): Transcriptional induction of the murine c-rel gene with serum and phorbol-12-myristate-13-acetate in fibroblasts. *Mol Cell Biol* 9: 5239–5243

Bull P, Morley KL, Hoekstra MF, Hunter T, Verma IM (1990): The mouse c-rel protein has an N-terminal regulatory domain and a C-terminal transcriptional trans-activation domain. *Mol Cell Biol* 10: 5473–5485

Capobianco AJ, Gilmore TD (1991): Repression of a the chicken c-rel promoter by v-Rel in chicken embryo fibroblasts is not mediated through a consensus NF-κB binding site. *Oncogene* 6: 2203–2210

Capobianco AJ, Simmons DL, Gilmore TD (1990): Cloning and expression of a chicken c-rel cDNA: unlike p69v-rel, p68c-rel is a cytoplasmic protein in chicken embryonic fibroblasts. *Oncogene* 5: 257–265

Carrasco D, Ryseck R-P, Bravo R (1993): Expression of rel/B transcripts during lymphoid organ development: specific expression in dendritic antigen-presenting cells. *Development* 118: 1221–1231

Chang CC, Zhang J, Lombardi L, Neri A, Dalla-Favera R (1994): Mechanism of expression and role in transcriptional control of the proto-oncogene NF-κB-2/lyt-10. *Oncogene* 9:923–933

Chen Y-Y, Wang LC, Huang MS, Rosenberg N (1994): An active v-able protein tyrosine kinase blocks immunoglobulin light-chain gene rearrangement. *Genes Dev* 8: 688–697

Chiao PJ, Miyamoto S, Verma IM (1994): Autoregulation of IκB-α activity. *Proc Natl Acad Sci USA* 91: 28–32

Coleman TA, Kunsch C, Maher M, Ruben SM, Rosen CA (1993): Acquisition of NF-κB1-selective DNA binding by substitution of four amino acid residues from NF-κB1 into RelA. *Mol Cell Biol* 13: 3850–3859

Collins T (1993): Biology of Disease. Endothelial nuclear factor-κB and the initiation of the atherosclerotic lesion. *Lab Invest* 68: 499–506

Cordle SR, Donald R, Read MA, Hawiger J (1993): Lipopolysaccharide induces phosphorylation of MAD3 and activation of c-Rel and related NF-κB proteins in human monocytic THP-1 cells. *J Biol Chem* 268: 268: 11803–11810

Costello R, Lipcey C, Algarte M, Cerdan C, Baeuerle PA, Olive D, Imbert J (1993): Activation of primary human T-lymphocytes through CD2 plus CD28 adhesion molecules induces long-term nuclear expression of NF-κB. *Cell Growth Diff* 4: 329–339

Cressman DE, Taub R (1993): IκB alpha can localize in the nucleus but shows no direct transactivation potential. *Oncogene* 8: 2567–2573

Danoff TM, Lalley PA, Chang YS, Heeger PS, Neilson EG (1994): Cloning, genomic organization, and chromosomal localization of the scya5 gene encoding the murine chemokine RANTES. *J Immunol* 152: 1182

Davis N, Bargmann W, Lim M-Y, Bose H (1990): Avian reticuloendotheliosis virus-transformed lymphoid cells contain multiple pp59v-rel complexes. *J Virol* 64: 584–591

Davis N, Ghosh S, Simmons DL, Tempst P, Liou H, Baltimore D, Bose HR (1992): Rel-associated pp40: an inhibitor of the rel family of transcription factors. *Science* 253: 1268–1271

Dbaibo GS, Obeid LM, Hannun YA (1993): Tumor necrosis factor-alpha (TNF-α) signal transduction through ceramid. Dissociation of growth inhibitor effects of TNF-α from activation of nuclear factor-kappa B. *J Biol Chem* 268: 17762–17766

Deisher TA, Haddix TL, Montgomery KF, Pohlman TH, Kaushansky K, Harlan JM (1993): The role of protein kinase C in the induction of VCAM-1 expression on human umbilical vein endothelial cells. *FEBS Lett* 331: 285–290

deMartin R, Vanhove B, Cheng Q, Hofer E, Csizmadia V, Winkler H, Bach FH (1993): Cytokine-inducible expression in endothelial cells of an IκB-α-like gene is regulated by NF-κB. *EMBO J* 12: 2773–2779

Devary Y, Rosette C, DiDonato JA, Karin M (1993): NF-κB activation by ultraviolet light not dependent on a nuclear signal. *Science* 261: 1442–1445

Diaz-Meco MT, Berra E, Municio MM, Sanz L, Lozano J, Dominguez I, Diaz-Golpe V, Lera MTLd, Alcami J, Paya CV, Arenzana-Seisdedos F, Virelizier J-L, Moscat J (1993): A dominant negative protein kinase c zeta subspecies blocks NF-κB activation. *Mol Cell Biol* 13: 4770–4775

Diehl JA, McKinsey TA, Hannink M (1993): Differential pp40/IκB-β inhibition of DNA binding by rel proteins. *Mol Cell Biol* 13: 1769–1778

Dobrzanski P, Ryseck R-P, Bravo R (1993): Both N- and C-terminal domains of RelB are required for full transactivation: role of the N-terminal leucine zipper-like motif. *Mol Cell Biol* 13: 1572–1482

Doerre S, Sista P, Sun S-C, Ballard DW, Greene WC (1993): The c-rel protooncogene product represses NF-κB p65-mediated transcriptional activation of the long terminal repeat of type 1 human immunodeficiency virus. *Proc Natl Acad Sci USA* 90: 1023–1027

Dokter WHA, Dijkstra AJ, Koopmans SB, Stulp BK, Keck W, Halie MR, Vellenga E (1994): G(Anh)MTetra, a natural bacterial cell wall breakdown product, induces interleukin-1β and interleukin-6 expression in human monocytes. *J Biol Chem* 269:4201–4206

Dressler KA, Mathias S, Kolesnick RN (1992): Tumor necrosis factor-alpha activates the sphinjonyelin signal transduction pathway in a cell-free system. *Science* 255: 1715–1718

Drew P, Ozato K (1994): personal communication

Du W, Maniatis T (1992): An ATF/CREB binding site is required for virus induction of the human interferon beta gene. *Proc Natl Acad Sci USA* 89: 2150–2154

Du W, Thanos D, Maniatis T (1993): Mechanisms of transcriptional synergism between distinct virus-inducible enhancer elements. *Cell* 74: 887–898

Duyao MP, Buckler AJ, Sonenshein GE (1990): Interaction of an NF-κB-like factor with a site upstream of the c-myc promoter. *Proc Natl Acad Sci USA* 87: 4727–4731

Duyao MP, Kessler DJ, Spicer DB, Batholomew C, Cleveland JL, Siekevitz M, Sonenshein GE (1992): Transactivation of the c-myc promoter by human T cell leukemia virus type 1 tax is mediated by NF-κB. *J Biol Chem* 267: 16288–16291

Dyer RB, Collaco CR, Niesel DW, Herzog NK (1993): Shigella flexneri invasion of HeLa cells induces NF-κB DNA-binding activity. *Infect Immun* 61: 4427–4433

Eck SL, Perkins ND, Carr DP, Nabel GJ (1993): Inhibition of phorbol ester-induced cellular adhesion by competitive binding of NF-κB B in vivo. *Mol Cell Biol* 13: 6530–6506

Embretson J, Zupancic M, Ribas JL, Burke A (1993): Massive covert infection of helper T lymphocytes and macrophages by HIV during the incubation period of AIDS. *Nature* 362: 359–362

Fan CM, Maniatis T (1991): Generation of p50 subunit of NF-κB by processing of p105 through an ATP-dependent pathway. *Nature* 354: 395–398

Feuillard J, Gouy H, Bismuth G, Lee LM (1991): NF-kappa B activation by tumor necrosis factor alpha in the Jurkat T cell line is independent of protein kinase A, protein kinase C, and Ca(2 +)-regulated kinases. *Cytokine* 3: 257–265

Feuillard J, Korner M, Fourcade C, Costa A (1994): Visualization of the endogenous NF-κB p50 subunit in the nucleus of follicular dendritic cells in germinal centers. *J Immunol* 152: 12–21

Finco TS, Baldwin AS (1993): κB site dependent induction of gene expression by diverse inducers of nuclear factor κB requires Raf-1. *J Bio Chem* 24: 17676–17679

Fracchiolla NS, Lombardi L, Slaina M, Migliazzi A, Baldini L, Berti E, Cro L, Polli E, Maiolo AT, Neri A (1993): Structural alterations of the NF-κB transcription factor lyt-10 in lymphoid malignancies. *Oncogene* 8: 2839–2845

Frantz B, Nordby EC, Bren G, Steffan N, Paya CV, Kincaid RL, Tocci MJ, O'Keefe SJ, O'Neill EA (1994): Calcineurin acts in synergy with PMA to inactivate IκB/MAD3, an inhibitor of NF-κB. *EMBO J* 13: 861–870

Franzoso G, Siebenlist U (1994): unpublished observations

Franzoso G, Bours V, Park S, Tomita-Yamaguchi M, Kelly K and Siebenlist U (1992): The candidate oncoprotein Bcl-3 is an antagonist of p50/NF-κB-mediated inhibition. *Nature* 359: 339–342

Franzoso G, Bours V, Azarenko V, Park S, Tomita-Yamaguchi M, Kanno T, Brown K, Siebenlist U (1993): The oncoprotein Bcl-3 can facilitate NF-κB-mediated transactivation by removing inhibiting p50 homodimers from select κB sites. *EMBO J* 12: 3893–3901

Franzoso G, Bours V, Siebenlist U (1994): unpublished observation

Fujita T, Nolan GP, Ghosh S, Baltimore D (1992): Independent modes of transcriptional activation by the p50 and p65 subunits of NF-κB. *Genes Dev.* 6: 775–787

Fujita T, Nolan GP, Liou H-C, Scott ML, Baltimore D (1993): The candidate proto-oncogene bcl-3 encodes a transcriptional coactivator that activates through NF-κB p50 homodimers. *Genes Dev* 7: 1354–1363

Fujita T, Reis LFL, Watanabe N, Kimura Y, Taniguchi T, Vilcek J (1989): Induction of the transcription factor IRF-1 and IFN-β mRNAs by cytokines and activators of second-messenger pathways. *Proc Natl Acad Sci USA* 86: 9936–9940

Ganchi PA, Sun S-C, Greene WC, Ballard DW (1992): IκB/MAD-3 masks the nuclear localization signal of NF-κB p65 and requires the transactivation domain to inhibit NF-κB p65 DNA binding. *Mol Biol Cell* 3: 1339–1352

Ganchi PA, Sun SC, Greene WC, Ballard DW (1993): A novel NF-κB complex containing p65 homodimers: implications for transcriptional control at the level of subunit dimerization. *Mol Cell Biol* 13: 7826–7835

Gay NJ, Ntwasa M (1993): The Drosophila ankyrin repeat protein cactus has a predominantly alpha-helical secondary structure. *FEBS Lett* 355: 155–160

Geng Y, Zhang B, Lotz M (1993): Protein tyrosine kinase activation is required for lipopolysaccharide induction of cytokines in human blood monocytes. *J Immunol* 151: 6692–6700

Ghosh S, Baltimore D (1990): Activation in vitro of NF-κB-γ phosphorylation of its inhibitor IκB. *Nature* 344: 678–682

Ghosh S, Gifford AM, Riviere LR, Tempst P, Nolan GP, Baltimore D (1990): Cloning of the p50 DNA binding subunit of NF-κB: homology to rel and dorsal. *Cell* 62: 1019–1029

Gilmore TD (1992): Role of rel family genes in normal and malignant lymphoid cell growth. *Cancer Surveys* 15: 69–87

Gilmore TD, Morin PJ (1993): The IκB proteins: members of a multifunctional family. *Trends Genet* 9: 427–433

Goldfeld AE, McCaffrey PG, Strominger JL, Rao A (1993): Identification of a novel cyclosporin-sensitive element in the human tumor necrosis factor alpha gene promoter. *J Exp Med* 178: 1365–1379

Gonzalez-Crespo S, Levine M (1994): Related target enhancers for dorsal and NF-κB signaling pathways. *Science* 264: 255–258

Govind S, Steward R (1991): Dorsovental pattern formation in Drosophila: signal transduction and nuclear targeting. *Trends Gen* 7: 119–125

Grassman R, Dengler C, Muller-Fleckenstein I, Fleckenstein B, McGuire K, Dokhelar MC, Sodroski JG, Haseltine WA (1989): Transformation of continuous growth of primary human T lymphocytes by human T-cell leukemia virus type I X-region genes transduced by a Herpesvirus saimiri vector. *Proc Natl Acad Sci USA* 86: 3351–3355

Grilli M, Jason J-S, Lenardo MJ (1993): NF-κB and rel-participants in a multiform transcriptional regulatory system. *Int Rev Cytol* 143: 1–62

Grimm S, Baeuerle PA (1993): The inducible transcription factor NF-κB: structure-function relationship of its protein subunits. *Biochem J* 290: 297–308

Gross V, Zhang B, Geng Y, Villiger PM, Lotz M (1993): Regulation of interleukin-6 (IL-6) expression: evidence for a tissue-specific role of protein kinase C. *J Clin Immunol* 13: 310–320

Grove M, Plumb M (1993): C/EBP, NF-κB, and c-Ets family members and transcriptional regulation of the cell specific and inducible macrophage inflammatory protein 1 alpha immediate-early gene. *Mol Cell Biol* 13: 5276–5289

Grumont RJ, Gerondakis S (1989): Structure of a mammalian c-rel protein deduced from the nucleotide sequence of murine cDNA clones. *Oncogene Res* 4: 1–8

Grumont RJ, Gerondakis S (1990): Murine c-rel transcription is rapidly induced in T cells and fibroblasts by mitogenic agents and the phorbol ester 12-O-tetradecanoylphorbol-13-acetate. *Cell Growth Differ* 1:345–350

Gunter KC, Irving SG, Zipfel PF, Siebenlist U, Kelley K (1989): Cyclosporin A-mediated inhibition of mitogen-induced gene transcription is specific for the mitogenic stimulus and cell type. *J Immunol* 142: 3286–3291

Hannibal MC, Markovitz DM, Clark N, Nabel GJ (1993): Differential activation of human immunodeficiency virus type 1 and 2 transcription by specific T-cell activation signals. *J Virol* 67: 5035–5040

Hannink M, Temin HM (1989): Transactivation of gene expression by nuclear and cytoplasmic rel proteins. *Mol Cell Biol* 9: 4323–4336

Hannink M, Temin HM (1990): Structure and autoregulation of the c-rel promoter. *Oncogene* 5: 1843–1850

Hansen SK, Baeuerle PA, Blasi F (1994): Purification, reconstitution, and IκB association of the c-Rel-p65 (RelA) complex, a strong activator of transcription. *Mol Cell Biol* 14: 2593–2603

Hansen SK, Nerlov C, Zabel U, Verde P, Johnsen M, Baeuerle PA, Blasi F (1992): A novel complex between the p65 subunit of NF-κB and c-Rel binds to a DNA element involved in the phorbol ester induction of the human urokinase gene. *EMBO J* 11: 205–213

Harada H, Fujita T, Miyamoto M, Kimura Y, Maruyama M, Furia A, Miyata T, Taniguchi T (1989): Structurally similar but functionally distinct factors, IRF-1 and IRF-2, bind to the same regulatory elements of IFN and IFN-inducible genes. *Cell* 58: 729–739

Harada H, Takahashi E-I, Itoh S, Harada K, Hori T-A (1994): Structure and regulation of the human interferon regulatory factor (IRF-1) and IRF-2 genes: implications for a gene network in the interferon system. *Mol Cell Biol* 14: 1500–1509

Haskill S, Beg AA, Tompkins SM, Morris JS, Yurochko AD, Sampson-Johannes A, Mondal K, Ralph P, Baldwin AS (1991): Characterization of an immediate-early gene induced in adherent monocytes that encodes IκB-like activity. *Cell* 65: 1281–1289

Hatada EN, Naumann M, Scheidereit C (1993): Common structural constituents confer IκB activity to NF-κB p105 and IκB/MAD-3. *EMBO J* 12: 2781–2788

Hatada EN, Nieters N, Wulczyn FG, Naumann M, Meyer R, Nucifora G, McKeithan TW, Scheidereit C (1992): The ankyrin repeat domains of the NF-κB precursor p105 and the protocogene bcl-3 acts as specific inhibitors of NF-κB DNA binding. *Proc Natl Acad Sci USA* 89: 2489–2493

Hay RT (1993): Control of nuclear factor-κB DNA-binding activity by inhibitory proteins containing ankyrin repeats. *Biochem Soc Trans* 21: 926–930

Hayashi T, Ueno Y, Okamoto T (1993): Oxidoreductive regulation of NF-κB. Involvement of a cellular reducing catalyst thioredoxin. *J Biol Chem* 268: 11380–11388

Henkel T, Zabel U, vanZee K, Muller JM, Fanning E, Baeuerle PA (1992): Intramolecular masking of the nuclear localization signal and dimerization domain in the precursor for the p50 NF-κB subunit. *Cell* 68: 1121–1133

Henkel T, Machleidt T, Alkalay I, Kronke M (1993): Rapid proteolysis of IκB-α is necessary for activation of transcription factor NF-κB. *Nature* 365– 182–185

Hirai H, Fujisawa J, Suzuki T, Ueda K, Muramatsu M, Tsuboi A, Arai N, Yoshida M (1992): Transcriptional activator tax of HTLV-1 binds to the NF-κB precursor p105. *Oncogene* 7: 1737–1742

Hiscott J, Marois J, Garoufalis J, D'Addario M (1993): Characterization of a functional NF-κB site in the human interleukin 1 beta promoter: evidence for a positive autoregulatory loop. *Mol Cell Biol* 13: 6231–6240

Hohmann H-P, Brockhaus M, Baeuerle PA, Remy R (1990a): Expression of the types A and B tumor necrosis factor (TNF) receptors is independently regulated, and both receptors mediate activation of the transcription factor NF-κB. *J Biol Chem* 265: 22409–22017

Hohmann HP, Remy R, Poschl B, vanLoon AP (1990b): Tumor necrosis factors-α and -β bind to the same two types of tumor necrosis factor receptors and maximally activate the transcription factor NF-κB at low receptor occupancy and within minutes after receptor binding. *J Biol Chem* 265: 15183–14188

Hohmann H-P, Remy R, Scheidereit C, vanLoon APGM (1991): Maintenance of NF-κB activity is dependent on protein synthesis and the continuous presence of external stimuli. *Mol Cell Biol* 11: 259–266

Hoyos B, Ballard DW, Bohnlein E, Siekevitz M, Greene WC (1989): κB-specific DNA binding proteins: role in the regulation of human interleukin-2 gene expression. *Science* 244: 457–460

Hrdlickova R, Nehyba J, Humphries EH (1994): v-rel induces expression of three avian immunoregulatory surface receptors more efficiently than c-rel. *J Vorol* 68: 308–319

Hrdlickova R, Nehyba J, Humphries EH (1994b): In vivo evolution of c-rel oncogenic potential. *J Virol* 68: 2371–2382

Hultmark D (1993): Immune reactions in Drosophila and other insects: a model for innate immunity. *Trends Genet* 9: 178–193

Hultmark D (1994): Ancient relationships. *Nature* 367: 116–117

Iademarco MF, McQuillan JJ, Rosen GD, Dean DC (1992): Characterization of the promoter for vascular cell adhesion molecule-1 (VCAM-1). *J Biol Chem* 267: 16323–16329

Inoue J-I, Kerr LD, Ransone LJ, Bengal E, Hunter T, Verma IM (1991): c-rel activates but v-rel suppresses transcription from κB sites. *Proc Natl Acad Sci USA* 88: 3715–3719

Inoue JI, Kerr LD, Kakizuka A, Verma IM (1992a): IκB-γ, a 70 kd protein identical to the C-terminal half of p100 NF-κB: a new member of the IκB family. *Cell* 68: 1109–1120

Inoue J, Kerr LD, Rashid D, Davis N, Bose HR, Verma IM (1992b): Direct association of pp40/IκB-β with rel/NF-κB transcription factors: role of ankyrin repeats in the inhibition of DNA binding activity. *Proc Natl Acad Sci USA* 89: 4333–4337

Inuzuka M, Ishikawa H, Kumar S, Gelinas C, Ito Y (1994): The viral and cellular Rel oncoproteins induce the differentiation of P19 embryonal carcinoma cells. *Oncogene* 9: 133–140

Ip YT, Levine M (1992): The role of the dorsal morphogen gradient in Drosophila embryogenesis. *Semin Devel Biol* 3: 15–23

Ip YT, Kraut R, Levine M, Rushlow C (1991): The dorsal morphogen is a sequence-specific DNA-binding protein that interacts with a long-range repression element in Drosophila. *Cell* 64: 439–446

Ip YT, Rach M, Engstrom Y, Kadalayil L, Cai H, Gonzalex-Crespo S, Tateri K, Levein M (1993): Dif, a dorsal-related gene that mediates an immune response in Drosophila. *Cell* 75: 753–763

Ishikawa H, Asano M, Kanda T, Kumar S, Gelinas C, Ito Y (1993): Two novel functions associated with the Rel oncoproteins: DNA replication and cell-specific transcriptional activation. *Oncogene* 8: 2889–2896

Isoda K, Roth S, Nusslein-Volhard C (1992): The functional domains of the Drosophila morphogen dorsal: evidence from the analysis of mutants. *Genes Develop* 6: 619–630

Israël A (1992): The rel/NF-κB family of transcription factors: a novel mechanisms to control gene expression (editorial). *Pathol Biol* 40: 212–214

Iwasaki T, Uehara Y, Graves L, Rachie N, Bomsztyk K (1992): Herbimycin A blocks IL-1-induced NF-κB DNA-binding activity in lymphoid cell lines. *Febs Lett* 298: 240–244

Jamieson C, McCaffrey PG, Rao A, Sen R (1991): Physiologic activation of T cells via a T-cell receptor induces NF-κB. *J Immunol* 147: 416–420

Jiang J, Levine M (1993): Binding affinities and cooperative interactions with bHLH activators delimit threshold responses to the dorsal gradient morphogen. *Cell* 72: 741–752

Johnson DR, Pober JS (1994): HLA class I Heavy-chain gene promoter elements mediating synergy between tumor necrosis factor and interferons. *Mol Cell Biol* 14: 1322–1332

Joseph CK, Byun HS, Bittman R, Kolesnick RN (1993): Substrate recognition by ceramide-activated protein kinase. Evidence that kinase activity is proline-directed. *J Biol Chem* 268: 20002–20006

Joshi-Barve SS, Rangnekar VV, Sells SF, Rangnekar VM (1993): Interleukin-1-inducible expression of gro-β via NF-κB activation is dependent upon tyrosine kinase signalling. *J Biol Chem* 268: 18018–18029

Kaltschmidt B, Baeuerle PA, Kaltschmidt C (1993): Potential involvement of the transcription factor NF-κB in neurological disorders. *Mol Aspects Med* 14: 171–190

Kamens J, Richardson P, Mosialos G, Brent R, Gilmore TD (1990): Oncogenic transformation by v-Rel requires an amino-terminal activation domain. *Mol Cell Biol* 10: 2840–2847

Kang SM, Tran AC, Grilli M, Lenardo MJ (1992): NF-κB subunit regulation in nontransformed CD4+ T lymphocytes. *Science* 256: 1452–1456

Kanno T, Brown K, Franzoso G, Siebenlist U (1994a): Kinetic analysis of Human T-cell Leukemia Virus type I Tax-mediated activation of NF-κB. *Mol Cell Biol* 14: in press

Kanno T, Franzoso G, Siebenlist U (1994b): HTLV-I Tax Mediated activation of NF-κB from novel p100 (NF-κB₂)-inhibited cytoplasmic reservoirs. *Proc Natl Acad Sci USA* 91: in press

Kaszubska W, vanHuijsduijnen RH, Ghersa P, DeRaemy-Schenk AM (1993): Cyclic AMP-independent ATF family members interact with NF-κB and function in the activation of the E-selection promoter in response to cytokines. *Mol Cell Biol* 13: 7180–7190

Kelly K, Davis P, Mitsuya H, Irving S, Wright J, Grassman R, Fleckenstein B, Wano Y, Greene W, Siebenlist U (1992): A high proportion of early response genes are constitutively activated in T cells by HTLV-1. *Oncogene* 7: 1463–1470

Kerr LD, Duckett CS, Wamsley P, Zhang Q, Chiao P, Nabel G, McKeithan TW, Baeuerle PA, Verma I (1992): The protooncogene BCL-3 encodes an IκB protein. *Genes Dev* 6: 2352–2363

Kerr LD, Inoue J-I, Davis N, Link E, Baeuerle PA, Bose HR, Verma IM (1991): The Rel-associated pp40 protein prevents DNA binding of Rel and NF-κB: relationship with IκB-β and regulation by phosphorylation. *Genes Development* 5: 1464–1476

Kerr LD, Ransone LJ, Wamsley P, Schmitt MJ, Boyer TG, Zhou Q, Berk AJ, Verma IM (1993): Association between proto-oncoprotein Rel and TATA-binding protein mediates transcriptional activation by NF-κB. *Nature* 365: 412–419

Kessler DJ, Duyao M, Spicer DB, Sonenshein GE (1992): NF-κB-like factors mediate interleukin 1 induction of c-myc gene transcription in fibroblasts. *J Exp Med* 176: 787–792

Kieran M, Blank V, Logeat F, Vandekerchove J, Lottspeich F, LeBail O, Urban MB, Kourilsky P, Baeuerle PA, Israël A (1990): The DNA binding subunit of NF-κB is identical to factor KBF1 and homologous to the rel oncogene product. *Cell* 62: 1007–1018

Kitajima I, Shinohara T, Bilakovics J, Brown DA (1993): Ablation of transplanted HTLV-I tax-transformed tumors in mice by antisense inhibition of NF-κB. *Science* 259: 1523

Klug CA, Gerety SJ, Shah PC, Chen Y-Y, Rice NR, Rosenbern, Singh H (1994): The v-abl tyrosine kinase negatively regulates NF-κB/Rel factors and blocks kappa gene transcription in pre-B lymphocytes. *Genes Dev* 8:678–687

Koong AC, Chen EY, Giaccia AJ (1994): Hypoxia causes the activation of nuclear factor kappa B through the phosphorylation of I kappa B alpha on tyrosine residues. *Cancer Res* 54: 1425–1430

Kowalik TF, Wing B, Haskill JS, Azizkhan JC, Baldwin AS, Huang E-S (1993): Multiple mechanisms are implicated in the regulation of NF-κB activity during human cytomegalovirus infection. *Proc Natl Acad Sci USA* 90: 1107–1111

Kralova J, Schatzle JD, Bargmann W, Bose HR (1994): Transformation of avian fibroblasts overexpressing the c-rel proto-oncogene and a variant of c-rel lacking 40 C-terminal amino acids. *J Virol* 68: 2073–2083

Kretzschmar M, Meisterernst M, Scheidereit C, Li G, Roeder RG (1992): Transcriptional regulation of the HIV-1 promoter by NF-κB in vitro. *Genes Dev.* 6: 761–774

Krikos A, Laherty CD, Dixit VM (1992): Transcriptional activation of the tumor necrosis factor alpha-inducible zinc finger protein, A20, is mediated by kappa B elements. *J Biol Chem* 267: 17971–17976

Kuang AA, Novak KD, Kang SM, Bruhn K, Lenardo MJ (1993): Interaction between NF-κB- and serum response factor binding elements activates an interleukin-2 receptor alpha-chain enhancer specifically in T lymphocytes. *Mol Cell Biol* 13: 2536–2545

Kumar S, Gelinas C (1993): IκB α-mediated inhibition of v-Rel DNA binding requires direct interaction with the RXXRXRXXC Rel/κB DNA-binding motif. *Proc Natl Acad Sci USA* 90: 8962–8966

Kumar S, Rabson AB, Gelinas C (1992): The RxxRxRxxC motif conserved in all Rel/κB proteins is essential for the DNA-binding activity and redox regulation of the v-Rel oncoprotein. *Mol Cell Biol* 12: 3094–3106

Kunsch C, Rosen CA (1993): NF-κB subunit-specific regulation of the interleukin-8 promoter. *Mol Cell Biol* 13: 6137–6146

Kunsch C, Ruben SM, Rosen CA (1992): Selection of optimal κB Rel DNA-binding motifs: interaction of both subunits of NF-κB with DNA is required for transcriptional activation. *Mol Cell Biol* 12: 4412–4421

Lalmanach-Girard AC, Chiles TC, Parker DC, Rothstein TL (1993): T cell-dependent induction of NF-κB in B cells. *J Exp Med* 177: 1215–1219

La Rosa FA, Pierce JW, Sonenshein GE (1994): Differential regulation of the c-myc oncogene promoter by the NF-κB rel family of transcription factors. *Mol Cell Biol* 14: 1039–1044

LeBail O, Schmidt-Ullrich R, Israël A (1993): Promoter analysis of the gene encoding the IκB-α/MAD3 inhibitor of NF-κB: positive regulation by members of the rel/NF-κB family. *EMBO J* 12: 5043–5049

LeClair KP, Blanar MA, Sharp PA (1992): The p50 subunit of NF-κB associates with the NF-IL6 transcription factor. *Proc Natl Acad Sci USA* 89: 8145–8149

Lee-Huang S, Lin JJ, Kung HF, Huang PL (1993): The human erythropoietin-encoding gene contains a CAAT box, TATA boxes and other transcriptional regulatory elements in its 5' flanking region. *Gene* 128: 227–236

Leiden JM, Wang CY, Petryniak B, Markovitz DM (1992): A novel Ets- related transcription factor, Elf-1, binds to human immunodeficiency virus type 2 regulatory elements that are required for inducible trans activation in T cells. *J Virol* 66: 5890–5897

Lenardo M, Siebenlist U (1994): Bcl-3-mediated nuclear regulation of the NF-κB trans-activating factor. *Immunol Today* 15: 145–146

Lernbecher T, Muller U, Wirth T (1993): Distinct NF-κB/Rel transcription factors are responsible for tissue-specific and inducible gene activation. *Nature* 365: 767–770

Li S, Sedivy JM (1993): Raf-1 protein kinase activates the NF-κB transcription factor by dissociating the cytoplasmic NF-κB-IκB complex. *Proc Natl Acad Sci USA* 90: 9247–9251

Liao F, Andalibi F, deBeer FC, Fogelman AM, Lusis AJ (1993): Genetic control of inflammatory gene induction and NF-κB-like transcription factor activation in response to an atherogenic diet in mice. *J Clin Invest* 91: 2572–2479

Lichtenstein M, Keini G, Cedar H, Bergman Y (1994): B cell-specific demethylation: a novel role for the intronic kappa chain enhancer sequence. *Cell* 76: 913–923

Lin YC, Brown K, Siebenlist U (1994): unpublished observations

Lindholm P, Reid RL, Brady JN (1992): Extracellular Tax-1 protein stimulates tumor necrosis factor-β and immunoglobulin κ light chain expression in lymphoid cells. *J Virol* 66: 1294–1302

Link E, Kerr LD, Schreck R, Zabel U, Verma I, Baeuerle PA (1992): Purified IκB-β is inactivated upon dephosphorylation. *J Biol Chem* 267: 239–246

Liou HC, Baltimore D (1993): Regulation of the NF-κB/rel transcription factor and IκB inhibitor system. *Curr Opin Cell Biol* 5: 477–487

Liou HC, Nolan GP, Ghosh S, Fujita T, Baltimore D (1992): The NF-κB p50 precursor, p105, contains an internal IκB-like inhibitor that preferentially inhibits p50. *EMBO J* 11: 3003–3009

Liu J, Sodeoka M, Lane WS, Verdine GL (1994): Evidence for a non-alpha-helical DNA-binding motif in the Rel homology region. *Proc Natl Acad Sci USA* 91: 908–912

Logeat F, Israël N, Ten R, Blank V, LeBail, Kourilsky P, Israel A (1991): Inhibition of transcription factors belonging to the rel/NF-κB family by a transdominant negative mutant. *EMBO J* 10: 1827–1832

Lowenstein CJ, Alley EW, Raval P, Snowman AM, Snyder SH, Russell SW, Murphy WJ (1993): Macrophage nitric oxide synthase gene: two upstream regions mediate induction by interferon gamma and lipopolysaccharide. *Proc Natl Acad Sci USA* 90: 9730–9734

Lu D, Thompson JD, Gorski GK, Rice NR, Mayer MG, Yunis JJ (1991): Alterations at the rel locus in human lymphoma. *Oncogene* 6: 1235–1241

Mathias S, Dressler KA, Kolesnick RN (1991): Characterization of a ceramide-activated protein kinase: stimulation by tumor necrosis factor a. *J Biol Chem* 88: 10009–10013

Mathias S, Younes A, Kan CC, Orlow I, Joseph C, Kolesnick RN (1993): Activation of the spingomyelin signaling pathway in intact EL4 cells and in a cell-free system by IL-1β. *Science* 259: 519–522

Matsusaka T, Fujikawa K, Nishio Y, Mukaida N (1993): Transcription factors NF-IL6 and NF-κB synergistically activate transcription of the inflammatory cytokines, interleukin 6 and interleukin 8. *Proc Natl Acad Sci USA* 90: 10193–10197

Matthews JR, Kaszubska W, Turcatti G, Wells TN, Hay RT (1993a): Role of cysteine 62 in DNA recognition by the P50 subunit of NF-κB. *Nucleic Acids Res* 21: 1727–1734

Matthews JR, Wakasugi N, Virelizier J-L, Yodoi J, Hay RT (1992): Thioredoxin regulates the DNA binding activity of NF-κB by reduction of a disulfide bond involving cysteine 62. *Nucl Acids Res* 30: 3821–3830

Matthews JR, Watson E, Buckley S, Hay RT (1993b): Interaction of the C-terminal region of p105 with the nuclear localisation signal of p50 is required for inhibition of NF-κB DNA binding activity. *Nucleic Acids Res* 21: 4516–4523

McDonnell PC, Kumar S, Rabson AB, Gelinas C (1992): Transcriptional activity of rel family proteins. *Oncogene* 7: 163–170

Meichle A, Schutze S, Hensel G, Brunsing D, Kronke M (1990): Protein kinase C-independent activation of nuclear factor κB by tumor necrosis factor. *J Biol Chem* 265: 8339–8343

Mellits KH, Hay RT, Goodburn S (1993): Proteolytic degradation of MAD3 (IκB alpha) and enhanced processing of the NF-κB precursor p105 are obligatory steps in the activation of NF-κB. *Nucleic Acids Res* 21: 5059–5066

Menon SD, Qin S, Guy GR, Tan YH (1993): Differential induction of nuclear NF-κB by protein phosphatase inhibitors in primary and transformed human cells. *J Biol Chem* 268: 26805–26812

Mercurio F, Didonato J, Rosette C, Karin M (1992): Molecular cloning and characterization of a novel Rel/NF-κB family member displaying structural and functional homology to NF-κB p50–p105. *DNA Cell Biol* 11: 523–537

Mercurio F, Didonato JA, Rossette C, Karin M (1993): p105 and p98 precursor proteins play an active role in NF-κB-mediated signal transduction. *Genes Dev.* 7: 705–718

Messer G, Weiss EH, Baeuerle PA (1990): Tumor necrosis factor beta (TNF-β) induces binding of the NF-κB transcription factor to a high-affinity κB element in the TNF-β promoter. *Cytokine* 2: 389–397

Meyer R, Hatada EN, Hohmann HP, Haiker M, Bartsch C, Rothlisberger U, Lahm HW, Schlaeger EJ, vanLoon APGM, Schiedereit C (1991): Cloning of the DNA-binding subunit of human nuclear factor κB: the level of its mRNA is strongly regulated by phorbol ester or tumor necrosis factor a. *Proc Natl Acad Sci USA* 88: 966–970

Meyer M, Schreck R, Baeuerle PA (1993a): H_2O_2 and antioxidants have opposite effects on activation of NF-κB and AP-1 in intact cells: Ap-1 as secondary antioxidant-responsive factor. *EMBO J* 12: 2005–2015

Meyer M, Schreck R, Muller J, Baeuerle PA (1993b): Redox control of gene expression by eukaryotic transcription factors NF-κB, AP-1 and SRF/TCF. In: *Oxidative Stress, Cell Activation and Viral Infection*, Packer L, Pasquier C, eds. Basel: Birkhauser Verlag

Michaely P, Bennett V (1992): The ANK repeat: a ubiquitous motif involved in macromolecular recognition. *Trends Cell Biol* 2: 127–129

Miyamoto S, Chiao PJ, Verma IM (1994): Enhanced IκBα degradation is responsible for constitutive NF-κB activity in mature murine B-cell lines. *Mol Cell Biol* 14: 3276–3282

Miyamoto M, Fujita T, Kimura Y, Maruyama M, Harada H, Sudo Y, Miyata T, Taniguchi T (1988): Regulated expression of a gene encoding a nuclear factor, IRF-1, that specifically binds to IFN-β gene regulatory elements. *Cell* 54: 903–913

Molitor JA, Walker WH, Doerre S, Ballard DW, Greene WC (1990): NF-κB: a family of inducible and differentially expressed enhancer-binding proteins in human T cells. *Proc Natl Acad Sci USA* 87: 10028–10032

Moore PA, Ruben SM, Rosen CA (1993): Conservation of transcriptional activation functions of the NF-κB p50 and p65 subunits in mammalian cells and Saccharomyces cerevisiae. *Mol Cell Biol* 13: 1666–1674

Morrison LE, Boehmelt G, Beug H, Enrietto PJ (1992): Expression of v-rel by a replication-competent virus in chicken embryo fibroblasts. *Oncogene* 6: 1657–1666

Muller JM, Ziegler-Heitbrock JHW, Baeuerle PA (1993): Nuclear factor κB, a mediator of lipopolysaccharide effects. *Immunobiol* 187: 233–256

Muroi M, Suzuki T (1993): Role of protein kinase A in LPS-induced activation of NF-κB proteins of a mouse macrophage-like cell line, J774. *Cellular Signaling* 5: 289–298

Nabel G, Baltimore D (1987): An inducible transcription factor activates expression of human immunodeficiency virus in T cells. *Nature* 326: 711–713

Nakayama K, Shimizu H, Mitomo K, Watanabe T (1992): A lymphoid cell-specific nuclear factor containing c-Rel-like proteins preferentially interacts with inter-leukin-6 κB-related motifs whose activities are repressed in lymphoid cells. *Mol Cell Biol* 12: 1736–1746

Narayanan R, Higgins KA, Perez JR, Coleman TA, Rosen CA (1993): Evidence for differential functions of the p50 and p65 subunits of NF-κB with a cell adhesion model. *Mol Cell Biol* 13: 3802–3810

Naumann M, Wulczyn FG, Scheidereit C (1993): The NF-κB precursor p105 and the proto-oncogene product Bcl-3 are IκB molecules and control nuclear transloca-tion of NF-κB. *EMBO J* 12: 213–222

Nehyba J, Hrdlickova R, Humphries EH (1994): Evolution of the oncogenic potential of v-rel: rel-induced expression of immunoregulatory receptors correlates with tumor development and in vitro transformation. *J Virol* 68: 2039–2050

Neiman PE, Thomas SJ, Loring G (1991): Induction of apoptosis during normal and neoplastic B-cell development in the bursa of Fabricius. *Proc Natl Acad Sci USA* 88: 5857–5861

Neish AS, Williams AJ, Palmer HJ, Whitley MZ, Collins T (1992): Functional analysis of the human vascular cell adhesion molecule 1 promoter. *J Exp Med* 176: 1583–1593

Nerenberg M, Hinrichs SH, Reynolds RK, Khoury G, Jay G (1987): The tat gene of human T-lymphotropic virus type 1 induces messenchymal tumors in transgenic mice. *Science* 237: 1324–1329

Neri A, Chang CC, Lombardi L, Salina M, Corradini P, Maiolo AT, Chaganti RSK, Dalla-Favera R (1991): B cell lymphoma-associated chromosomal translocation involves candidate oncogene lyt-10, homologous to NF-κB p50. *Cell* 67: 1075–1087

Niederman TMJ, Garcia JV, Hastings WR, Luria S, Ratner L (1992): Human immunodeficiency virus type 1 nef protein inhibits NF-κB induction in human T cells. *J Virol* 66: 6213–6219

Nielsch U, Zimmer SG, Babiss LE (1991): Changes in NF-kappa B and ISGF3 DNA binding activities are responsible for differences in MHC and beta-IFN gene expression in Ad5-versus Ad12-transformed cells. *Embo J* 10: 4169–4175

Nolan GP, Baltimore D (1992): The inhibitory ankyrin and activator Rel proteins. *Curr Opin Genet Dev* 2: 211–220

Nolan GP, Fujita T, Bhatia K, Huppi K, Liou H-C, Scott ML, Baltimore D (1993): The bcl-3 proto-oncogene encodes a nuclear IκB-like molecule that preferentially interacts with NF-κB p50 in a phosphorylation-dependent manner. *Mol Cell Biol* 13: 3557–3566

Nolan GP, Ghosh S, Liou H-C, Tempst P, Baltimore D (1991): DNA binding and IκB inhibition of the cloned p65 subunit of NF-κB, a rel-related polypeptide. *Cell* 64: 961–969

Norris JL, Manley JL (1992): Selective nuclear transport of the Dorsophila morphogene dorsal can be established by a signaling pathway involving the transmembrane protein Toll and protein kinase A. *Genes Devel* 6: 1654–1667

Ohmori Y, Hamilton TA (1993): Cooperative interaction between interferon (IFN) stimulus response element and κB sequence motifs controls IFN-γ- and lipopolysaccharide-stimulated transcription from the murine IP-10 promoter. *J Biol Chem* 268: 6677–6688

Ohno H, Takimoto G, McKeithan TW (1990): The candidate proto-oncogene bcl-3 is related to genes implicated in cell lineage determination and cell cycle control. *Cell* 60: 991–997

Olashaw NE, Kowalik TF, Huang ES, Pledger WJ (1992): Induction of NF-κB-like activity by platelet-derived growth factor in mouse fibroblasts. *Mol Biol Cell* 3: 1131–1139

Osborn L, Kunkel S, Nabel GJ (1989): TNF-α and interleukin 1 stimulate the human immunodeficiency virus enhancer by activation of the NF-κB. *Proc Natl Acad Sci USA* 86: 2336–2340

Pantaleo G, Graziosi C, Demarest JF, Butini L (1993a): HIV infection is active and progressive in lymphoid tissue during the clinically latent stage of disease. *Nature* 362: 355–358

Pantaleo G, Graziosi C, Fauci AS (1993b): New concepts in the immunopathogenesis of human immunodeficiency virus infection. *N Engl J Med* 328: 327–335

Parhami F, Fang ZT, Fogelman AM, Andalibi A (1993): Minimally modified low density lipoprotein-induced inflammatory responses in endothelial cells are mediated by cyclic adenosine monophosphate. *J Clin Invest* 92: 471–478

Paya CV, Ten RM, Bessia C, Alcami J, Hay RT, Virelizier J-L (1992): NF-κB-dependent induction of the NF-κB p50 subunit gene promoter underlies self-perpetuation of human immunodeficiency virus transcription in monocytic cells. *Proc Natl Acad Sci USA* 89: 7826–7830

Perkins ND, Edwards NL, Duckett CS, Agranoff AB (1993): A cooperative interaction between NF-κB and Sp1 is required for HIV-1 enhancer activation. *EMBO J* 12: 3551–3558

Perkins ND, Schmid RM, Duckett CS, Leung K, Rice NR, Nabel GJ (1992): Distinct combinations of NF-κB subunits determine the specificity of transcriptional activation. *Proc Natl Acad Sci USA* 89: 1529–1533

Pierce JW, Lenardo M, Baltimore D (1988): An oligonucleotide that binds nuclear factor NF-κB acts as a lymphoid-specific and inducible enhancer element. *Proc Natl Acad Sci USA* 85: 1482–1486

Plaksin D, Baeuerle P, Eisenbach L (1993): KBF-1 (p50 NF-κB homodimer) acts as a repressor of H-2Kb gene expression in metastatic tumor cells. *J Exp Med* 177: 1651–1662

Ranganathan PN, Khalili K (1993): The transcriptional enhancer element, κB, regulates promoter activity of the human neurotropic virus, JCV, in cells derived from the CNS. *Nucleic Acids Res* 21: 1959–1964

Ray KP, Kennard N (1993): Interleukin-1 induces a nuclear form of transcription factor NF kappa B in human lung epithelial cells. *Agents Actions* 38: C61–3

Ray A, Prefontaine KE (1994): Physical association and functional antagonism between the p65 subunit of transcription factor NF-κB and the glucocorticoid receptor. *Pro Natl Acad Sci USA* 91: 752–756

Read MA, Whitley MZ, Williams AJ, Collins T (1994): NF-κB and IκB-α: an inducible regulatory system in endothelial activation. *J Exp Med* 179: 503–412

Reis LFL, Harada H, Wolchok JD, Taniguchi T, Vilcek J (1992): Critical role of a common transcription factor, IRF-1, in the regulation of IFN-β and IFN-inducible genes. *EMBO J* 11: 185–193

Rice NR, Ernst MK (1993): In vivo control of NF-κB activation by IκB-α. *EMBO J* 12: 4685–4695

Rice NR, Gilden RV (1988): The rel oncogene. In: *The Oncogene Handbook*, Reddy EP, Skalka AM, Curran T, eds. Amsterdam: Elsevier Sci

Rice NR, MacKichan ML, Israel A (1992): The precursor of NF-κB p50 has IκB-like functions. *Cell* 71: 243–253

Richardson PM, Gilmore TD (1991): vRel is an inactive member of the Rel family of transcriptional activating proteins. *J Virol* 65: 3122–3230

Riviere Y, Blank V, Kourilsky P, Israel A (1991): Processing of the precursor of NF-κB by the HIV-1 protease during acute infection. *Nature* 350: 622–625

Ron D, Brasier AR, Habener JF (1990): Transcriptional regulation of hepatic angiotensinogen gene expression by the acute-phase response. *Mol Cell Endocrinol* 74: C97–104

Ron D, Brasier AR, Habener JF (1991): A new family of large nuclear proteins that recognize nuclear factor kappa B-binding sites through a zinc finger motif. *Mol Cell Biol* 11: 2887–2895

Ross I, Buckler-White AJ, Rabson AB, Ingland G, Martin MA (1991): Contribution of NF-κB and SP1 binding motifs to the replicative capacity of human immunodeficiency virus type 1: distinct patterns of viral growth are determined by T cell types. *J Virol* 65: 4350–4358

Roulston A, Beauparlant P, Rice N, Hiscott J (1993): Chronic human immunodeficiency virus type 1 infection stimulates distinct NF-κB B/rel DNA binding activities in myelomonoblastic cells. *J Virol* 67: 5235–5246

Roulston A, D'Addario M, Boulerice F, Caplan S, Wainberg MA, Hiscott J (1992): Induction of monocytic differentiation and NF-κB-like activities by human immunodeficiency virus 1 infection of myelomonoblastic cells. *J Exp Med* 175: 751–763

Ruben SM, Dillon PJ, Schreck R, Henkel T, Chen CH, Maher M, Baeuerle PA, Rosen CA (1991): Isolation of a rel-related human cDNA that potentially encodes the 65-kD subunit of NF-κB. *Science* 251: 1490–1493

Ruben SM, Klement JF, Coleman TA, Maher M, Chen CH, Rosen CA (1992): I-Rel:

a novel rel-related protein that inhibits NF-κB transcriptional activity. *Genes Dev.* 6: 745–760

Ryseck RP, Bull P, Takamiya M, Bours V, Siebenlist U, Dobrzanski P, Bravo R (1992): RelB, a new rel family transcription activator that can interact with p50-NF-κB. *Mol Cell Biol* 12: 674–684

Ryter SW, Gomer CJ (1993): Nuclear factor κB binding activity in mouse L1210 cells following photofrin II-mediated photosensitization. *Photochem Photobiol* 58: 753–756

Saklatvala J, Rawlinson LM, Marshall CJ, Kracht M (1993): Interleukin-1 and tumour necrosis factor activate the mitogen activated protein (MAP) kinase kinase in cultured cells. *FEBS Lett* 334: 189–192

Sambucetti LC, Cherrington JM, Wilkinson GWG, Mocarski ES (1989): NF-κB activation of the cytomegalovirus enhancer is mediated by a viral transactivator and by T cell stimulation. *EMBO J* 8: 4251–4258

Sarkar S, Gilmore TD (1993): Transformation by the vRel oncoprotein requires sequences carboxy-terminal to the Rel homology domain. *Oncogene* 8: 2245–2252

Scheinman RI, Beg AA, Baldwin AS (1993): NF-κB p100 (lyt-10) is a component of H2TF1 and can function as an IκB-like molecule. *Mol Cell Biol* 13: 6089–6101

Schieven GL, Kirihara JM, Myers DE, Ledbetter JA, Uckun FM (1993): Reactive oxygen intermediates activate NF-κB in a tyrosine-kinase dependent mechanisms and in combination with vanadate activate the p56 lck and p59 fyn tyrosine kinase in human lymphocytes. *Blood* 82: 1212–1220

Schmidt A, Hennighausen L, Siebenlist U (1990): Inducible nuclear factor binding to the kappa B elements of the human immunodeficiency virus enhancer in T cells can be blocked by cyclosporin A in a signal-dependent manner. *J Virol* 64: 4037–4041

Schmitz ML, Baeuerle PA (1991): The p65 is responsible for the strong transcription activation potential of NF-κB. *EMBO J* 10: 3805–3817

Schmitz ML, Henkel T, Baeuerle PA (1991): Proteins controlling the nuclear uptake of the NF-κB, rel and dorsal. *Trends Cell Biol* 1: 130–137

Schreck R, Albermann K, Baeuerle PA (1992a): NF-κB: an oxidative stress-responsive transcription factor of eukaryotic cells (a review). *Free Rad Res Comms* 17: 221–237

Schreck R, Bevec D, Dukor B, Baeuerle PA, Chedid L, Bahr GM (1992b): Selection of a muramyl peptide based on its lack of activation of nuclear factor-κB as a potential adjuvant for AIDS vaccines. *Clin Exp Immunol* 90: 188–193

Schreck R, Grassman R, Fleckenstein B, Baeuerle PA (1992c): Antioxidants selectively suppress activation of NF-κB by human T-cell leukemia virus type I tax protein. *J Virol* 66: 6288–6293

Schreck R, Meier B, Maennel DN, Droge W, Baeuerle A (1992d): Dithiocarbamates as potent inhibitors of nuclear factor κB activation in intact cells. *J Exp Med* 175: 1181–1194

Schreck R, Rieber P, Baeuerle PA (1991): Reactive oxygen intermediates as apparently widely used messengers in the activation of the NF-κB transcription factor and HIV-1. *EMBO J* 10: 2247–2258

Schreck R, Zorbas H, Winnacker EL, Baeuerle PA (1990): The NF-κB transcription factor induces DNA binding which is modulated by its 65-kD subunit. *Nucl Acids Res* 18: 6497–6502

Schulze-Osthoff K, Bakker AC, Vanhaesebroeck B, Beyaert R, Jacob WA, Fiers W

(1992): Cytotoxic activity of tumor necrosis factor is mediated by early damage to mitochondrial functions _ evidence for the involvement of mitochondrial adical generation. *J Biol Chem* 267: 5317–5322

Schulze-Osthoff K, Beyaert R, Van-dervoorde V, Haegeman G, Fiers W (1993): Depletion of the mitochondrial electron transport abbrogates the cytotoxic and gene induction effects of toxic and gene induction effects of TNF. *EMBO J* 12: 3095–3104

Schutze S, Pothoff K, Machleidt T, Bercovic D, Wiegmann K, Kronke M (1992): TNF activates NF-κB by phosphatidylcholine-specific phospholipase C-induced "acidic" sphingomyelin breakdown. *Cell* 71: 765–776

Scott ML, Fujita T, Liou HC, Nolan GP, Baltimore D (1993): The p65 subunit of NF-κB regulates IκB by two distinct mechanisms. *Genes Dev* 7: 1266–1276

Segars JH, Nagata T, Bours V, Medin IA, Franzoso G, Blanco JCG, Drew PD, Becker KG, An J, Tang T, Stephany DA, Neel B, Siebenlist U, Ozato K (1993): Retinoic acid induction of major histocompatibility class complex I genes in NTera-2 embryonal carcinoma cells involves induction of NF-κB (p50-p-65) and retinoic acid beta-retinoid x receptor beta heterodimers. *Mol Cell Biol* 13: 6157–6169

Sen R, Baltimore D (1986a): Multiple nuclear factors interact with the immunoglobulin enhancer sequences. *Cell* 46: 705–716

Sen R, Baltimore D (1986b): Inducibility of κ immunoglobulin enhancer-binding protein NF-κB by a posttranslational mechanism. *Cell* 47: 921–928

Shattuck RL, Wood LD, Jaffe GJ, Richmond A (1994): MGSA/GRO transcription is differentially regulated in normal retinal pigment epithelial and melanoma cells. *Mol Cell Biol* 14: 791–802

Shelton CA, Wasserman SA (1993): pelle encodes a protein kinase required to establish dorsoventral polarity in the Drosophila embryo. *Cell* 72: 515–525

Shirakawa F, Mizel SB (1989): In vitro activation and nuclear translocation of NF-κB catalyzed by cyclic AMP-dependent protein kinase and protein kinase C. *Mol Cell Biol* 9: 2424–2430

Shu HB, Agranoff AB, Nabel EG, Leung K (1993): Differential regulation of vascular cell adhesion molecule 1 gene expression by specific NF-κB subunits in endothelial and epithelial cells. *Mol Cell Biol* 13: 6283–6289

Smith MR, Greene WC (1991): Molecular biology of type I human T-cell leukemia virus (HTLV-I) and adult T-cell leukemia. *J Clin Invest* 87: 761–766

Sokoloski JA, Sartorelli AC, Rosen CA, Narayanan R (1993): Antisense oligonucleotides to the p65 subunit of NF-κB block CD11b expression and alter adhesion properties of differentiated HL-60 granulocytes. *Blood* 82: 625–632

St. Johnston D, Nusslein-Volhard C (1992): The origin of pattern and polarity in the Drosophila embryo. *Cell* 68: 201–219

Staudt LM, Lenardo MJ (1991): Immunoglobulin gene transcription. *Annu Rev Immunol* 9: 373–398

Stein B, Baldwin AS (1993): Distinct mechanisms for regulation of the interleukin-8 gene involve synergism and cooperativity between C/EBP and NF-κB. *Mol Cell Biol* 13: 7191–7198

Stein B, Baldwin AS, Ballard DW, Greene WC, Angel P, Herrlich P (1993a): Cross-coupling of the NF-κB p65 and Fos/Jun transcription factors produces potentiated biological function. *EMBO J* 12: 3879–3891

Stein B, Cogswell PC, Baldwin AS (1993b): Functional and physical associations between NF-κB and C/EBP family members: a rel domain b-ZIP interaction. *Mol Cell Biol* 13: 3964–3974

Stephens RM, Rice NR, Hiebsch RR, Bose HR, Gilden RV (1983): Nucleotide sequence of v-rel: the oncogene of the reticuloendotheliosis virus. *Proc Natl Acad Sci USA* 80: 6229–6232

Steward R (1987): Dorsal, an embryonic polarity gene in Drosophila is homologous to the vertebrate proto-oncogene, c-rel. *Science* 238: 692–694

Stylianou E, O'Neill LA, Rawlinson L, Edbrooke MR (1992): Interleukin 1 induces NF-κB through its type I but not its type II receptor in lymphocytes. *J Biol Chem* 267: 15836–15841

Sun S-C, Ganchi PA, Ballard DW, Greene WC (1993): NF-κB controls expression of inhibitor IκBa: evidence for an inducible autoregulatory pathway. *Science* 259: 1912–1915

Sun S-C, Ganchi PA, Beraud C, Ballard DW, Greene WC (1994): Autoregulation of the NF-κB transactivator RelA (p65) by multiple cytoplasmic inhibitors containing ankyrin motifs. *Proc Natl Acad Sci USA* 91: 1346–1350

Suzuki T, Hirai H, Fujisawa J, Fujita T, Yoshida M (1993): A trans-activator Tax of human T-cell leukemia virus type 1 binds to NF-κB p50 and serum response factor (SRF) and associates with enhancer DNAs of the NF-κB site and CArG box. *Oncogene* 8: 2391–2397

Ten RM, Blank V, Le Bail O, Kourilsky B, Israel A (1993): Two factors, IRF-1 and KBF1/NF-κB, cooperate during induction of MHC class I gene expression by interferon α/β or Newcastle disease virus. *C R Acad Sci III* 316: 496–501

Ten RM, Paya CV, Israël N, LeBail O, Mattei M-G, Virelizier J-L, Kourilsky P, Israël A (1992): The characterization of the promoter of the gene encoding the p50 subunit of NF-κB indicates that it participates in its own regulation. *EMBO J* 11: 195–203

Tewari M, Dobrzanski P, Mohn KL, Cressman DE, Hsu J-C, Bravo R, Taub R (1992): Rapid induction in regenerating liver of RL/IF-1 (an IκB that inhibits NF-κB, RelB-p50, and c-Rel-p50) and PHF, a novel κB site-binding complex. *Mol Cell Biol* 12: 2898–2908

Thanos D, Maniatis T (1992): The high mobility group protein HMG I(Y) is required for NF-κB-dependent virus induction of the human IFN-β gene. *Cell* 71: 777–789

Thevenin C, Kim S-C, Rieckmann P, Fujiki H, Norcross MA, Sporn MB, Kehrl JH (1991): Induction of nuclear factor-κB and the human immunodeficiency virus long terminal repeat by okadaic acid, a specific inhibitor of phosphatases I and 2A. *New Biologist* 2: 793–800

Toledano MB, Leonard WJ (1991): Modulation of transcription factor NF-κB binding activity by oxidation-reduction in vitro. *Proc Natl Acad Sci USA* 88: 4328–4332

Toledano MB, Ghosh D, Trinh F, Leonard WJ (1993): N-terminal DNA-binding domains contribute to differential DNA-binding specificities of NF-κB p50 and p65. *Mol Cell Biol* 13: 852–860

Trede NS, Castigli E, Geha RS, Chatila T (1993): Microbial superantigens induce NF-κB in the human monocytic cell line THP-1. *J Immunol* 150: 5604–5613

Uckun FM, Schieven GL, Tuel-Ahlgren LM, Dibirdik I, Myers D, Ledbetter JA, Song CW (1993): Tyrosine phosphorylation is a mandatory proximal step in radiation-induced activation of the protein kinase C signaling pathway in human B-lymphocyte precursors. *Proc Natl Acad Sci USA* 90: 252–256

Ueberla K, Lu YC, Chung E, Haseltine WA (1993): The NF-κB p65 promoter. *J AIDS Res* 6: 227–230

Urban MB, Baeuerle PA (1990): The 65-kD subunit of NF-κB is a receptor for IκB and a modulator of DNA-binding specificity. *Genes Develop* 4: 1975–1984

Verweij CL, Geerts M, Aarden LA (1991): Activation of interleukin-2 transcription via the T-cell surface molecule CD28 is mediated through an NF-kB-like response element. *J Biol Chem* 266: 14179–14182

Voraberger G, Schafer R, Stratowa C (1991): Cloning of the human gene for intercellular adhesion molecule 1 and analysis of its 5′ regulatory region. Induction by cytokines and phorbol ester. *J Immunol* 147: 2777–2786

Walker WH, Stein B, Ganchi PA, Hoffman JA, Kaufman PA, Ballard DW, Hannink M, Greene WC (1992): The v-rel oncogene: insights into the mechanism of transcriptional activation, repression and transformation. *J Virol* 66: 5018–5029

Wasserman SA (1993): A conserved signal transduction pathway regulating the activity of the rel-like proteins dorsal and NF-κB. *Mol Biol Cell* 4: 767–771

Watanabe M, Muramatsu M, Hirai H, Suzuki T (1993): HTLV-I encoded Tax in association with NF-κB precursor p105 enhances nuclear localization of NF-κB p50 and p65 in transfected cells. *Oncogene* 8: 2949–2958

Wilhelmsen KC, Eggleton K, Temin HM (1984): Nucleic acid sequence of the oncogene v-rel in reticuloendotheliosis virus strain T and its cellular homolog, the protooncogene c-rel. *J Virol* 52: 172–182

Wulczyn FG, Naumann M, Scheidereit C (1992): Candidate proto-oncogene bcl-3 encodes a subunit-specific inhibitor of transcription factor NF-κB. *Nature* 358: 597–599

Xie QW, Kashiwabara Y, Nathan C (1994): Role of transcription factor NF-κB/Rel in induction of nitric oxide synthase. *J Biol Chem* 269: 4705–5708

Xu X, Prorock C, Ishikawa H, Maldonado E (1993): Functional interaction of the v-Rel and c-Rel oncoproteins with the TATA-binding protein and association with transcription factor IIB. *Mol Cell Biol* 13: 6733–6741

Yang Z, Costanzo M, Golde W, Kolesnick RN (1993): Tumor necrosis factor activation of the shingomyelin pathway signals nuclear factor kappa B translocation in tact HL-60 cells. *J Biol Chem* 268: 20520–20523

Zabel U, Baeurle PA (1990): Purified human IκB can rapidly dissociate the complex of the NF-κB transcription factor with its cognate DNA. *Cell* 61: 255–265

Zabel U, Henkel T, dosSantosSilva M, Baeuerle P (1993): Nuclear uptake control of NF-κB by MAD-3, and IκB protein present in the nucleus. *EMBO J* 12: 201–211

Zhang Y, Broser M, Rom WN (1994): Activation of the interleukin-6 by Mycobacterium tuberculosis and lipopolysaccharide is mediated by nuclear factors NF-IL-6 and NF-kappa B. *Proc Natl Acad Sci USA* 91: 2225–2229

Ziegler-Heitbrock HW, Sternsdorf T, Liese J, Belohradsky B, Weber C, Wedel A, Shreck R, Bauerle P, Strobel M (1993): Pyrrolidine dithiocarbamate inhibits NF-κB mobilization and TNF production in human monocytes. *J Immunol* 151: 6986–6993

Zuniga-Pflucker JC, Schwartz ML, Lenardo MY (1993): Gene transcription in differentiating immature T cell receptor (neg) thymocytes resembles antigen-activated mature T cells. *Medicine* 178: 1139–1149

5

PPAR : a Key Nuclear Factor in Nutrient / Gene Interactions?

BÉATRICE DESVERGNE AND WALTER WAHLI

Introduction

Retinoids as well as steroid and thyroid hormones are small lipophilic molecules that exert an intricate array of combinatorial effects during embryogenesis, cellular differentiation, and homeostasis in the adult organism. Complexity in the signalling pathway of these hormones results from the functional association of low affinity cytoplasmic hormone binding proteins and high affinity nuclear hormone receptors. The latter interact with polymorphic response elements linked to target genes and mediate the hormonal response at the transcriptional level.

Structural and functional analysis of the nuclear hormone receptors revealed that they belong to a superfamily of factors whose members are related to each other to different extents (Gronemeyer, 1992; Parker, 1993; Wahli and Martinez, 1991). Their most conserved region contains two so-called zinc fingers that constitute the core of the DNA binding domain which specifically recognizes hormone response elements. This conservation was and is still exploited to isolate additional members of the superfamily by cross-hybridization screening of cDNA libraries, and it now appears that the family is much more diverse than originally thought. As a consequence of this isolation strategy, several proteins which are authentic members of the superfamily are still in search of a ligand, and they are called orphan receptors for this reason. In fact, the possibility remains open that some of them function as constitutive ligand-independent transcriptional regulators. However, this is most likely the exception since the homology of the hormone binding domain in orphan receptors with that of known ligand-dependent receptors suggests that the orphans are activated by ligands. The possibility that molecules so far not considered as bona fide hormones are ligands of members of the superfamily raises fascinating questions as

INDUCIBLE GENE EXPRESSION, VOLUME 1
P.A. Baeuerle, Editor
© 1995 Birkhäuser Boston

to the origin of the superfamily and the diversity of pathways it may control. Along this line of thought, metabolic substrates, nutrients or xenobiotics could correspond to ligands of orphan receptors. Conceptually, such a regulatory system would resemble certain types of gene control by environmental agents or metabolic intermediates in yeast and bacteria. Transposed to higher organisms, the idea can be best illustrated by the liver, which receives most of its blood supply directly from the gut, via the large portal vein, while lipids absorbed by the intestinal mucosa reach the liver after having entered the blood circulation via the lymphatic ducts. As a result, hepatocytes are exposed to frequent dramatic changes in the level and composition of nutrients, or to various toxic substances. They respond to these stimuli by the activation or repression of genes encoding proteins involved in different metabolic pathways or detoxifying systems. So far, the proteins that recognize nutrients or xenobiotics and transduce the signal for transcriptional gene regulation are poorly characterized. Nevertheless, it is conceivable that certain of these intracellular receptors are members of the nuclear receptor superfamily since from a general point of view, the activation, for instance of detoxifying cytochrome P-450 genes by xenobiotics, appears to be very similar to that of steroid hormone target genes.

This prediction has been substantiated by the discovery of the peroxisome proliferator activated receptors (PPARs) (Green and Wahli, 1994; Keller and Wahli, 1993). These receptors have been named according to their capacity to be activated by many compounds which share in common the property of inducing peroxisome proliferation especially in rodent liver. As described below, PPARs are involved in the control of genes encoding lipid metabolism-associated proteins and are activated by physiological concentrations of fatty acids, or by fibrate hypolipidemic drugs and other peroxisome proliferators such as certain plasticizers and herbicides.

Peroxisome Proliferation as Response to a Multiplicity of Signals

Peroxisomes are ubiquitous cytoplasmic organelles with a diameter of 0.2 to 1 μm, surrounded by a single membrane delimiting the matrix compartment, which comprises the bulk of peroxisomal enzymes. These enzymes are involved in catabolic as well as anabolic pathways, particularly in lipid metabolism, such as the degradation of fatty acids and their derivatives via β-oxidation and the synthesis of ether lipids, cholesterol and dolichols. The main substrates of peroxisomal β-oxidation are very long-chain fatty acids, dicarboxylic fatty acids, 2-methyl branched fatty acids, prostaglandins, bile acid intermediates and xenobiotics. The oxidative degradation of polyamines, purines, D-amino acids and 2-L-hydroxy acids also occurs in peroxisomes. All these oxidation reactions, as well as the deactivation of superoxide anions, lead to the formation of hydrogen peroxide which is disposed of by catalase, an abundant peroxisomal enzyme (Mannaerts and Van Veldhoven, 1993; Osmundsen et al, 1991).

Hepatic and renal peroxisomes in rodents respond with a massive proliferation to various xenobiotics, therefore named peroxisome proliferators. In this process, the induction of synthesis of peroxisomal membrane and matrix proteins is followed by an increase in the size and content of the peroxisomes which then divide to form daughter organelles (Small, 1993). In particular, this proliferation is accompanied by a dramatic increase of the mRNAs, and consequently of the corresponding proteins, involved in peroxisomal β-oxidation (Figure 5.1) (Lazarow and deDuve, 1976; Rao and Reddy, 1987). In rodents, a sustained exposure to peroxisome proliferators causes hepatomegaly followed by hepatocarcinogenesis.

The first chemical to be identified as a peroxisome proliferator in mouse and rat was clofibrate (Hess et al, 1965), a hypolipidemic drug whose administration reduces the serum level of triglycerides and cholesterol, therefore limiting the risk of coronary heart disease in hyperlipidemic patients (Sitori et al, 1977). Subsequently, all other fibric acid derivatives used as hypolipidemic drugs were also found to be peroxisome proliferators (Lock et al, 1989). In addition to these drugs, a wide variety of compounds, for which no obvious common structural property can be delineated, induce peroxisome proliferation (Figure 5.2). They can be categorized as nonfibrate hypolipidemic drugs, industrial plasticizers such as some phthalate and adipate esters, herbicides such as 2,4,5-trichlorophenoxyacetic acid, and leukotriene antagonists (Lock et al, 1989; Nemali et al, 1989; Reddy and Lalwani, 1983). Interestingly, they all have hypolipidemic properties.

Natural factors, such as high-fat diets, also induce reversibly peroxisome proliferation in rodents (Flatmark et al, 1988; Neat et al, 1980), suggesting that this phenomenon represents a response to metabolic stimuli. Peroxisome proliferation is preferentially induced when the diet contains a high proportion of very-long-chain fatty acids known to be poorly oxidized via the mitochondrial β-oxidation pathway, such as partially hydrogenated fish oil (Norum et al, 1989; Flatmark and Christiansen, 1993). However, the induction of peroxisome proliferation is not restricted to a single type of fatty acids, and a broad range of metabolizable and nonmetabolizable fatty acids is effective. In addition to dietary factors, fatty acid overloads due to metabolic disturbances such as

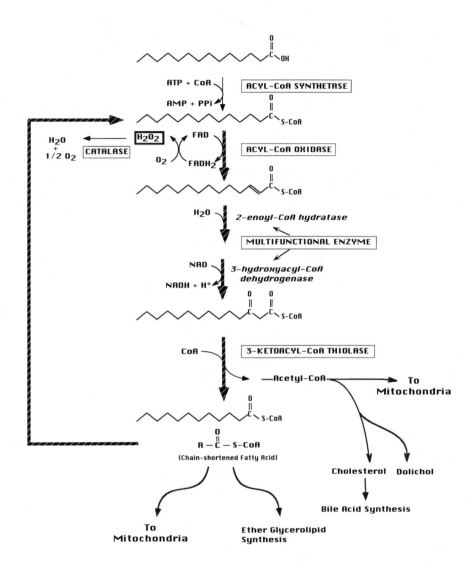

Figure 5.1 The peroxisomal pathway of fatty acid β-oxidation. Fatty acids are activated to fatty acid CoA esters by the acyl-CoA synthetase located in the peroxisomal membrane. They can then enter the β-oxidation pathway in the peroxisomal matrix where they are subjected to a series of four reactions leading to the shortening of the fatty acid chain length by two carbon atoms and to the concomitant liberation of one molecule of acetyl-CoA. These reactions are catalyzed by the three core enzymes of the β-oxidation pathway, the acyl-CoA oxidase, the enoyl-CoA hydratase/ 3-hydroxyacyl-CoA dehydrogenase (multifunctional enzyme) and the thiolase.

starvation (Orellana et al, 1992) and diabetes (Hori et al, 1981), also increase peroxisomal β-oxidation.

Peroxisomes are present in all eukaryotic cells from yeast to plants and higher vertebrates, as expected for an organelle that fulfils several important functions. However, only a subset of animal species undergoes peroxisome proliferation in response to peroxisome proliferators and develops the subsequent processes of hepatomegaly, hyperplasia and hepatocarcinogenesis if the treatment is maintained. Mouse and rat are most responsive,

Chemical class	Examples	Structural feature
Fibrate derivatives	Clofibrate, Bezafibrate, Ciprofibrate Clobuzarit, Fenofibrate, Nafenopin *(hypolipidaemic drugs)*	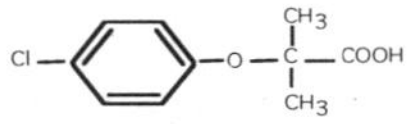 Chlofibric acid
Other xenobiotics	Pirinixic acid (Wy-14,643) Tibric acid, Tiadenol *(hypolipidaemic drugs)* Ly 171883 *(leukotriene receptor antagonist)* Dehydroepinadrosterone * *(steroid)* Acetylsalicylic acid * *(prostaglandin synthesis inhibitor)*	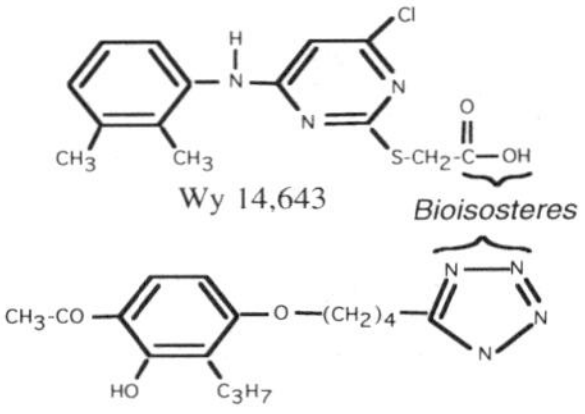 Wy 14,643 Bioisosteres LY 17 1883
Herbicides	Fomesafen, Lactofen, 2,4-Dichlorophenoxyacetic acid 2,4,5-Trichlorophenoxyacetic acid and related compounds	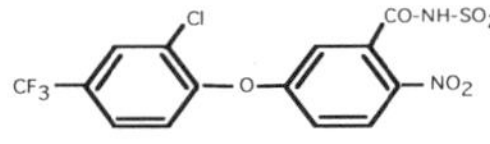 Fomesafen
Plasticizers	Di-(2-ethylhexyl)phtalhate Di-(isononyl)phtalhate and other phtalhate esters Di-(2-ethylhexyl)adipate (DEHA)	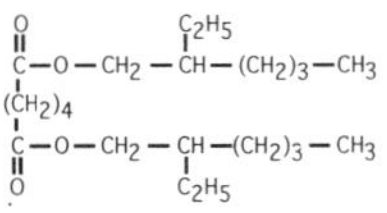 DEHA
Solvents and industrial compounds	Perchloroethylene, Trichloroethylene, Trichloroacetic acid * Perchloro-n-octanoic acid and related compounds	$ClCH = CCl_2$ Trichloroethylene
Dietary fat	Long-chain and very long chain, polyunsaturated or monounsaturated fatty acids	

Figure 5.2 Classes of compounds acting as peroxisome proliferators. Compounds causing peroxisome proliferation in vivo but not in primary cultures of rat hepatocytes are indicated by an asterisk. Thus, it is thought that peroxisome proliferation is induced indirectly by the compounds marked by the asterisk.

hamster is intermediate, and guinea pig, dog and primates are either very weakly responsive or nonresponsive (Lock et al, 1989; Orton et al, 1984; Reddy and Lalwani, 1983). The situation is less clear in human where solely the most potent fibrates seem to induce only a marginal peroxisome proliferation (Lock et al, 1989). As yet, very little is known on the basic mechanisms underlying the considerable susceptibility differences among species regarding peroxisome proliferation and carcinogenic action of peroxisome proliferators. Not only the level of the response but also its nature can vary enormously. There are examples where stimulation of peroxisomal fatty acid β-oxidation, peroxisome proliferation and hepatocarcinogenesis are uncoupled. In both *Rana esculenta* and *Xenopus laevis*, two amphibian species, clofibrate stimulates peroxisomal β-oxidation, but peroxisome proliferation is observed only in *Rana* (Ciolek and Dauça, 1991). Similarly, the carcinogenic potencies of various peroxisome proliferators in rodents differ considerably. For example, prolonged treatment with the hypolipidemic compound pirinixic acid (Wy-14,463) has a 100% liver tumour incidence, as compared to only 10% with the plasticizer di-(2-ethylhexyl) phthalate which produces only slightly less peroxisome proliferation than pirinixic acid (Marsman et al, 1988).

Recent research efforts tried to define the molecular link between peroxisome proliferators and the stimulation of peroxisomal fatty acid β-oxidation, peroxisome proliferation and hepatocarcinogenesis, based on the similarity of responses to fatty acids and other peroxisome proliferators. It has been proposed that soluble receptors would induce genes involved in these processes. The first indication for such an activation mechanism has been the detection of a nafenopin-binding protein in rat liver cytosol (Lalwani et al, 1983). Such a binding activity also has been found in kidney extracts. However, direct binding of peroxisome proliferators to the purified cytosolic protein has not been confirmed. Furthermore, its ubiquitous expression at high levels makes it unlikely to be a mediator of peroxisome proliferator action. Since peroxisome proliferators control genes encoding peroxisomal as well as microsomal β-oxidation enzymes in a tissue-specific manner and at the transcriptional level, the existence of a transcription factor based mechanism of action of peroxisome proliferators has been proposed. This hypothesis includes the possibility that the biological mediator of peroxisome proliferator action might be a member of the nuclear hormone receptor superfamily (Green, 1992). This has led to the identification of nuclear receptors that can be activated by peroxisome proliferators and fatty acids and which indeed belong to the steroid/thyroid/retinoid nuclear receptor superfamily (Dreyer et al, 1992; Issemann and Green, 1990; Issemann et al, 1993; Keller et al, 1993a; Göttlicher et al, 1992).

Different Types of Peroxisome Proliferator Activated Receptors

There are at least three types of PPARs : α, β and γ, all of which can be activated by fatty acids and peroxisome proliferators. Similarly to other nuclear receptors, the amino acid sequences of the PPARs can be divided into distinct regions (A to F) based on the relatedness among themselves and with other members of the superfamily (Figure 5.3) (Parker, 1993; Wahli and Martinez, 1991). The three types of PPARs have been cloned in *Xenopus laevis*, mouse and human, taking into account that the mouse and human PPAR NUCI are likely to be of the β-type (see below) (Dreyer et al, 1992; Issemann and Green, 1990; Chen et al, 1993; Zhu et al, 1993; Greene et al, 1994; Schmidt et al, 1992; Sher et al, 1993). In addition the α type has also been found in rat (Göttlicher et al, 1992). Interestingly, the amino acid sequence conservation of a particular type, α, β or γ, is greater across species than that observed for the three PPAR types in a given species (Figure 5.3). The same holds true for the other members of the superfamily RARs and RXRs, where three types α, β and γ also exist (Leid et al, 1992).

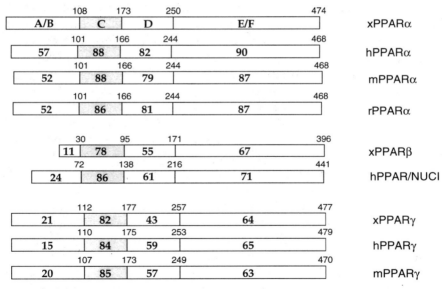

Figure 5.3 List and comparison of the known PPARs. Amino acid sequences of the PPARs have been subdivided into domains A–E and aligned to the corresponding domains of xPPARα. The amino acid sequences are represented by open bars. The numbers above the bars indicate the last amino acid of each corresponding domain. Numbers within the bars give the sequence similarities in the five different domains of the receptors expressed as per cent amino acid identity relative to xPPARα. The highly conserved DNA binding domain is highlighted by shading.

The phylogenetic tree of PPARs (Figure 5.4A) is based on sequence comparisons of the central conserved portion of the ligand binding domain. This tree indicates that PPARα, PPARβ and PPARγ are encoded by different loci. The situation remains to be clarified for NUCI. Two of the three methods used suggest that it is the homolog of xPPARβ, but the third one indicates that it may represent an independent locus, closely related to the β locus (Figure 5.4B). Analysis of further β-like PPAR homologues when they become available, for instance from birds, is required to determine whether NUCI belongs to the β subtype or indeed, represents a different receptor as has been suggested recently (Chen et al, 1993).

With regard to the whole superfamily, PPARs belong to the first of the three subfamilies of nuclear receptors along with the receptors of thyroid hormone (TR), retinoic acid (RAR) and the two orphan receptors Rev-ErbAα($=$ear1) and E75, which are the closest relatives of the PPARs (Laudet et al, 1992; Dreyer et al, 1993). Globally, two different periods can be recognised in the evolution of this subfamily. During the first period, which predates the arthropod/vertebrate dichotomy (approximately 500 million years ago) (Knoll, 1992), the ancestral TR, RAR and PPAR appeared. The second period corresponds to the duplication of the ancestral TR gene into two genes TRα and TRβ, as well as of the ancestral RAR gene into three genes RARα, RARβ and RARγ. Similarly, the three known PPAR loci appeared during this second period.

It is possible to compare the speed of evolution within the PPAR, RAR and TR groups of genes. In each of these groups, mammalian and *Xenopus* homologs of the same gene, which have been separated for the same time, have been characterized. Assuming that amphibians and mammals separated 400 million years ago, the speed of divergence of the homologs after the separation of the two lineages can be estimated. Based on the percentage of amino-acid sequence differences in the conserved central region of the ligand binding domain, the PPAR genes have evolved approximately two to threefold faster than the TR or the RAR genes (Figure 5.4). It is not known whether the duplication events within the TR, RAR or PPAR group of genes occurred at the same time, although several arguments including the chromosomal location of TR, RAR and PPAR genes are in favor of the hypothesis of such a "big bang" of gene duplication at the appearance of the early vertebrates (Keese and Gibbs, 1992).

The chromosomal localization of the human genes encoding PPARα and PPARγ has been defined. They map on different chromosomes. The hPPARγ gene is on chromosome 3 at position 3p25, close to RARβ and TRβ at positions 3p24 and 3p21, respectively (Drabkin et al, 1988; Greene et al, 1994; Mattei et al, 1991). This localization may have

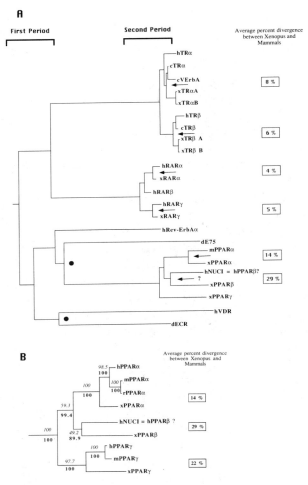

Figure 5.4 Phylogeny of the PPARs. A) Phylogenetic tree connecting the members of the thyroid, retinoid, vitamin D, and PPAR subfamily. This tree has been generated by comparison of the central conserved portion of the ligand binding domains, which comprises the Ti (TI) and dimerization (DM) domains of these receptors (Forman and Samuels, 1990). The length of the horizontal branches represents the divergence of the sequences and is not proportional to time. A long branch, for instance, could correspond to a short period of time if the genes evolved very rapidly. Dark circles and arrows indicate the dichotomy between vertebrate and invertebrate genes and *Xenopus* and mammalian genes respectively. The boxed percentages indicate amino acid differences between the mammalian and *Xenopus* Ti-DM sequences, which have been calculated using the Clustal alignment algorithm. The tree has been calculated using the Fitch least square algorithm (Dreyer et al, 1993). B) Fitch tree of the PPARs. This tree is based on sequence comparisons of the C, D and E domains of all PPARs known to date. Identical topologies are given by two methods of calculation: Distance Matrix (NJ) and Parsimony (PAUP or PROTPARS). The number in each branch corresponds to the bootstrap estimate on the parsimony tree (italic) or the NJ tree (bold) (a 100% means that in repeated computer simulations, the branching depicted is observed in all occurrences). The boxed percentages are as in A. h = human; r = rat; m = mouse; c = chicken; x = *Xenopus*; d = *Drosophila*.

interesting implications since 3p deletions are commonly seen in a variety of carcinomas, whereas the 3p25-p21 deletion has been observed, but infrequently, in patients with chronic lymphoproliferative disorders. So far, however, there is no proof that disruption of hPPARγ contributes to any human malignancy (Green et al, 1994). The hPPARα gene has been mapped on chromosome 22 slightly telomeric to a linkage group of six genes and genetic markers located in the general region 22q12-q13.1 (Sher et al, 1993). This location is different from that of RARα and γ on chromosome 17q21.1 and 12q13 (Mattei et al, 1991), respectively and of TRα on chromosome 17q21 (Dayton et al, 1984). Thus, it appears that PPARα is on a chromosome to which no RAR nor TR loci have been mapped.

Structure of the PPAR Genes

Useful information concerning the degree of relatedness between genes that are members of a same family or superfamily is the degree of similarity in their genomic organization since position and number of introns in a given gene are important indicators of its evolution in the context of the gene family to which it belongs (Laudet et al, 1992).

There are eight exons in the mPPARα gene spanning at least 30 kilobases with two noncoding exons comprising most of the 5′-untranslated region (Gearing et al, 1994). The first noncoding exon of mPPARα is differentially spliced to give at least two distinct mRNAs, a situation similar to that of the RAR genes where differential splicing in the 5′-untranslated region also occurs. The coding region, whose organization has also been determined for the xPPARβ (Krey et al, 1993) is comprised of six exons (Figure 5.5). The third intron, the first to interrupt the coding region, is between the sequences encoding the N-terminal domain (exon 3) and the first zinc finger of the DNA binding domain (exon 4). Its position corresponds to that found in the RARγ gene (Lehmann et al, 1991). The fourth intron separates the regions encoding the two zinc fingers. An intron is also found at this same position in the Rev-ErbAα/TR/RAR genes (Laudet et al, 1991; Lazar et al, 1989; Lehmann et al, 1991; Miyajima et al, 1989; Shi et al, 1992). The position is precisely conserved in xPPARβ, but it occurs one nucleotide upstream in mPPARα. The exon encoding the second zinc finger ends at a canonical position conserved amongst all nuclear hormone receptor genes even in the COUP-TF gene, which has only two introns (Ritchie et al, 1990). Similarly, domain D is encoded by a single exon as is the case in the majority of the genes for other members of the superfamily.

More interestingly, the E or ligand binding domain of xPPARβ and

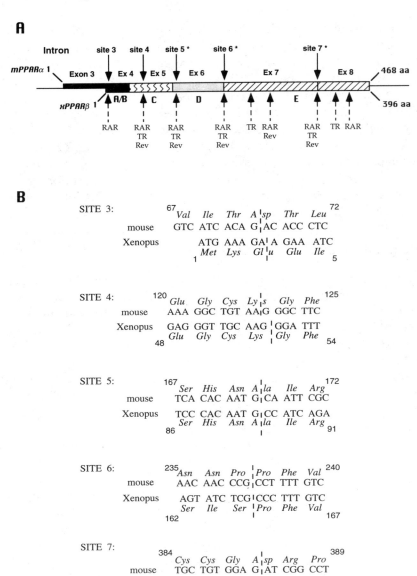

Figure 5.5 Genomic organization of the mouse PPARα and the *Xenopus* PPARβ coding regions. A) Location of the intron sites on the mPPARα and xPPARβ cDNAs (solid arrows). Asterisks indicate intron sites common to all vertebrate nuclear hormone receptors, and the broken arrows the relative position of the intron sites in the TR, RAR, and Rev-erbAα(Rev) receptors. The functional domains of the receptors are given (A–E). B) The nucleotide and amino acid sequences spanning the splice sites in the coding region of the mPPARα and xPPARβ are compared. The broken lines indicate the positions of the intron sites.

mPPARα is encoded by only two exons, a unique feature among the superfamily members. The splice site between these two exons is located close to the end of the coding sequence. This position is conserved in all nuclear receptors with the exception of the *Drosophila* E75 gene, where it is lacking. The presence of only a single intron in the E domain of xPPARβ and mPPARα makes these genes different from their closest relative, the Rev-ErbAα gene, which possess an additional intron in this domain. Thus, xPPARβ and mPPARα are structurally intermediate between two homologous genes, the E75 *Drosophila* gene which contains no intron in this domain (Segraves and Hogness, 1990), and the human Rev-ErbAα gene that contains two (Lazar et al, 1989; Miyajima et al, 1989). In short, the structure of the PPAR genes is unique, but their closest relatives based on exon/intron organization are the E75, Rev-ErbAα, TR and RAR genes. This confirms membership to a same subfamily as determined previously by sequence comparisons.

The degree of divergence between the mPPARα and the xPPARβ is relatively high as it is in general between the α-type and β-type PPARs (Figure 5.3). In contrast, the exon junctions are relatively well conserved indicating homologous positions of the introns in the two genes (Figure 5.5). Furthermore it reveals a constraint on these locations most likely resulting from the requirements of the splicing machinery.

The 5'-flanking region of the mPPARα gene is reminiscent of that of other nuclear hormone receptor genes. There is no TATA nor CCAAT elements close to the transcription initiation sites, but there are seven putative Sp1 binding sites or GC boxes and the whole 5'-flanking region is GC rich (Gearing et al, 1994). The promoters of the androgen, thyroid hormone, glucocorticoid, retinoic acid and progesterone receptor genes have a similar structural organization.

Expression of PPAR Messenger RNAs

The expression of the *Xenopus* PPARs, whose cDNAs have been isolated from ovary (α and β) and liver (γ) cDNA libraries, have been studied during oogenesis, embryogenesis and in adult organs. xPPARα and to a greater extent xPPARβ mRNAs accumulate already in early oogenesis, and the pool of maternal transcripts persists in the embryos up to gastrula stages. A replacement of the maternal transcripts by zygotic transcripts of the same types is detected during or after gastrulation. In adult *Xenopus* organs, xPPARα and xPPARβ are ubiquitously expressed (Dreyer et al, 1993; Dreyer et al, 1992; Keller et al, 1993b). In contrast, xPPARγ mRNA is not detected during oogenesis, with the exception of a shorter transcript that cannot encode a full-length receptor. In adult *Xenopus*, xPPARγ has a relatively restricted expression with the highest levels in fat body and kidney and a moderate level in liver. Human tissues also express two different PPARγ, which correspond to the full length mRNA and, as in *Xenopus*, to a version too short to encode a functional receptor. Both transcripts are detected in colon, bladder, kidney, skeletal muscle, liver, spleen, placenta, stomach and in hematopoietic cells. The two transcripts were also found in fetal kidney, liver and lung. Only the long transcript is detected in cultured normal primary bone marrow stromal cells and in a variety of human leukemia cell lines. Finally, only the short form is found in normal neutrophils, peripheral blood lymphocytes and in circulating leukemic cells from patients with AML, ALL and CML (Greene et al, 1994).

In mouse, PPARα transcripts are detected only in liver and in brown adipose tissue from the fetal period (mouse gestation day 16) onwards into adulthood. Postnatally, mPPARα is also expressed in the heart, kidney and weakly in skeletal muscle, small intestine, testis and thymus (Beck et al, 1992; Issemann and Green, 1990). In adult rats analyzed with the human probe for NUCI (β-type PPAR), high level expression is found in heart, lung, kidney, spleen, ovaries and low level expression in skin and bone cells (Schmidt et al, 1992). Compared to mPPARα, which is highly expressed in liver, the level of NUCI transcripts is at its lowest in this organ.

The differences in expression of PPARs suggest that they have specific regulatory roles in different organs. However, the ubiquitous expression of xPPARα and xPPARβ indicates that PPARs may also be involved more generally in the regulation of basal cellular functions as is also suggested by the roles of the enzymes whose genes are regulated by these receptors (see below). A detailed expression analysis of the different types of PPARs in different tissues by in situ hybridization using specific probes or by immunocytochemistry with specific antibodies is required to assess the extent of expression specificity of each of the different PPARs.

So far, there is little evidence that PPARs are directly involved in cell differentiation, with the exception of cultured 3T3-L1 cells that can be induced to differentiate into adipocytes. Continued exposure of 3T3-L1 cells to peroxisome proliferators leads to adipose conversion, during which PPAR as well as its heterodimerization partner (see below) are stimulated (Chawla and Lazar, 1994). The correlation between the potency of various peroxisome proliferators to activate PPAR and their ability to induce adipose conversion suggests that PPARs are mechanistically involved in the differentiation process, but their precise role remains to be elucidated. As mentioned above, PPARs are also expressed in a variety of nonadipose tissues where they undoubtedly play a different role.

Structural Characteristics of PPARs as Transcription Factors

As mentioned above, PPAR cDNAs have been isolated by virtue of the conserved nature of the sequences encoding the DNA binding domain of nuclear hormone receptors. The structural similarity between members of the superfamily extends over the whole molecule, organized in structural modules. In the past, extensive structure-function analyses have been performed on the glucocorticoid receptor and estrogen receptor, and much of the information gained has helped to formulate and test the hypothesis according to which structural similarities between nuclear receptors imply similarities in function. These studies, besides allowing the display of common features, have revealed differences defining unique characteristics of each of the receptors, as will be presented below for PPARs.

PPARs are constitutively nuclear receptors, as revealed by immuno-cytochemical analyses of endogenous receptors, and of transiently expressed receptors in cells transfected with PPAR expression vectors. Therefore, their cytoplasmic-nuclear translocation is independent of exogenous activators (Dreyer et al, 1993; Braissant and Wahli, 1994). Considering the fact that PPARs are activated by fatty acids (see below), the possibility that endogenous fatty acids induce nuclear translocation cannot be excluded. However, since addition of exogenous activators is required for full transcriptional induction by the nuclear PPARs, it would imply that nuclear translocation needs less activator than transcriptional activation, which is unlikely. No obvious constitutive nuclear localisation signal (NLS) similar to the one described in the GR, or to those postulated in other nuclear hormone receptors, can be detected by sequence comparison (Dingwall and Laskey, 1991). This could indicate that the NLS of PPARs could consist of several, dispersed pro-signals that only mutagenesis could diagnose, as described for PR and ER (Ylikomi et al, 1992).

The DNA binding domain is the best conserved structure among all members of the nuclear hormone receptor superfamily and is formed of two zinc fingers folded in a single globular domain. Several subdomains have been delineated using functional and structural analyses of various members of the superfamily. The P box corresponds to the C-terminal knuckle of the first zinc finger and determines specific contacts between the nuclear receptor and DNA (Luisi et al, 1991; Mader et al, 1989; Umesono and Evans, 1989). The PPARs possess the same P box primary sequence as TR, VDR, and RAR (Figure 5.6). Consequently, it was predicted and later confirmed that PPARs recognize, on the DNA, a hormone response element which comprises the hexameric AGGTCA

A

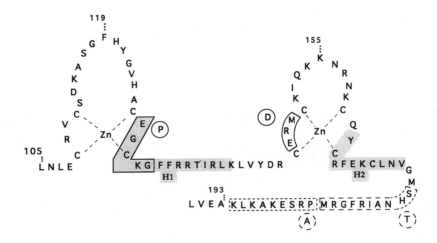

B

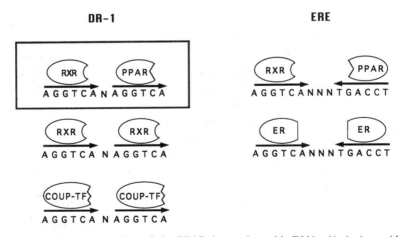

Figure 5.6 Schematic representation of the PPAR interaction with DNA. A) Amino acid sequence and secondary structure of the DNA-binding domain of xPPARα. Boxed sequences correspond to the various subdomains described in the text. Putative A and T boxes are given in dotted lines. Sequences in a grey background form α-helical structures (H1 and H2), as demonstrated for both the glucocorticoid and the estrogen receptors. B) Diagram representing the complexes bound to PPAR response element (DR-1) and to estrogen response elements (ERE). PPARs bind preferentially to a DR-1 element as heterodimers with RXR that, by analogy to other RXR heterodimers, has been drawn on the 5'-half of the element. A RXR homodimer or a COUP-TF homodimer can also bind to a DR-1 response element. The PPAR/RXR heterodimer can interact with the estrogen response element (ERE), usually recognized by an estrogen receptor (ER) homodimer.

half-site motif, like the other members of this P box sub-class. The D box consists of the amino acids of the first knuckle of the second zinc finger and has been proposed as a dimerization surface involved in half-site spacing recognition (Hirst et al, 1992). Only three amino acids compose the PPAR D box whereas in almost all other nuclear receptors it contains five (Figure 5.6). As yet, no specific function has been attributed to this rather unique PPAR D box. The T box and the A box, located immediately downstream of the second zinc finger, have been defined in RXR, the 9-cis retinoic acid receptor, and in NGF1-B, respectively. The T box contributes to RXR homodimerization (Lee et al, 1993; Wilson et al, 1992), and the A box is essential for monomer binding of NGF1-B to its response element (Wilson et al, 1992). Functional data on the characteristics and role of the putative A and T boxes in PPARs are at present missing (Figure 5.6).

Dimerization is essential for the function of most of the nuclear receptors. As mentioned, some of the DNA binding domain elements are involved in dimer formation. They have been analysed in detail for TR/RXR and RAR/RXR heterodimers (Desvergne, 1994). Again, such studies need now to be considered for PPAR-containing complexes. Another major dimerization element is part of the E domain in which nine heptad repeats are very well conserved among hormone receptors, a primary structure reminiscent of the leucine zipper sequence mediating c-fos/c-jun heterodimerization (Forman et al, 1989). The heptad repeats are present in PPARs as well as in RXRs and are likely to be involved in a symmetrical contact between these heterodimerization partners.

The preferential binding of most nuclear hormone receptors as dimers is reflected at the level of DNA in the structure of the response element characterized by two half-sites, each bearing the consensus hexameric sequence AGGTCA or a variation thereof. *Sensus stricto* steroid receptors bind only as homodimers to elements in which the half-sites are organized in a palindromic array (Martinez and Wahli, 1991). Other receptors, like TRs and RARs, recognize response elements diversely organized as palindromes, inverted palindromes or direct repeats to which they bind preferentially as heterodimers with RXR (Desvergne, 1994). In the case of PPARs, the response element found in native promoters (see below) and then studied as synthetic consensus element, is formed of a direct repeat of the AGGTCA half-site, with a one nucleotide spacer between the half elements (DR-1) (Figure 5.6). The complex formed in vitro on such a response element is a PPAR-RXR heterodimer (Gearing et al, 1993; Issemann et al, 1993; Keller et al, 1993a; Kliewer et al, 1992; Krey et al, 1994a). The strongest activation of PPRE-controlled gene requires the presence of the two activators, a peroxisome proliferator and 9-cis retinoic acid, for PPAR and RXR, respectively. Although in vitro gel retardation assays indicate a synergistic interaction between PPAR and RXR for binding as heterodimers to the PPRE (DR-1), the transcriptional activation mediated by PPAR and RXR in cotransfection experiments is additive (Keller et al, 1993a; Gearing et al, 1993; Issemann et al, 1993). Thus, it is not clear whether, in vivo, PPAR-RXR heterodimers are the only complexes formed on the PPRE or if, alternatively, homodimers also occur, since RXR homodimers are known to bind the DR-1 element (Zhang and Pfahl, 1993). Ultimately, transfection experiments with dominant negative PPAR and RXR mutants that still form heterodimers but do not stimulate transcription, or transfection experiments with cells deficient in endogenous PPAR and RXR are needed to answer the question of which PPAR and/or RXR-containing complexes are functionally relevant in vivo. It is of interest to note that all nuclear receptors that bind to a direct repeat element preferentially do so as heterodimer with RXR which exclusively binds the 5' half-site of the elements (Desvergne, 1994). With the exception of COUP-TF which binds as homodimer, all belong to the same subfamily. Together, these results indicate that RXR plays a particular role in the convergence of the retinoid signalling pathway with that of various other hormones, or peroxisome proliferators and fatty acids, as far as PPARs are involved.

PPARs, while binding to only one type of direct repeat, e.g. with a spacing of one nucleotide between the repeated half sites, also bind to the palindromic estrogen response element (ERE) AGGTCANNNT-GACCT, and mediate peroxisome proliferator stimulation of a heterologous ERE driven promoter (Keller and Wahli, 1994). The ability of EREs to function as PPREs in native promoters and the physiological conditions allowing interactions of PPAR and EREs remains to be assessed. Nevertheless, knowing that at least in vitro, it is the PPAR/RXR heterodimer that binds to the ERE, the potential for the convergence of these pathways, estrogen, retinoids, peroxisome proliferators-fatty acids is of particular biological interest.

The Puzzling Activation of the PPARs

Binding of a specific ligand is considered as the prime event leading to the activation of a nuclear hormone receptor. However, for several members of the steroid/thyroid receptor superfamily no ligand is known. For this reason, as already mentioned, these receptors are called orphan receptors. Very likely, the ligand for some of them will be found in the future, as it has been the case for 9-cis retinoic acid which was identified as the ligand of RXR long after the isolation of this receptor. However, other orphans such as NGF1-B or Ftz-F1 may function as constitutive transcription factors that do not require a ligand-dependent activation process (Wilson et al, 1991; Ellinger-Ziegelbauer et al, 1994). Similarly, positive transcriptional activation of a target gene is observed with xPPARα in absence of activators. However, this effect is minor or absent with the other PPARs, and the addition to the culture medium of peroxisome proliferators leads to a substantial increase in the expression of the responsive target gene with all PPARs, xPPARα included (Dreyer et al, 1993; Tugwood et al, 1992). The nature of the mechanism by which these various substances activate PPARs is still unclear, but several observations discussed below may give some insight into the activation mechanism.

Class of fatty acids			PPAR activation	
Polyunsaturated fatty acids	Eicosapentaenoic acid	C20:5ω3	+	Arachidonic Acid
	Docosahexaenoic acid	C22:6ω3	+	
	Linolenic acid	C18:3ω3	+	
	Linoleic acid	C18:2ω6	+	ETYA
	Arachidonic acid	C20:4ω6	+	
	5,8,11,14-eicosatetraynoic acid (ETYA)		+	
Monounsaturated fatty acids	Petroselinic acid	C18:1ω12	+	
	Oleic acid	C18:1ω9	+	Oleic Acid
	Elaidic acid	C18:1ω9(*trans*)	+	
	Erucic acid	C22:1ω9	−	
	Nervonic acid	C24:1ω9	−	
Saturated fatty acids	Caproic acid	C6	(+)	
	Caprylic acid	C8	(+)	
	Capric acid	C10	+	Palmitic Acid
	Lauric acid	C12	+	
	Myristic acid	C14	+	
	Palmitic acid	C16	+	
	Stearic acid	C18	+	
Other particular fatty acids	*3-thia fatty acids*: Tetradecylthioacetic acid [CH₃CH₂(CH₂)₁₂ SCH₂COOH]		+	
	Dicarboxilic fatty acids: Dodecanedioic	C12	−	Hexadecanedioic acid
	Hexadecanedioic	C16	+	

Figure 5.7 Activation of PPARs by fatty acids. Cells were cotransfected with a PPAR responsive reporter gene and PPAR expression vectors. The various fatty acids were added to the culture medium at concentrations varying from 50μm to 150μm. +, (+) and − correspond to molecules that induce an activation, a weak activation or no activation, respectively.

Most peroxisome proliferators are capable of activating the PPARs. As previously mentioned, high fat diets, similarly to peroxisome proliferators, induce peroxisome proliferation. Thus, natural fatty acids are good candidates as direct and physiologically relevant PPAR activators, if not ligands (Figure 5.7). In transient expression assays measuring the stimulation of a PPAR responsive gene, fatty acids with a chain length of at least 10 carbons at concentrations between 50–100μm activate PPARs from different species. Fatty acids with a shorter chain length are much less active in general (Issemann et al, 1993; Keller et al, 1993a; Schmidt et al, 1992; Sher et al, 1993; Göttlicher et al, 1992). Furthermore, the position or number of unsaturated double-bonds have no major effect upon activity with the exception of the xPPARα, which appears to have a preference for polyunsaturated rather than monounsaturated or saturated fatty acids. No difference in activation has been seen between ω-3 and ω-6 fatty acids, in spite of the observation that ω-3 fatty acids, similar to hypolipidemic drugs, are beneficial in lowering blood lipid concentrations (Nestel, 1990). Therefore, it appears that no one fatty acid is an exclusive PPAR activator or ligand. Interestingly, nervonic acid and erucic acid, very long chain monounsaturated fatty acids which are exclusively β-oxidized in peroxisomes, are not able to activate PPARs. In good correlation with this finding but in contrast to other fatty acids, they slow down the β-oxidation process (Flatmark et al, 1983). Since peroxisome proliferators are known to stimulate dicarboxylation of fatty acids, dicarboxylic fatty acids have been tested for their capability to activate PPARs. Surprisingly, dodecanedioic acid is inactive whereas hexadecanedioic acid is one of the most potent activators reported so far. This difference in activation potency may be explained by a difference in the rapidity by which the fatty acids are metabolized. Indeed, thiol-substituted fatty acids that are unable to be metabolized by β-oxidation or the synthetic arachidonic acid analogue 5-,8-,11-,14-eicosatetraynoic acid (ETYA), whose alkyne bonds make it metabolically inert, are amongst the strongest activators. Consistent with this result, molecules derived from arachidonic acid metabolism (prostaglandins, thromboxanes and leukotrienes) are not active. Accordingly, common inhibitors of the known eicosanoid-generating pathways do not abrogate activation by arachidonic acid. Together, all these results support the suggestion that strong activity or weak activity is due to slow or rapid cellular metabolism of the corresponding fatty acids and that unmetabolized fatty acids or their CoA-esters are the activators of PPARs (Keller et al, 1993a; Issemann et al, 1993).

Although not all of the xenobiotics defined as peroxisome proliferators have been tested as PPAR activators, the fact that they stimulate in vivo the activity of enzymes whose encoding genes are PPAR responsive, strongly suggests that most of them are PPAR activators. Among the exceptions there is the natural steroid dehydroepiandrostenedione (DHEA) and acetylsalicylic acid, which are likely to induce peroxisome proliferation by an indirect mechanism (Hertz et al, 1991). While peroxisome proliferators encompass many classes of chemicals (Figure 5.2), they do have some common characteristics such as a lipophilic backbone and an acidic function or are similar in their three-dimensional structure. For instance, the tetrazole function in leukotriene antagonists that stimulate peroxisome proliferation and peroxisomal β-oxidation and the carboxilic function in fibrates are bioisosteres, i.e. they have chemical and physical similarities resulting in broadly similar biological properties. Moreover, models of the three-dimensional organization of peroxisome proliferators suggest that their compact conformation resembles that of oleic acid or possibly other fatty acids (Eacho et al, 1993; Feller and Intrasuksri, 1993; Lake and Lewis, 1993).

Would, therefore, all these various compounds bind directly to PPARs? Interestingly, fatty acids and some peroxisome proliferators are structurally close enough to both directly interact with the liver fatty acid binding protein (FABP) (Cannon and Eacho, 1991; Khan and Sorof, 1994). The direct binding of fatty acids or fatty acyl-CoA to PPARs would occur with PPAR recognition determinants on the acidic function or CoA group and with extra stability provided by hydrophobic interactions with the lipophilic fatty acid backbone (Green and Wahli, 1994). Regarding this hypothesis, it is noteworthy that fatty acids need to be activated by esterification with an acetyl-CoA before being oxidized via the β- as well as ω-oxidation pathways. Furthermore, xenobiotics other than peroxisome proliferators, which contain a carboxilic function, are metabolized via the formation of CoA thioesters (Caldwell, 1984). It is therefore conceivable that the carboxyl group containing peroxisome proliferators can also be activated to a CoA thioester and interact with PPARs as fatty acyl-CoA would do. The above mechanism is also compatible with the substrate overload hypothesis which has been proposed for peroxisome proliferation independently of the discovery and characterization of PPARs (Lock et al, 1989). According to this hypothesis, an excess influx of fatty acids or fatty acyl-CoA into the liver induces the cytochrome P450IVA1 ω-oxidation which converts long chain fatty acids into long-chain dicarboxylic acids. The accumulation of the latter, poorly oxidised in the mitochondria, leads to induction of peroxisomal β-oxidation enzymes. In support of this model, clofibrate-mediated increase in P450IVA1 activity precedes that of peroxisomal β-oxidation enzymes (Kaikaus et al, 1993).

As yet, there is no direct evidence that acyl-CoA thioesters or their dicarboxilic acid derivatives are ligands for PPARs, and other activation mechanisms need to be carefully investigated. For example, peroxisome proliferators and fatty acids could induce the synthesis of a unique PPAR ligand, or they could trigger the release of an unknown second messenger activating PPAR. Alternatively, they could all be metabolized to a common ligand. Thus, determining whether peroxisome proliferators and fatty acids or their metabolites are PPAR ligands remains an important challenge to allow a better understanding of the complex lipid metabolic reactions they appear to modulate.

Peroxisome Proliferator Activated Receptor Target Genes

Peroxisome proliferators induce several enzymes important in intracellular fatty acid metabolism. For defining a link between peroxisome proliferators, activation of PPARs and transcriptional induction of the genes encoding these enzymes, it is crucial to determine a direct implication of these receptors in the regulatory process. Since stimulation of peroxisomal fatty acid β-oxidation is one of the key effects of peroxisome proliferators, genes encoding enzymes of this pathway represent prime candidate target genes of PPARs. The rate-limiting and specificity-defining enzyme of the pathway is acyl-CoA oxidase which is of additional interest because the oxidation reaction it catalyzes produces hydrogen peroxide. The oxidative stress resulting from elevated hydrogen peroxide levels is possibly linked to the carcinogenic effect of peroxisome proliferators. The promoter region and upstream sequences of the rat acyl-CoA oxidase gene have been examined for peroxisome proliferator response elements in transfection experiments. Two PPREs located between -570 and -559 and between -215 and -202 upstream of the transcription initiation site have been identified and tested in their natural promoter context as well as upstream of heterologous promoters (Osumi et al, 1991; Dreyer et al, 1992; Tugwood et al, 1992; Krey et al, 1994). As mentioned above, these regulatory sequences can be defined as DR-1 like elements comprised of two AGGTCA half-sites which are characteristic of receptors having the same P box as PPARs. In the acyl-CoA oxidase promoter, these consensus half-sites are found in the antisense orientation so that the sequence read on the coding strand is a DR-1 composed of two TGACCT (Figure 5.8)

More recently, additional PPREs closely related to the acyl-CoA oxidase PPRE have been found in regulatory sequences of the peroxisomal β-oxidation multifunctional enzyme (enoyl-CoA hydratase/3-

GENE	LOCALISATION OF THE ENZYME ACTIVITY	FUNCTION	RESPONSE ELEMENT
ACO (-570/-558)	peroxisome	1st step in fatty acid β-oxidation	CCCGAACGTGACCTTTGTCCTGGTCC
(-214/-202)			GGGTTTCTTGACCTTCTACCTTGCTC
HD (-2939/-2927)	peroxisome	2d and 3rd step in fatty acid β-oxidation	TGACCTATTGAACTATTACCTACATT
1C-ACS (-123/-106)	peroxisomal membrane ?	Activation of fatty acids by acylation	GATTCATGTGACTGATGCCCTGAAGA
CYP4A6 Z (-650/-662)	microsome	ω-hydroxylation involved in the formation of dicarboxilic acids	CCCTCAACTTTGCCCTAGTTCAGTGT
X (-728/-740)			TTGGACCCTGGCCTTTGTCCTACTTG
MTHMGS (-104/-92)	mitochondrial	Liver ketogenesis (Acetyl CoA metabolism)	TTGTTCTGAGACCTTTGGCCCAGTTT
L-FABP (-68/-56)	cytosolic	Cytosolic binding site for fatty acids	ACAATCACTGACCTATGGCCTATATT
ME (-328/-340)	cytosolic	Malate decarboxilation providing NADPH for fatty acid synthesis	GGAGGGGATCAACTTTGACCCAGAAT
CONSENSUS			TGACCT$\frac{T}{A}$TGNCCT

Figure 5.8 Target genes of PPPARs. Identified PPAR target genes are listed along with the subcellular localization and the function of the proteins they encode. The sequence and position of the PPREs in the promoter of these genes are indicated. Coordinates given in parentheses correspond to the first and last nucleotide of the DR-1 elements whose half-site motifs are indicated by arrows. Conserved nucleotides are highlighted by shading. Hexamer motifs resembling the consensus half-site present in proximity of the DR-1 are marked by dotted arrows. ACO: fatty acyl-CoA oxidase (see Figure 5.1); HD: enoyl-CoA hydratase/3-hydroxyacyl-CoA dehydrogenase (see Figure 5.1); ACS (C1): fatty acyl-CoA synthase (C1 promoter) (see Figure 5.1); CYP4A6: Cytochrome P450 CYP4A6 (fatty acid ω-hydroxylase); MTHMGS: mitochondrial 3-hydroxy-3-methylglutaryl CoA synthase; L-FABP: liver fatty acid binding protein; ME: malic enzyme.

hydroxyacyl-CoA dehydrogenase) (Zhang BW et al, 1992; Bardot et al, 1993; Krey et al, 1993), the rabbit cytochrome P450 CYP4A6 gene encoding a microsomal ω-fatty acid hydroxylase (Krey et al, 1993; Muerhoff et al, 1992), the rat fatty acid binding protein gene (Issemann et al, 1992), the rat long chain acyl CoA synthetase gene (Schoonjans and Auwerx, 1994), the mitochondrial HMG-CoA synthase gene (Rodriguez et al, 1994) and the malic enzyme gene (Baes et al, 1994; IJpenberg et al, 1994) (Figure 5.8). Since the expression of all these genes is affected by peroxisome proliferators in vivo, these findings indicate that PPARs mediate many effects of these compounds. Furthermore, the products of all target genes known so far are part of lipid metabolism pathways in different compartments of the cell: cytosol, microsomes, mitochondria and peroxisomes. Comparative analysis of the PPREs of these genes confirms the organisation of the response element as a DR-1. Interestingly, the so-called spacing nucleotide is always a T or an A, while the third nucleotide of the second half-site, well conserved in other hormone response elements, is indifferently occupied by A, G, T or C in PPREs.

In addition to the identified PPAR target genes, several other genes encoding enzymes positively or negatively regulated by peroxisome proliferators are likely to be controlled by the PPARs. For example, peroxisome proliferators modulate the level of expression of carnitine acyltransferase, carnitine octanoyltransferase, carnitine palmitoyltransferase, 2,4-dienoyl-CoA reductase, liver lipoprotein lipase, apolipoprotein AI, apolipoprotein AIV, hepatic lipase and transthyretin, only to mention a few (Auwerx, 1992; Motojiama et al, 1992; Osmundsen et al, 1991). Further analysis will determine if the promoters of negatively and positively regulated genes contain the same PPRE, in which case specific combinations of transcription factors or special interactions between them would lead to inhibition or stimulation of transcription. Alternatively, putative negative PPREs having a structure different from positive known PPRE may be involved.

Functional Interactions between PPARs and other Transcription Factors

There are several ways by which PPARs could interact with other transcription factors, either members of the nuclear hormone receptor superfamily or other transcriptional activators. For simplicity only three types of functional interactions with other members of the superfamily are mentioned here. First, interaction by heterodimerization is examplified by the PPAR/RXR heterodimers as already discussed above. Indeed, the dual regulation resulting from this association is demonstrated by the fact that peroxisomal β-oxidation genes as well as PPRE-containing chimeric reporter genes are also induced by retinoic acid (Hertz and Bar-Tana, 1992; Keller et al, 1993a) implying a role for RXR. Since several nuclear hormone receptors are capable of forming functional heterodimers with RXR, competition for the RXR partner must exist between PPAR and other receptors in cells expressing several types of these receptors and in which the amount of RXR is the limiting factor. So far, there is no report of heterodimerization between PPAR and a member of the superfamily different from RXR, but this possibility remains open. Second, functional interaction can occur in form of a competition between different receptors for the DR-1 hormone response element. RXR homodimers are able to bind to DR-1 elements (Zhang X-k et al, 1992) but their role in natural promoters is not well assessed. Another example of competition is illustrated by the chicken ovalbumin upstream promoter transcription factor (COUP-TF) which recognizes several differently spaced direct repeat motifs to which it binds as a homodimer. It appears to act as a repressor of the induction of target genes by VDR, TR, and RAR by competing with them for their binding sites (Cooney et al, 1993; Cooney et al, 1992). Similarly, COUP-TF1 also binds to the PPRE, as tested with the multifunctional enzyme gene PPRE, and it antagonizes the action of PPARs (Miyata et al, 1993). Thus, members of the COUP-TF family may also play a role in lipid homeostasis by modulating the PPAR-mediated signalling of fatty acids, hypolipidemic drugs or other xenobiotics and may emerge as possible central regulators of several hormone-responsive pathways. Third, PPARs could also compete with the estrogen receptor for binding to EREs. As previously mentioned, the physiological importance of this putative fatty acid-estrogen interference mechanism needs to be further documented.

So far, little is known about the functional interactions of PPARs with other transcriptional regulators as they may occur on natural promoters. However, interactions with other transcription factors such as CTF/NF-1, Sp1 and AP1, which also modulate transcriptional activity, may occur as described for the estrogen or glucocorticoid receptors. These latter interactions result in both positive and negative regulation of target promoters. We have recently analysed the importance of such interactions for the activity of the acyl-CoA oxidase gene promoter. This PPAR target promoter is TATA-less and, in addition to the two PPREs, contains at least six GC boxes which can bind Sp1, a configuration suggesting a cooperation of PPAR and Sp1 for the control of acyl-CoA oxidase expression. This functional interaction has been demonstrated in *Drosophila* SL-2 cells devoid of the Sp1 factor, by transfection of expression vectors for PPAR, RXR and Sp1, alone or in combination. Little expression is obtained in absence of Sp1 whose presence induces a strong synergistic interaction with the PPAR/RXR heterodimer (Krey, et al, 1994b). Interestingly, in addition to the acyl-CoA oxidase gene, the gene encoding the multifunctional enzyme is also controlled by TATA-less promoter containing Sp1 sites. Along the same line of thought, the promoter of the mPPARα gene has no TATA nor CCAAT elements but comprises seven putative Sp1 binding sites. It is not yet known if this promoter is itself regulated by PPAR.

Conclusions

The data accumulated so far are in favor of a model in which PPARs are the mediators of the signalling actions of fatty acids, hypolipidemic drugs and other peroxisome proliferators (Figure 5.9). According to this model,

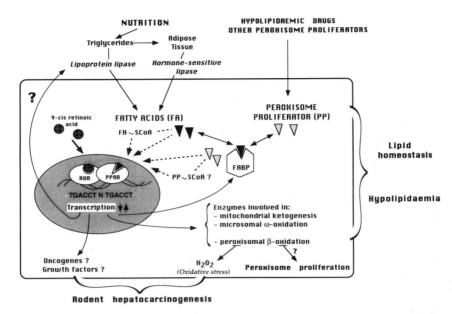

Figure 5.9 Model of the peroxisome proliferator and fatty acid signaling action. Free fatty acids are released from circulating triglycerides upon action of the lipoprotein lipase. In the target cell cytoplasm, fatty acids or peroxisome proliferators (PP) are bound to the fatty acid binding protein (FABP) and enter the nucleus, possibly after esterification, and activate PPARs. PPARs, as heterodimers with RXR, bind to a DR-1 response element within the promoter of target genes. The resulting effect is a modulation, positive or negative, of the expression of the responsive genes. This results in lipid homeostasis in the normal situation, or in hypolipidaemia, peroxisome proliferation and hepatocarcinogenesis (rodents) in pharmacological situations.

and in analogy to other receptors that are members of the superfamily, PPARs are directly activated by these compounds. The receptors then regulate the expression of genes by interacting with specific response elements associated with these target genes. Alternatively, peroxisome proliferators that bind to the cellular fatty acid binding protein (FABP) (Cannon and Eacho, 1991; Khan and Sorof, 1994), displace the fatty acids whose increased intracellular levels may activate the PPARs. However, since fatty acids and peroxisome proliferators compete for binding to FABP, it is conceivable that they also compete for direct binding to PPARs. There are obvious parallels between this model and the mode of action of retinoic acid and possibly thyroid hormones. Retinoic acid and thyroid hormones bind to cellular binding proteins, CRABP and CTBP (Hashizume et al, 1989), respectively, and to nuclear hormone receptors, the retinoic acid receptors (RAR) and the thyroid hormone receptors (TR). Interestingly, the three types of nuclear receptors, PPAR, RAR and TR are related members of the same subfamily and therefore are thought to be derived from a common ancestor. In parallel, FABP and CRABP are also related (Jones et al, 1988) and thus, may originate from a common ancestral gene. Since the primary structure of CTBP is not known as yet, its affiliation can not be determined. Thus, the three aforementioned signalling pathways may present a homologous coevolution pattern between, on one hand, cytoplasmic proteins thought to regulate cellular free fatty acid, retinoic acid or thyroid hormone concentrations and, on the other hand, the nuclear receptors, PPAR, RAR and TR which mediate the biological action of fatty acids, retinoic acid and thyroid hormones through control of gene activity. In this respect, it is not surprising that these three receptors share some common functional properties such as a constitutive nuclear localisation, a response element structured as a direct repeat and a preference for heterodimerization with RXR. Together, this argues in favor of fatty acids or their activated CoA-esters as natural ligands of PPARs, just like retinoic acid and T3 directly bind to their receptors. However, this remains to be demonstrated.

If the effects of peroxisome proliferators described herein are all mediated by PPARs, these receptors represent a unique possibility for understanding more about peroxisome proliferation and nonmutagenic hepatocarcinogenesis in rodents. The oxidative stress hypothesis proposes that hydrogen peroxide, produced by the increase in peroxisomal fatty acid β-oxidation accumulates because the level of catalase, which destroys it, is not increased in proportion. This results in oxidative damage of DNA and possibly tumor initiation (Reddy and Lalwani, 1983). In favor of an alternative mechanism, compounds leading to a similar level of peroxisome proliferation such as the hypolipidemic drug pirinixic acid (Wy-14,643) and the plasticizer di(2-ethyhexyl) phthalate (DEHP) have a weak and strong carcinogenic potency which correlates with their low and high mitogenic effects, respectively (Marsman et al, 1988). This suggests that the carcinogenicity of peroxisome proliferators depends on their role in growth and differentiation. In this process, PPARs could act by altering the expression of relevant genes such as oncogenes, or genes encoding growth factors and their receptors. In agreement with this hypothesis, peroxisome proliferators stimulate the expression of several proto-oncogenes, but so far a direct action of PPARs in this induction has not been described (Latruffe et al, 1993). Since there are marked differences among species in their responsiveness to peroxisome proliferators with respect to carcinogenesis, a thorough examination of the function of PPARs in humans is important to assess the hazard these compounds may represent. More interestingly, understanding the molecular bases of these differences may reveal crucial steps in the carcinogenic process.

The initial interest in peroxisome proliferators and particularly the fibrate class of hypolipidemic drugs was due to their capacity to lower serum triglyceride levels (Havel and Kane, 1973). Cholesterol also is lowered albeit with less efficiency. Therefore, these compounds are preferentially used in patients with severe hypertriglyceridemia which represents a major risk factor for the development of atherosclerosis and its consequences with respect to coronary heart disease. Possible mechanisms of their mode of action are through an increase in lipoprotein lipase activity which lowers the blood level of triglycerides and increases the intracellular level of fatty acids. The action on cholesterol might be through a decrease in its synthesis or an increased conversion of cholesterol to bile acids (Grundy et al, 1972; Sodhi et al, 1971). However, a direct link between the receptors and the expression of potential PPAR target genes involved in these pathways has not yet been established. With therapeutic goals in mind, identification of the ligand molecules, possibly the hypolipidemic drugs themselves or their activated form as mentioned above, will help to understand more about the structure function relationship of PPAR. Such analyses should improve the design not only of new hypolipidemic drugs but also of herbicides, plastizicers or leukotriene antogonists devoid of carcinogenic effects.

One of the fascinating fields now beginning to open is the key role that peroxisome proliferator activated receptors appear to play in lipid metabolism and homeostasis. All target genes identified and discussed herein are involved in fatty acid catabolism rather than in the lipogenic pathways, indicating that they may occupy a key position in a general control system that copes with an overload of fatty acids. This may occur after normal food intake or, more particularly, with high fat diets and pathological conditions, such as diabetes, leading to high serum lipid concentrations. The function of PPARs is likely to be important also during development or early life, especially at stages of lipid metabolism adjustments resulting from changes in nutritional regimens (Girard et al, 1994). If it is confirmed that fatty acids, or perhaps their CoA esters, are natural ligands of PPARs, it would imply that nutritional fatty acids act like retinoids, steroid or thyroid hormones in their control of gene expression. We propose that PPARs are key control elements in the nutrient/gene interactions, which regulate gene expression for the control of tissue fuel selection with respect to the substrate competition between fatty acids and glucose. Indeed, glucose after its phosphorylation to glucose-6-phosphate can activate transcription of glycolytic genes on one hand and lipogenic genes on the other hand, a phenomenon that is insulin-dependent or independent according to the cell type (Vaulont and

Kahn, 1994). If our proposal is correct, fatty acids should have an inhibitory effect on lipogenic enzyme gene expression. Indeed, the first illustration of this proposal is that a diet enriched in polyunsaturated fatty acids inhibits the fatty acid synthase gene expression in liver (Girard et al, 1994). It is now of interest to clarify whether PPARs are directly involved in the repression of this gene and possibly other lipogenic and glycolytic genes. Conversely, genes mainly involved in fatty acid catabolism that are stimulated by fatty acids would be negatively regulated by high glucose levels.

In conclusion, fatty acids as major dietary constituents, participate in concert with several hormones in the regulation of gene expression in response to food intake or nutritional changes. We think that PPARs are one of the central regulators of these nutrient/gene interactions.

Acknowledgments

We thank J. Auwerx, J-Å Gustafsson, M. Greene, D. Haro, M. Lazar for communicating results prior to publication; V. Laudet for help with the preparation of the evolutionary trees; E. Farmer, H. Keller, G. Krey for discussion of the manuscript. The work done in the authors' laboratory was supported by the Etat de Vaud and the Swiss National Science Foundation.

References

Auwerx J (1992): Regulation of gene expression by fatty acids and fibric acid derivatives : An integrative role for peroxisome proliferator activated receptors. *Horm Res* 38: 269–277

Baes M, Castelein H, Declercq PE (1994): The malic enzyme promoter contains multiple recognition sites for nuclear hormone receptors. *J Cell Biochem* 18B: 361

Bardot O, Aldridge TC, Latruffe N, Green S (1993): PPAR-RXR heterodimer activates a peroxisome proliferator response element upstream of the bifunctional enzyme gene. *Biochem Biophys Res Commun* 192: 37–45

Beck F, Plummer S, Senior PV, Byrne S, Green S, Brammar WJ (1992): The ontogeny of peroxisome-proliferator-activated receptor gene expression in the mouse and rat. *Proc Royal Soc Lond [Biol]* 247: 83–87

Braissant O, Wahli W (1994): unpublished observation

Caldwell J (1984): Xenobiotic acyl-coenzymes A critical intermediates in the biochemical pharmacology and toxicology of carboxylic acids. *Biochem Society Trans* 12: 9–11

Cannon JR, Eacho PI (1991): Interaction of LY171883 and other peroxisome proliferators with fatty-acid-binding protein isolated from rat liver. *Biochem J* 280: 387–391

Chawla A, Lazar MA (1994): Peroxisome proliferator and retinoid signaling pathways co-regulate preadipocyte phenotype and survival. *Proc Natl Acad Sci USA* 91: 1786–1790

Chen F, Law SN, O'Malley BW (1993): Identification of two mPPAR related receptors and evidence for the existence of five subfamily members. *Biochem Biophys Res Comm* 196: 671–677

Ciolek E, Dauça M (1991): The effect of clofibrate on amphibian hepatic peroxisomes. *Biol Cell* 71: 313–320

Cooney AJ, Leng XH, Tsai SY, O'Malley BW, Tsai MJ (1993): Multiple mechanisms of chicken ovalbumin upstream promoter transcription factor-dependent repression of transactivation by the vitamin-D, thyroid hormone, and retinoic acid receptors. *J Biol Chem* 268: 4152–4160

Cooney AJ, Tsai SY, O'Malley BW, Tsai MJ (1992): Chicken ovalbumin upstream promoter transcription factor (COUP-TF) dimers bind to different GGTCA response elements, allowing COUP-TF to repress hormonal induction of the Vitamin-D(3), Thyroid hormone, and Retinoic acid receptors. *Mol Cell Biol* 12: 4153–4163

Dayton AI, Selden JR, Laws G, Dorney DJ, Finan J, Tripputi P, Emanuel BS, Roveera G, Nowell PC, Croce C (1984): A human c-*erb*A oncogene homologue is closely proximal to the chromosome 17 breakpoint in acute promyelocytic leukemia. *Proc Natl Acad Sci USA* 81: 4495–4499

Desvergne B (1994): How do thyroid hormone receptors bind to structurally diverse response elements? *Mol Cell Endocrinol*: 100: 125–131

Dingwall C, Laskey RA (1991): Nuclear Targeting Sequences - A Consensus. *Trends Biochem Sci* 16: 478–481

Drabkin H, Kao F-T, Hartz J, Hart I, Gazdar A, Weinberger C, Evans R, Gerber M (1988): Localization of human ERBA2 to the 3p22-3p24.1 region of chromosome 3 and variable deletion in small cell lung cancer. *Proc Natl Acad Sci USA* 85: 9258–9262

Dreyer C, Keller H, Mahfoudi A, Laudet V, Krey G, Wahli W (1993): Positive regulation of the peroxisomal β-oxidation pathway by fatty acids through activation of peroxisome proliferator activated receptors (PPAR). *Biol Cell* 77: 67–76

Dreyer C, Krey G, Keller H, Givel F, Helftenbein G, Wahli W (1992): Control of the peroxisomal beta-oxidation pathway by a novel family of nuclear hormone receptors. *Cell* 68: 879–887

Eacho PI, Foxworthy PS, Herron DK (1993): Tetrazole substituted acetophenone peroxisome proliferators: structure-activity relationships and effects on hepatic lipid metabolism. In: *Peroxisomes: Biology and Importance in Toxicology and Medicine*, Gibson G, Lake B, eds. London: Taylor & Francis

Ellinger-Ziegelbauer H, Hihi AK, Laudet V, Keller H, Wahli W, Dreyer C (1994): FTZ-F1-related orphan receptors in *Xenopus laevis*: transcriptional regulators differentially expressed during early embryogenesis. *Mol Cell Biol* 14:2786–2797

Feller DR, Intrasuksri U (1993): Structural requirements for peroxisome proliferation by phenoxyacetic and fatty acid analogues in primary cultures of rat hepatocytes. In: *Peroxisomes: Biology and Importance in Toxicology and Medicine*, Gibson G, Lake B, eds. London: Taylor & Francis

Flatmark T, Christiansen EN (1993): Modulation of peroxisomal biogenesis and lipid metabolizing enzymes by dietary factors. In: *Peroxisomes: Biology and Importance in Toxicology and Medicine*, Gibson G, Lake B eds. London: Taylor & Francis

Flatmark T, Christiansen EN, Kryvi H (1983): Evidence for a negative modulating effect of erucic acid on the peroxisomal beta-oxidation enzyme system and biogenesis in rat liver. *Biochem Biophys Acta* 753: 460–466

Flatmark T, Nilsson A, Krames J, Eikhom T-S, Fukami MH, Kryvi H, Christiansen EN (1988): On the mechanism of induction of the enzyme systems for peroxisomal *β*-oxidation of fatty acids in rat liver by diets rich in partially hydrogenated fish oil. *Biochem Biophys Acta* 962: 122–130

Forman BM, Samuels HH (1990): Interactions among a subfamily of nuclear hormone receptors : the regulatory zipper model. *Mol Endocrinol* 4: 1293–1301

Forman BM, Yang C-R, Au M, Casanova J, Ghysdael J, Samuels HH (1989): A domain containing leucine-zipper-like motifs mediate novel *in vivo* interactions between the thyroid hormone and retinoic acid receptors. *Mol Endocrinol* 3: 1610–1626

Gearing KL, Crickmore A, Gustafsson JÅ (1994): Structure of the mouse peroxisome proliferator activated receptor α gene. *Biochem Biophysic Res Comm*: 199: 255–263

Gearing KL, Göttlicher M, Teboul M, Widmark E, Gustafsson JA (1993): Interaction of the peroxisome-proliferator-activated receptor and retinoid X receptor. *Proc Natl Acad Sci USA* 90: 1440–1444

Girard J, Perdereau D, Foufelle F, Prip-Buus C, Ferré P (1994): Regulation of lipogenic enzyme expression by nutrients and hormones. *FASEB J* 8: 36–42

Göttlicher ME, Widmark E, Li Q, Gustafsson JA (1992): Fatty acids activate a chimera of the clofibric acid-activated receptor and the glucocorticoid receptor. *Proc Natl Acad Sci USA* 89: 4653–4657

Green S (1992): Receptor-mediated mechanisms of peroxisome proliferators. *Biochem Pharmacol* 43: 393–401

Green S, Wahli W (1994): Peroxisome proliferator activated receptors: finding the orphan a home. *Mol Cell Endocrinol* 100: 149–153

Greene ME, Blumberg B, McBride OW, Yi HF, Kronquist K, Kwan K, Hsieh L, Greene GL, Nimer SD (1994): personal communication

Gronemeyer H (1992): Control of transcription activation by steroid hormone receptors. *FASEB J* 6: 2524–2529

Grundy SM, Ahrens EH, Salen G, Nestel SPH, Nestel PJ (1972): Mechanisms of action of clofibrate on cholesterol metabolism in patients with hyperlipidemia. *J Lipid Res* 13: 531–551

Hashizume K, Miyamoto T, Ichikawa K, Sakurai A, Ohtsuka H, Kobayashi M, Nishii Y, Yamada T (1989): Evidence for the presence of two active forms of cytosolic 3,5,3'-triiodo-L-thyronine (T3)-binding protein (CTBP) in rat kidney. *J Biol Chem* 264: 4864–4871

Havel RJ, Kane JP (1973): Drugs and lipid metabolism. *Annu Rev Pharmacol* 13: 287–308

Hertz R, Bar-Tana J (1992): Induction of peroxisomal beta-oxidation genes by retinoic acid in cultured rat hepatocytes. *Biochem J* 281: 41–43

Hertz R, Aurbach R, Hashimoto T, Bar-Tana J (1991): Thyromimetic effect of peroxisomal proliferators in rat liver. *Biochem J* 274: 745–751

Hess R, Staubli W, Reiss W (1965): Nature of the hepatomegalic effect produced by ethyl-chlorophenoxy-isobutyrate in the rat. *Nature* 208: 856–859

Hirst MA, Hinck L, Danielsen M, Ringold GM (1992): Discrimination of DNA response elements for thyroid hormone and estrogen is dependent on dimerization of receptor DNA binding domains. *Proc Natl Acad Sci USA* 89: 5527–5531

Hori S, Ishii H, Suga T (1981): Changes in peroxisomal fatty acid oxidation in diabetic rat liver. *J Biochem* 90: 1691–1696

IJpenburg A, Desvergne B, Wahli W (1994): unpublished observation

Issemann I, Green S (1990): Activation of a member of the steroid hormone receptor superfamily by peroxisome proliferators. *Nature* 347: 645–650

Issemann I, Prince RA, Tugwood JD, Green S (1992): A role for fatty acids and liver fatty acid binding protein in peroxisome proliferation? *Biochem Soc Trans* 20: 824–827

Issemann I, Prince RA, Tugwood JD, Green S (1993): The peroxisome proliferator activated receptor: retinoid X receptor heterodimer is activated by fatty acids and fibrate hypolipidemic drugs. *J Molec Endocrinol* 11: 37–47

Jones TA, Bergfors T, Sedzik J, Unge T (1988):The three-dimensional structure of P2 myelin protein. *EMBO J* 7: 1597–1604

Kaikaus RM, Chan WK, Lysenko N, Ray R, De Montellano PRO, Bass NM (1993): Induction of peroxisomal fatty acid beta-oxidation and liver fatty acid-binding protein by peroxisome proliferators - mediation via the cytochrome P-450IVA1 omega-hydroxylase pathway. *J Biol Chem* 268: 9593–9603

Keller H, Dreyer C, Medin J, Mahfoudi A, Ozato K, Wahli W (1993a): Fatty acids and retinoids control lipid metabolism through activation of peroxisome proliferator-activated receptor-retinoid X receptor heterodimers. *Proc Natl Acad Sci USA* 90: 2160–2164

Keller H, Mahfoudi A, Dreyer C, Hihi AK, Medin J, Ozato K, Wahli W (1993b): Peroxisome proliferator activated receptors and lipid metabolism. *Ann NY Acad Sci* 684: 157–173

Keller H, Wahli W (1994): unpublished observation

Keller H, Wahli W (1993): Peroxisome proliferator-activated receptors: A link between endocrinology and nutrition? *Trends Endocrinol Metab* 4: 291–296

Keese PK, Gibbs A (1992): Origins of genes: 'Big bang' or continuous creation? *Proc Natl Acad Sci USA* 89: 9489–9493

Khan SH, Sorof S (1994): Liver fatty acid-binding protein: specific mediator of the mitogenesis induced by two classes of carcinogenic peroxisome proliferators. *Proc Natl Acad Sci USA* 91: 848–852

Kliewer SA, Umesono K, Noonan DJ, Heyman RA, Evans RM (1992): Convergence of 9-Cis retinoic acid and peroxisome proliferator signalling pathways through heterodimer formation of their receptors. *Nature* 358: 771–774

Knoll AH (1992): The early evolution of eukaryotes – a geological perspective. *Science* 256: 622–627

Krey G, Keller H, Mahfoudi A, Medin J, Ozato K, Dreyer C, Wahli W (1993): *Xenopus* peroxisome proliferator activated receptors: genomic organization, response element recognition, heterodimer formation with RXR and activation by fatty acids. *J Steroid Biochem Mol Biol* 47: 65–73

Krey G, Keller H, Mahfoudi A, Wahli W (1994a): PPARs : nuclear hormone receptors controlling peroxisomal fatty acid β-oxidation. In: *Peroxisomal Disorders in Relation to Functions and Biogenesis of Peroxisomes*, Wansers RJA, Schutgens RBH, Tabak HF, eds. Amsterdam: Elsevier Science bv

Krey G, Mahfoudi A, Wahli W (1994b): unpublished observation

Lake BG, Lewis DFV (1993): Structure-activity relationships for chemically induced peroxisome proliferation in mammalian liver. In: *Peroxisomes: Biology and Importance in Toxicology and Medicine*, Gibson G, Lake B, eds. London: Taylor & Francis

Lalwani ND, Fahl WE, Reddy JK (1983): Detection of a nafenopin-binding protein in a rat liver cytosol associated with the induction of peroxisome proliferation by hypolipidemic compounds. *Biochem Biophys Res Commun* 116: 389–393

Latruffe N, Bugaut M, Bournot P, Benteja M, Ramirez LC, Cherakaoui Malki M (1993): Molecular basis of gene regulation by peroxisome proliferators. In: *Peroxisomes: Biology and Importance in Toxicology and Medicine*, Gibson G, Lake B, eds. London: Taylor & Francis

Laudet V, Begue A, Henryduthoit C, Joubel A, Martin P, Stehelin D, Saule S (1991): Genomic organization of the human thyroid hormone receptor-alpha (c-erbA-1) gene. *Nucleic Acids Res* 19: 1105–1112

Laudet V, Hanni C, Coll J, Catzeflis F, Stehelin D (1992): Evolution of the nuclear receptor gene superfamily. *EMBO J* 11: 1003–1013

Lazar MA, Hodin RA, Darling DS, Chin WW (1989): A novel member of the thyroid/steroid hormone receptor family is encoded by the opposite strand of the rat c-*erbA*α transcriptional unit. *Mol Cell Biol* 9: 1128–1136

Lazarow P, deDuve C (1976): A fatty acyl-CoA oxidizing system in the rat liver peroxisomes: enhancement by clofibrate, a hypolipidemic drug. *Proc Natl Acad Sci USA* 73: 2042–2046

Lee MS, Kliewer SA, Provencal J, Wright PE, Evans RM (1993): Structure of the retinoid X receptor α DNA binding domain: A helix required for homodimeric DNA binding. *Science* 260: 1117–1121

Lehmann JM, Hoffmann B, Pfahl M (1991): Genomic organization of the retinoic acid receptor gamma-gene. *Nucleic Acids Res* 19: 573–578

Leid M, Kastner P, Chambon P (1992): Multiplicity generates diversity in the retinoic acid signalling pathways. *Trends Biochem Sci* 17: 427–433

Lock EA, Mitchell AM, Elcombe CR (1989): Biochemical mechanisms of induction of hepatic peroxisome proliferation. *Ann Rev Pharmacol Toxicol* 29: 145–163

Luisi BV, Xu WX, Otwinowski Z, Freedman LP, Yamamoto KR, Sigler PB (1991): Crystallographic analysis of the interaction of the glucocorticoid receptor with DNA. *Nature* 352: 497–505

Mader S, Kumar V, de Verneuil H, Chambon P (1989): Three amino acids of the oestrogen receptor are essential to its ability to distinguish an oestrogen from a glucocorticoid-responsive element. *Nature* 338: 271–274

Mannaerts GP, Van Veldhoven PP (1993): Role of peroxisomes in mammalian metabolism. In: *Peroxisomes: Biology and Importance in Toxicology and Medicine*, Gibson G, Lake B, eds London: Taylor & Francis

Marsman DS, Cattley RC, Conway JG, Popp JA (1988): Relationship of hepatic peroxisome proliferation and replicative DNA synthesis to the hepatocarcinogenicity of the peroxisome proliferators di(2-ethyl-hexil)phthalate and [4-chloro-6-(2,3-xylidino)-2-pyrimidinylthio]acetic acid (Wy 14,643) in rats. *Cancer Res* 48: 6739–6744

Martinez E, Wahli W (1991): Characterization of hormone response elements. In: *Nuclear Hormone Receptors*, Parker MG, ed. London: Harcourt Brace Jovanovitch

Mattei MG, Rivière M, Krust A, Ingvarsson S, Vennstrom B, Islam MQ, Levan G,

Kautner P, Zelent A, Chambon P (1991): Chromosomal assignment of retinoic acid receptor (RAR) genes in the human, mouse, and rat gnomes. *Genomics* 10: 1061–1069

Miyajima NR, Horiuchi R, Shibuya Y, Fukushige SI, Matsubara KI, Toyoshima K, Yamamoto T (1989): Two erbA-homologs encoding proteins with different T3 binding capacities are transcribed from opposite DNA strands of the same genetic locus. *Cell* 57: 31-39

Miyata KS, Zhang B, Marcus SL, Capone JP, Rachubinski RA (1993): Chicken Ovalbumin upstream promoter transcription factor (COUP-TF) binds to a peroxisome proliferator-responsive element and antagonizes peroxisome proliferator-mediated signaling. *J Biol Chem* 268: 19169–19172

Motojiama K, Goto S, Imanaka T (1992): Specific repression of transthyrethin gene expression in rat liver by a peroxisome proliferator clofibrate. *Biochem Biophys Res Comm* 188: 799–806

Muerhoff AS, Griffin KJ, Johnson EF (1992): The peroxisome proliferator-activated receptor mediates the induction of CYP4A6, a cytochrome-P450 fatty-acid omega-hydroxylase, by clofibric acid. *J Biol Chem* 267: 19051–19053

Neat CE, Thomassen S, Osmundsen H (1980): Induction of peroxisomal β-oxidation in rat liver by high-fat diets. *Biochem J* 186: 369–371

Nemali MR, Reddy MK, Usuda N, Reddy PG, Comeau LD, Rao MS, Reddy JK (1989): Differential induction and regulation of peroxisomal enzymes: predictive value of peroxisome proliferation in identifying certain nonmutagenic carcinogens. *Toxicol Appl Pharmacol* 97: 72–87

Nesel PJ (1990): Effects of n-3 fatty acids on lipid metabolism. *Annu Rev Nutr* 10: 149–167

Norum KR, Christiansen EN, Christopherson BO, Bremer J (1989): Metabolic and nutritional aspects of long chain fatty acids of marine origin. In: *The Role of Fat in Human Nutrition*, Vergroesen AJ, Crawford M, eds. London: Academic Press

Orellana M, Fuentes O, Rosenbluth H, Lara M, Valdez E (1992): Modulation of rat liver peroxisomal and microsomal fatty acid oxidation by starvation. *FEBS Letters* 310:193–196

Orton TC, Adam HK, Bentley M, Holloway B, Tucker MJ (1984): Species differences in the morphological response of the liver following chronic clofibrate administration. *Toxicol Appl Pharmacol* 73: 138–151

Osmundsen H, Bremer J, Pedersen JI (1991): Metabolic aspects of peroxisomal beta-oxidation. *Biochim Biophys Acta* 1085: 141–158

Osumi T, Wen JK, Hashimoto T (1991): Two cis-acting regulatory sequences in the peroxisome proliferator-responsive enhancer region of rat acyl-CoA oxidase gene. *Biochem Biophys Res Commun* 175: 866–871

Parker MG (1993): Steroid and related receptors. *Current Opinion in Cellular Biology* 5: 499–504

Rao MS, Reddy JK (1987): Peroxisome proliferation and hepatocarcinogenesis. *Carcinogenesis* 8: 631–636

Reddy JK, Lalwani ND (1983): Carcinogenesis by hepatic peroxisome proliferators: evaluation of the risk of hypolipidemic drugs and industrial plasticizers to humans. *CRC Crit Rev Toxicol* 12: 1–58

Ritchie HH, Wang L-H, Tsai S, O'Malley BW, Tsai MJ (1990): COUP-TF gene : a structure unique for the steroi/thyroid receptor family. *Nucleic Acids Res* 18: 6857–6862

Rodriguez JC, Gil-Gomez G, Hegardt FG, Haro D (1994): The peroxisome proliferator-activated receptor mediates the induction of the mitochondrial 3-hydroxy-3-methylglutaryl-CoA synthase gene by fatty acids. *J Biol Chem*: in press

Schmidt A, Endo N, Rutledge SJ, Vogel R, Shinar D, Rodan GA (1992): Identification of a new member of the steroid hormone receptor superfamily that is activated by a peroxisome proliferator and fatty acids. *Mol Endocrinol* 6: 1634–1641

Schoonjans K, Auwerx J (1994): personal communication

Segraves WA, Hogness DS (1990): The E75 ecdysone-inducible gene responsible for the 75B early puff in Drosophila encodes two new members of the steroid receptor superfamily. *Genes & Dev* 4: 204–219

Sher T, Yi HF, Mcbride OW, Gonzalez FJ (1993): cDNA cloning, chromosomal mapping, and functional characterization of the human peroxisome proliferator activated receptor. *Biochemistry* 32: 5598–5604

Shi Y-B, Yaoita Y, Brown DD (1992): Genomic organization and alternative promoter usage of the two thyroid hormone receptor β genes in Xenopus-laevis. *J Biol Chem* 267: 733–738

Sitori CR, Catapano A, Proletti R (1977): Therapeutic significance of hypolipidemic and antiatherosclerotic drugs. *Atherosclerosis Rev* 2: 113–153

Small GM (1993): Peroxisome biogenesis. In: *Peroxisomes: Biology and Importance in Toxicology and Medicine*, Gibson G, Lake B, eds. London: Taylor & Francis

Sodhi, HS, Kudchodkar BJ, Horlick L, Weder CH (1971): Effects of chlorophenoxyisobutyrate on the synthesis and metabolism on cholesterol in man. *Metabolism* 20: 348–359

Tugwood JD, Issemann I, Anderson RG, Bundell KR, McPheat WL, Green S (1992): The mouse peroxisome proliferator activated receptor recognizes a response element in the 5' flanking sequence of the rat acyl CoA oxidase gene. *EMBO J* 11: 433–439

Umesono K, Evans RM (1989): Determinants of target gene specificity for steroid/thyroid hormone receptors. *Cell* 57: 1139–1146

Vaulont S, Kahn A (1994): Transcriptional control of metabolic genes by carbohydrates. *FASEB J* 8: 28–35

Wahli W, Martinez E (1991): Superfamily of steroid nuclear receptors: positive and negative regulators of gene expression. *FASEB J* 5: 2243–2249

Wilson TE, Fahrner TJ, Johnston M, Milbrandt J (1991): Identification of the DNA binding site for NGF1-B by genetic selection in yeast. *Science* 252: 1296–1300

Wilson TE, Paulsen RE, Padgett KA, Milbrandt J (1992): Participation of non-zinc finger residues in DNA binding by two nuclear orphan receptors. *Science* 256: 107–110

Ylikomi T, Bocquel MT, Berry M, Gronemeyer H, Chambon P (1992): Cooperation of protosignals for nuclear accumulation of estrogen and progesterone receptors. *EMBO J* 11: 3681–3694

Zhang BW, Marcus SL, Sajjadi FG, Alvares K, Reddy JK, Subramani S, Rachubinski RA, Capone JP (1992): Identification of a peroxisome proliferator-responsive element upstream of the gene encoding rat peroxisomal Enoyl-CoA Hydratase/3-Hydroxyacyl-CoA Dehydrogenase. *Proc Natl Acad Sci USA* 89: 7541–7545

Zhang X-k, Hoffman B, V Tran P-B, Graupner G, Pfahl M (1992): Retinoid X receptor is an auxiliary protein for thyroid hormone and retinoic acid receptors. *Nature* 355: 442–446

Zhang X-k, Pfahl M (1993): Regulation of retinoid and thyroid hormone action through homodimeric and heterodimeric receptors. *Trends Endocrinol Metab* 4: 156–162

Zhu Y, Alvars K, Huang Q, Rao MS, Reddy JK (1993): Cloning of a new member of the peroxisome proliferator-activated receptor gene family from mouse liver. *J Biol Chem* 258: 26817–26820

6

Mechanism of Signal Transduction by the basic Helix-Loop-Helix Dioxin Receptor

Lorenz Poellinger

Introduction: Biological Effects of Dioxins and Structurally Related Environmental Contaminants

Dioxins (most notably 2,3,7,8-tetrachlorodibenzo-*p*-dioxin, TCDD, Figure 6.1) and related halogenated aromatic hydrocarbons (e.g. poly-chlorinated biphenyls and dibenzofurans) are a class of man-made pollutants which are ubiquitously present in the environment. They are of no commercial use but are formed as unwanted by-products during the production of certain herbicides, defoliants (e.g. Agent Orange) and insecticides. In addition, incomplete combustion of organic halogenated compounds in municipal and industrial incinerators is also a well-documented source of these compounds. Strikingly, dioxins have a biological half-life in humans of the order of a decade, and, due to their pronounced biological and chemical stability, they have become widespread environmental contaminants which can be expected to accumulate within the food chain and persist throughout the ecosystem in the future (Safe, 1990; Gallo et al, 1991).

Dioxins and related compounds give rise to a plethora of biochemical and toxic responses in experimental animal (particularly rodent) models, includ-ing immunosuppression, thymic involution, liver damage, severe epithelial disorders, birth defects, tumor promotion, and a dramatic wasting syndrome ultimately leading to death (Poland Knutson, 1982; Safe, 1986; 1990). In humans the most characteristic effect of dioxins is a hyperkeratotic and metaplastic response of the hair follicles and intrafollicular epidermis, leading to persistent acne-like lesions (Suskind, 1985). Although a number of recent epidemiological studies indicate an increasing number of cancer cases emerging from exposed populations, the biological effects of dioxins on humans are a matter of intense debate (Axelson, 1993; Bailar, 1991). However, exposure of both human and rodent cells to concentrations of

INDUCIBLE GENE EXPRESSION, VOLUME 1
P.A. Baeuerle, Editor
© 1995 Birkhäuser Boston

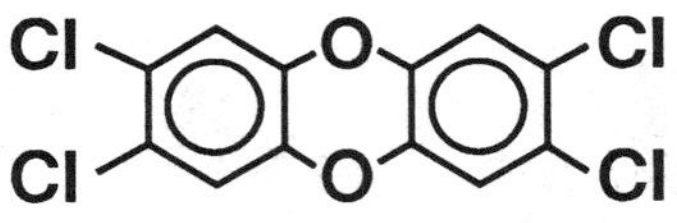

2,3,7,8-Tetrachlorodibenzo-*p*-dioxin

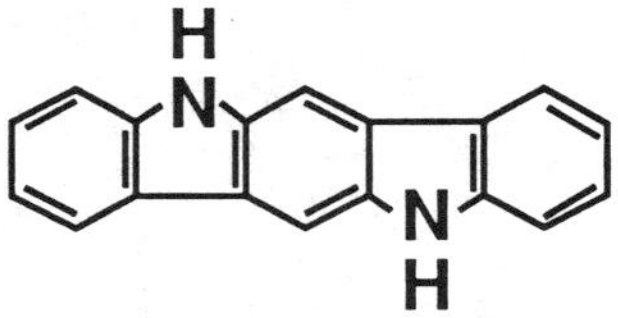

Indolo[3,2-*b*]carbazole

Figure 6.1 Examples of two different classes of ligands of the dioxin receptor: environmental contaminants (2,3,7,8-tetrachlorodibenzo-*p*-dioxin, TCDD), and ligands of dietary origin (indolo[3,2-*b*]carbazole, ICZ).

dioxins in the nM range results in very potent induction of transcription of a battery of genes encoding drug metabolizing enzymes including, for instance, cytochrome P-450IA1, glutathione *S*-transferase Ya and NADP(H):quinone reductase (Nebert and Gonzales, 1986; Fujii-Kuriyama et al, 1992; Poellinger et al, 1992; Whitlock, 1993). Interestingly, in certain target cells the dioxin receptor also appears to regulate the transcription of growth modulatory genes, i.e. the plasminogen activator inhibitor-2 and interleukin-1β genes (Sutter et al, 1991), in addition to inducing the expression of a battery of genes encoding drug metabolizing enzymes. Induction studies of drug metabolizing enzymes in different inbred highly responsive (e.g. C56BL) and less responsive (e.g. DBA2) strains of mice have documented responsiveness as an autosomal dominant trait (Poland and Knutson, 1982; Nebert and Gonzales, 1986) and suggested at an early stage the cytochrome P-450IA1 induction response is mediated by a receptor protein: the dioxin receptor (also termed aryl hydrocarbon receptor). The receptor model has been further substantiated using wild-type and mutant hepatoma cell lines (Hankinson, 1983; Whitlock, 1993), and the use of dioxin-responsive versus dioxin-resistant strains of mice has implicated the dioxin receptor not only in enzyme induction processes but also in other biological responses to dioxin, e.g. thymic involution, cleft palate formation and hepatic porphyria (Poland and Knutson, 1982; Safe, 1986; 1990).

The Dioxin Receptor: A Ligand-activated Nuclear Receptor

The dioxin receptor was originally detected using ligand binding assays, and found to be an intracellular protein able to bind dioxin (used here to refer specifically to TCDD) with saturable high affinity ($K_d \approx 1nM$) and specificity for planar aromatic congeners of dioxin as well as polocyclic aromatic hydrocarbons such as benzo(a)pyrene and 3-methylcholanthrene (Poland and Knutson, 1982). Noncovalent and covalent labeling studies (Poland et al, 1986; Wilhelmsson et al, 1986) as well as immuno-chemical experiments (Poland et al, 1991; Whitelaw et al, 1993b) have revealed a molecular weight of about 100 kDa for the receptor monomer which is present in low abundance (around 3,000 to 5,000 molecules per cell) in virtually all rodent tissues or human cells examined (Poellinger et al, 1992; Gradin et al, 1993). Although the receptor is phosphorylated (Berghard et al, 1993), the functional significance of this phosphorylation has not yet been clearly defined (see below for discussion). The receptor is a basic helix-loop-helix (bHLH) factor (Burbach et al, 1992; Ema et al, 1992), showing similarity not only to the broad class of bHLH transcription factors but also to the human factor Arnt (Hoffman et al, 1991) and the *Drosophila* proteins Per (Period) and Sim (Single-minded), all of which share a ≈ 250-amino-acid-long region of similarity with the dioxin receptor (Takahashi et al, 1992) (see Figure 6.2 for a schematic representation). This region of similarity (termed PAS for Per, Arnt and Sim) has no known function but has recently been reported to mediate homo-dimerization processes of the *Drosophila* factor Per which, unlike the other known members of the PAS family of factors (Figure 6.2), does not contain a bHLH motif (Huang et al, 1993).

The bHLH motif defines a superfamily of proteins that regulate cell type-specific transcription, as well as cell proliferation and transformation. Among these proteins are the Myc oncoproteins and their dimerization partner factors, e.g. Max (Prendergast and Ziff, 1992); the products of the *Drosophila achaete-scute* complex, which regulate neurogenesis; twist,

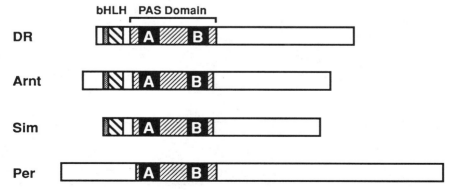

Figure 6.2 Schematic representation of the bHLH/PAS proteins dioxin receptor (DR), Arnt and Sim, and the PAS factor Per. Two hydrophobic repeat sequences (denoted A and B) within the PAS domain are indicated by solid black boxes.

which controls mesoderm formation; and daughterless, which participates in sex determination and formation of the peripheral nervous system in Drosophila (Jan and Jan, 1994). Similarly, a mammalian *achaete-scute* homolog has recently been shown in gene disruption experiments to be required for the early development of olfactory and autonomic neurons (Guillemot et al, 1993). In addition, the bHLH multigene family of regulatory factors comprises the four myogenic determination factors MyoD, myogenin, Myf5, and MRF4, all of which have been defined by their ability to convert fibroblasts to muscle, and to activate skeletal muscle-specific gene transcription when expressed ectopically in a variety of nonmuscle cells (Edmondson and Olson, 1993; Weintraub, 1993; Olson and Klein, 1994). bHLH factors are also involved in biological processes including lymphoid-specific transcription (Kadesh, 1993), more ubiquitous and constitutive gene transcription mechanisms (e.g. USF and AP-4) (Gregor et al, 1990; Hu et al, 1990), and centromere binding in yeast (Baker and Masison, 1990; Cai and Davis, 1990).

There are distinct classes of HLH factors which share combinations of the basic and HLH domains, and a conserved heptad leucine repeat or zipper (Z) motif. As schematically illustrated in Figure 6.3, these combinations result in the generation of HLH factors, which lack the basic domain and act as dominant negative regulators of their cognate bHLH partner proteins; e.g. Id, a dominant negative regulator of MyoD (Benezra et al, 1990); bHLH factors (e.g. MyoD, E12/E47), and bHLH/Z factors (e.g. Myc, Max, AP-4, TFE3 and USF) (Kadesh, 1993). In the case of bHLH factors, extensive mutagenesis has demonstrated that the HLH region is required for dimerization and that the adjacent basic region is required for DNA binding (Edmondson and Olson, 1992; Kadesh, 1993). In bHLH/Z factors

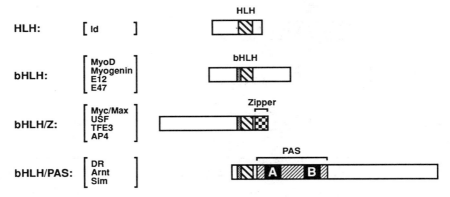

Figure 6.3 Different subclasses of bHLH factors. Examples of factors belonging to the different categories are given in brackets. Z, leucine heptad repeat (zipper).

both the HLH and the Z motifs are involved in protein oligomerization (Kadesh, 1993). Moreover, it appears that the Z region may promote higher order associations, since the minimal bHLH/Z domain of USF forms a bivalent homotetrameric structure in solution, whereas the minimal bHLH domain of USF forms a monovalent homodimer (Ferré-D'Amaré et al, 1994). Finally, in addition to stabilizing protein-protein interactions, the Z region in bfHLH/Z proteins may also play a role in determining dimerization specificity among different classes of these factors (Hu et al, 1990; Beckman and Kadesh, 1991). In contrast, an additional, distinct class of proteins is defined by those factors, notably the dioxin receptor, that possess the basic and HLH domains contiguous with the PAS homology region, here termed bHLH/PAS factors.

Recent structural analysis of the protein-DNA complex generated by homodimers of the bHLH/Z factors Max (Ferré-D'Amaré et al, 1993) and USF (Ferré-D'Amaré et al, 1994) have demonstrated DNA recognition by the basic region and the formation of a parallel four-helix bundle by the two helices in the HLH domain with the loops to the outside. Moreover, the basic region undergoes a folding transition from a random coil to an α-helical structure as it recognizes its cognate DNA sequence (Fischer et al, 1993; Ferré-D'Amaré et al, 1994). In X-ray crystallography studies the amino acids within the basic regions of Max and USF that establish contacts with their palindromic recognition sequence have been identified (Ferré-D'Amaré et al, 1993; 1994) (see Figure 6.4, amino acids indicated by a star; Figure 6.5A). These amino acids are strongly conserved both within the bHLH and bHLH/Z classes of HLH factors

BASIC	HELIX 1	LOOP	HELIX 2
mDR: AEGIKSNPSKRHR	DRLNTELDRLASLLP	--FPQDVINKLD	KLSVLRLSVSYLRAK
hDR: AEGIKSNPSKRHR	DRLNTELDRLASLLP	--FPQDVINKLD	KLSVLRLSVTYLRAK
Arnt: ARENHSEIERRRR	NKMTAYITELSDMVP	--TCSALARKPD	KLTILRMAVSHMKSL
Sim: MKEKSKNAARTRR	EKENTEFCELAKLLP	--LPAAITSQLD	KASVIRLTTSYLKMR
TFE3: KKDNHNLIERRRR	FNINDRIKELGTLIP	--KSSDPEMRWN	KGTILKASVDYIRKL
MyoD: RRKAATMRERRRL	SKVNEAFETLKRCTS	----SNPNQRLP	KVEILRNAIRYIEGL
cMyc: KRRTHNVLERQRR	NELKRSFFALRDQIP	---ELENNEKAP	KVVILKKATAYILSV
Max: KRAHHNALERKRR	DHIKDSFHSLRDSVP	----SLQGEKAS	RAQILDKATEYIQYM
USF: RRAQHNEVERRRR	DKINNWIVQLSKIIP	DCSMESTKSGQS	KGGILSKACDYIQEL

Figure 6.4 Partial sequence alignment of the bHLH domain of the mouse dioxin receptor (mDR) (Burbach et al, 1992; Ema et al, 1992), human dioxin receptor (hDR) (Itoh et al, 1993; Dolwick et al, 1993a) with human Arnt (Hoffman et al, 1991); Sim (Nambu et al, 1991); TFE3 (Beckman et al, 1990); MyoD (Lassar et al, 1989); cMyc (Prendergast et al, 1991); Max (Blackwood and Eisenman, 1991; Prendergast et al, 1991); and USF (Gregor et al, 1990). Conserved residues are highlighted, and the stars indicate amino acids of Max and USF which establish contacts with their palindromic E box recognition sequence, as determined by X-ray crystallography (Ferré-D'Amaré et al, 1993; 1994).

A   *E Box Motif:*

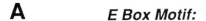

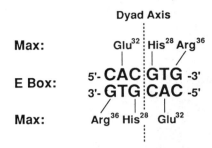

Dyad Axis

Max: Glu^{32} His^{28} Arg^{36}

E Box: 5'- CAC GTG -3'
          3'- GTG CAC -5'

Max: Arg^{36} His^{28} Glu^{32}

B   *XRE Sequences:*

Promoter/Enhancer:

Cytochrome P-450IA1: XRE-1:   GGCTCTTC **TCACGC** AACTCCGG

XRE-1:   CCCAGCTA **GCGTGA** CAGCACTG

Glutathione *S*-transferase Ya: CG **TCA**G**GC** ATGTT **GCGTG**C AT

NAD(P)H:Quinone Reductase: TTCCCCTT **GCGTGC** AAAGGC

C   *E Box versus XRE Motifs:*

E Box Core: CA**CGTG**
               GTGCAC

Dioxin Receptor Binding Core: T**CACG**C
                                 A**GTGC**G

Figure 6.5 Sequences dioxin receptor binding core motifs of (A) the two-fold symmetric E box; and (B) XRE sequences of the promoter/enhancer regions of the rat cytochrome P-450IA1 (Fujisawa-Sehara et al, 1987); rat glutathione S-transferase Ya (Paulson et al, 1990); and rat NAD(P)H:quinone reductase (Favreau and Pickett, 1991) genes. (C) Comparison of the E box motif and the core dioxin receptor binding core sequence of XREs. In panel A a schematic diagram is presented of contacts between nucleotides of the E box and amino acids of Max, as determined by X-ray crystallographic analysis of the Max-E-box complex (Ferré-D'Amaré et al, 1993).

(see Figure 6.4 for sequence alignment). Interestingly, they are also conserved within the basic region of bHLH/PAS factors, particularly Arnt (Figure 6.4). However, whereas most bHLH and bHLH/Z proteins bind to a common consensus element 5'-CANNTG-3' known as the E-box (Kadesh, 1993), the ligand-activated dioxin receptor fails to reconize this very sequence motif (Whitelaw et al, 1993b; Mason et al, 1994). In contrast it specifically binds to the core sequence 5'-TCACGC-3' which is conserved within dioxin or xenobiotic response elements (XREs) of dioxin-regulated promoters and enhancers (schematically represented in Figure 6.5B). Conversely, although the XRE core sequence is somewhat related to the twofold symmetrical E box motif CACGTG (Figure 6.5C) which constitutes a strong binding site for, among other bHLH factors, Myc/Max and USF (Ferré-D'Amaré et al, 1993; 1994), in vitro expressed bHLH factors (e.g. Max and USF) do not recognize the XRE target sequence (Poellinger, 1994). Moreover, in preliminary experiments we have hitherto failed to observe any dimerization of the dioxin receptor with selected members of the bHLH or bHLH/Z families of factors (Poellinger, 1994). However, in the absence of an extensive analysis addressing this issue, it is premature to speculate on any cross-dimerization mechanism of the dioxin receptor with any of the known bHLH or bHLH/Z factors. Given the background that the PAS region mediates homo-dimerization of the non-bHLH Per factor (Huang et al, 1993), it remains to be conclusively established whether the PAS region plays any role in the dimerization of the dioxin receptor, the stability of dimer complexes, and/or the DNA binding specificity of the dioxin receptor. Since the Z region has been implicated in dimerization specificity of bHLH/Z factors (Kadesh, 1993), it is an attractive possibility that the PAS region may determine specificity in the selection of dimerization partner factors and thus possibly modulate DNA binding specificity of the dioxin receptor.

The Dioxin Receptor Mediates Signal Transduction from the Cytoplasm to the Nucleus

In the absence of ligand, the dioxin receptor appears to be present in the cytoplasmic compartment of target cells in a latent, inactive (non-DNA binding) configuration. Although it has not been unambiguously established, it seems that dioxin may enter target cells by passive diffusion over the plasma membrane. Upon ligand binding the ligand-receptor complex becomes converted to a form that apparently translocates to the cell nucleus in vivo (Landers and Bunce, 1991; Poellinger et al, 1992; Whitlock, 1993).

The nuclear translocation process of the dioxin receptor has recently been documented by immunohistochemical techniques (Pollenz et al, 1994). Experimental evidence for the model of ligand-induced nuclear transloca- tion of the receptor has also been obtained by extracting the dioxin receptor from isolated pools of purified nuclei or cytosolic material prior to and subsequent to ligand treatment (Poland and Knutson, 1992; Whitlock, 1993). Importantly, strong experimental support for a cytoplasmic localiza- tion of the dioxin receptor in nonstimulated cells has been provided by enucleation experiments (Gudas et al, 1986). In addition to inducing the nuclear translocation step, the process of ligand binding initiates activation of the receptor to a DNA binding form, enabling the receptor to specifically recognize XREs of target promoters (Denison et al, 1988; Fujisawa-Sehara et al, 1988; Hapgood t al, 1989; Neuhold et al, 1989). Moreover, in vivo footprinting experiments have documented dioxin-induced protection of the XRE elements of the enhancer/promoter region cytochrome P-450IA1 gene, and experiments performed in mutant hepatoma cell lines have implicated the dioxin receptor in this process (Watson and Hankinson, 1992; Wu and Whitlock, 1993). Interestingly, cytosolic and nuclear forms of the receptor show considerable charge heterogeneity (Perdew and Hollen- back, 1990; Perdew, 1991), indicating that the receptor may become phosphorylated during the ligand-induced nuclear transport and/or recep- tor activation processes. The above model implicates the dioxin receptor directly in signal transduction. Thus, similar to the mechanism of action of several members of the steroid receptor superfamily including the gluco- corticoid receptor, the dioxin receptor mediates signal transduction by dioxin by performing at least two critical functions in the regulatory pathway: (1) it mediates specific recognition of the signal; and (2) it directly establishes a contact with cognate response elements of target genes. Furthermore the dioxin receptor, together with a great number of the various members of the steroid hormone receptor superfamily, functionally represents a gene regulatory protein which requires ligand-dependent conversion from a covert precursor to an active form. In the case of both the dioxin and glucocorticoid receptors this ligand-induced receptor activa- tion mechanism appears to correlate with ligand-induced nuclear import of the activated receptor form.

Modulation of Dioxin Receptor Function by The Molecular Chaperone hsp90 (90 kDa Heat Shock Protein)

Interestingly, the cytosolic, inducible form of dioxin receptor is stably associated with the 90 kDa heat shock protein, hsp90 (Denis et al, 1988a;

Perdew, 1988; Wilhelmsson et al, 1990), and is recovered as a $\approx 9S$, ≈ 300 kDa heteromeric complex (Wilhelmsson et al, 1986; 1990). Hsp90 is the most abundant constitutively expressed stress protein in the cytosol of eukaryotic cells (Lindquist and Craig, 1988), and it has recently been shown to chaperone protein folding in vitro, preventing protein aggregation and modulating protein activity (Miyata and Yahara, 1992; Wiech et al, 1992). The ≈ 300 kDa, hsp90-associated form of receptor does not bind DNA (Wilhelmsson et al, 1990). However, dissociation of hsp90 is sufficient to unmask the previously cryptic DNA binding activity of the receptor (Wilhelmsson et al, 1990), arguing that receptor function is repressed by protein-protein interaction with hsp90.

Our results indicate that hsp90 does not only repress receptor function by a possible steric interference mechanism. In addition, hsp90 seems to be required for efficient binding of ligand. Once dissociated from hsp90, it is not possible to form a stable receptor-ligand complex (Pongratz et al, 1992). These observations are consistent with the model that hsp90 acts as a molecular chaperone on the receptor determining the ability of the protein to assume and/or maintain a ligand binding conformation and thus facilitating subsequent functional responses of the receptor to the extracellular signal. Consistent with this model, we have shown that the dioxin receptor, upon artificially induced release of hsp90 in extracts from non-ligand-stimulated cells, shows constitutive, dioxin-nonresponsive DNA binding activity, in addition to being unable to bind ligand (Pongratz et al, 1992).

Regulation of nuclear receptor function by hsp90 is not unique for the dioxin receptor system. For instance, functional activities of the glucocorticoid receptor appear also to be modulated by interaction with hsp90 (Pratt et al, 1992; Pratt, 1993; Smith and Toft, 1993). It is possible to derepress the glucocorticoid receptor to a DNA binding state by hormone-induced release of hsp90 in vitro (Denis et al, 1988b). Strikingly, the inducible forms of both glucocorticoid and dioxin receptors are extracted from nonstimulated target cells as $\approx 9S$ hsp90-associated multiprotein complexes of about 300 kDa. In the case of the ≈ 300 kDa form of glucocorticoid receptor, it has been demonstrated to contain a dimer of hsp90 (Denis et al, 1987), suggesting that the glucocorticoid receptor interacts with hsp90 in a monomeric conformation. In further similarity to the dioxin receptor system (see above), induction of DNA binding activity of the glucocorticoid receptor by release of hsp90 is accompanied by a loss of high affinity ligand binding activity (Bresnick et al, 1989; Nemoto et al, 1990b). It appears therefore that hsp90 serves as a cellular chaperone molecule which, in addition to repressing receptor activity in nonstimulated cells, directly determines signal-responsiveness of distinct nuclear receptors (including the dioxin and glucocorticoid receptors) by mediating correct folding of the ligand binding domains of these proteins into a high affinity binding conformation. In support of this model, the glucocorticoid receptor exhibits a decreased hormone-responsiveness when expressed in mutant yeast strains with reduced levels of hsp90 (Picard et al, 1990). A yeast model system recently also has been used to isolate hsp90 mutants which decrease the function of steroid receptors, including the glucocorticoid receptor. Similar to the results obtained with reduced levels of hsp90, such hsp90 mutants negatively regulate the ability of the glucocorticoid receptor to be activated in response to hormone treatment (Bohen and Yamamoto, 1993).

Ligand-dependent Activation of the Dioxin Receptor

As outlined above, exposure to dioxin in vivo, or in vitro treatment with dioxin under high ionic strength conditions, leads to release of hsp90 and an activated dioxin receptor form with high affinity for XRE target sequences. We have reconstituted under cell-free conditions dioxin-dependent conversion of the cryptic receptor form to a DNA binding species using crude cytosolic extracts or partially purified protein preparartions from non-dioxin-treated cells (Nemoto et al, 1990a; Cut-hill et al, 1991). Activation of the cryptic or latent receptor in vitro is dose-dependent and stimulated by ligands in a manner that reflects their relative binding affinities for the receptor protein in vitro and their relative potencies to induce cytochrome P-450IA1 transcription in vivo (Cuthill et al, 1991).

To further reconstitute under cell-free conditions the ligand-dependent activation process, we have also investigated the DNA binding properties of the partially purified, hsp90-associated form of dioxin receptor. This form of receptor can bind ligand, and, in the absence of ligand, its DNA binding activity is repressed (Pongratz et al, 1992). Remarkably, in spite of its bona fide levels of ligand binding activity, it is not possible to activate its DNA binding function in response to ligand treatment in vitro, strongly arguing that the ligand-activated receptor requires an auxiliary factor for DNA binding activity (Whitelaw et al, 1993b). In complementation assays we have identified a distinct activity that strongly enhances the binding of the receptor to its target DNA element. This activity corresponds by functional and biochemical criteria to the bHLH/PAS factor Arnt (Whitelaw et al, 1993b; Mason et al, 1994). In fact, individually expressed or purified forms of dioxin receptor and Arnt do not show any detectable affinity for the XRE target sequence, whereas dimerization enables both proteins to specifically recognize cognate response elements (Reyes et al, 1992; Dolwick et al, 1993b; Matsushita et al, 1993; Whitelaw et al, 1993b; Mason et al, 1994).

Among proteins in the growing family of factors bearing the bHLH motif, heterodimerization processes appear to constitute a critical mechanism of regulation of the DNA binding activity of these factors. For instance, c-Myc heterodimerizes with Max to efficiently bind to the E-box target sequences (Prendergast and Ziff, 1992). In a similar fashion, the bHLH protein E12 appears to be a functional and physical partner protein of bHLH myogenic factors, including MyoD and myogenin, in the activation of muscle-specific gene expression (Edmondson and Olson, 1993). Thus, a strikingly distinct and restricted pattern of heterodimerization has been observed among these factor, even though they are capable of binding to very similar, if not identical, target DNA sequences in vitro.

Importantly, co-immunoprecipitation experiments have demonstrated that Arnt forms a strong physical complex with the ligand-activated dioxin receptor in solution, but it fails to heterodimerize with the ligand-free, hsp90-associated receptor form (Matsushita et al, 1993; Probst et al, 1993; Whitelaw et al, 1993b). The bHLH motif is required for dioxin receptor-Arnt interaction since deletion of this very motif abrogates functional interaction in vivo (Whitelaw et al, 1993b) as well a physical interaction in vitro (Mason et al, 1994). Dioxin receptor-Arnt interaction can also be documented in reconstitution experiments using a cytosolic extract from non-ligand-treated Hepa-1 hepatoma cells. This extract contains functional dioxin receptor and Arnt proteins (Hoffman et al, 1991). In the absence of dioxin, however, no DNA binding activity can be detected in this extract toward the receptor recognition sequence in the XRE-1 element of the cytochrome P-450IA1 promoter (Fujisawa-Sehara et al, 1987), as assessed by gel mobility shift experiments (Figure 6.6, lane 1). Exposure of the cytosolic extract to dioxin induces the formation of a protein-DNA complex that harbors both the dioxin receptor and Arnt partner factors, as examined by the use of antibodies against these two proteins. Whereas addition of preimmune serum does not affect the induced DNA binding activity, XRE complex formation is inhibited in the presence of receptor-specific antibodies, and, finally, addition of Arnt antibodies results in a supershift the protein-DNA complex (Figure 6.6, compare lanes 2–5). Thus, these data demonstrate that both the dioxin receptor and Arnt are recruited by dioxin into a complex with the XRE target sequence.

In agreement with these observations, the DNA binding form of ligand-activated dioxin receptor has a native molecular mass of about

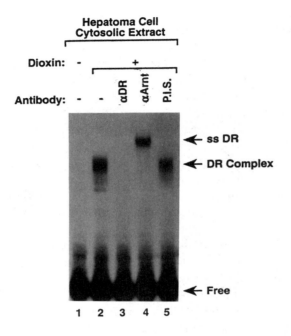

Figure 6.6 Reconstitution of ligand-induced activation of the cytoplasmic dioxin receptor form in vitro. Cytosol was prepared from untreated mouse hepatoma cells Hepa-1 and exposed in vitro to solvent alone (lane 1) or 5 nM dioxin (lanes 2–5) as described (Cuthill et al, 1991). The DNA binding activity or the receptor was monitored in a gel mobility shift assay using the XRE-1 sequence of the cytochrome P-450IA1 gene (Fujisawa-Sehara et al, 1987) as specific probe. The reactions were also incubated with polyclonal antibodies against the dioxin receptor (αDR), Arnt (αArnt) or preimmuneserum (P.I.S.), as indicated. The positions of unbound (Free) probe, the dioxin receptor-dependent protein-DNA complex (DR complex), and a receptor complex super-shifted by the antibodies (ss DR) are indicated.

200 kDa (Hapgood et al, 1989), strongly suggesting that the ligand-activated dioxin receptor complex is a heterodimer of the ≈ 100 kDa receptor and the ≈ 90 kDa Arnt factors. In summary, ligand-dependent activation of the dioxin receptor to a functional form appears to be a rather complex process involving several distinct and critical steps: (1) binding of ligand; (2) release of hsp90; and (3) subsequent dimerization with the bfHLH partner factor Arnt which promotes the DNA binding function of the receptor. A model summarizing our current understanding of the ligand-dependent activation process of the dioxin receptor is illustrated in Figure 6.7.

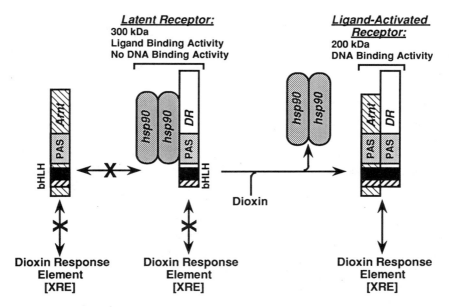

Figure 6.7 Model for ligand-dependent activation of the dioxin receptor into a DNA binding form (modified and adapted with permission from American Society for Microbiology from Whitelaw et al, 1993b).

Role of the bHLH/PAS Partner Factor Arnt in Signal Transduction by the Dioxin Receptor

Arnt was originally cloned as a factor that functionally complements a mutant, dioxin-nonresponsive subclone (c4) of the hepatoma cell line Hepa-1 (Hoffman et al, 1991). Interestingly, these mutant cells express a dioxin receptor phenotype which appears to be deficient in nuclear translocation but shows bona fide levels of ligand binding activity (Legraverend et al, 1982). In contrast, expression of Arnt restores dioxin-induced transcription of target genes (Hoffman et al, 1991; Whitelaw et al, 1993a) and dioxin-regulated nuclear translocation of the dioxin receptor in these cells (Hoffman et al, 1991). Arnt has therefore been postulated to govern nuclear translocation of the ligand-activated dioxin receptor form (Hoffman et al, 1991). However, it is formally possible that the failure to extract the ligand-activated dioxin receptor from nuclei of dioxin-treated, Arnt-deficient c4 cells may simply reflect the low intrinsic DNA binding activity of the receptor, and it remains to be examined by immunochemical techniques whether the cellular compartmentalization of the dioxin receptor is altered in an Arnt-free environment, i.e. in mutant Arnt-deficient cells. It will also be critical to determine the intracellular localization of Arnt in both nontreated and dioxin-exposed wild-type target cells, and to address whether Arnt-receptor dimerization occurs prior to or subsequent to nuclear transloca-tion of the ligand-activated dioxin receptor. The in vitro activated, DNA binding cytosolic dioxin receptor form is biochemically indistinguishable from the activated receptor form recovered in nuclear extracts from dioxin-stimulated cells (Cuthill et al, 1991), arguing that all the compo-nents necessary for generation of the active form of receptor are present in the cytosolic cell extract. On the other hand, the presence of Arnt in the cytosolic extract could reflect an artifact due to redistribution of nuclear proteins to the cytosol when exposed to the relatively large buffer volumes used during extract preparation.

In our efforts to reconstitute ligand-dependent activation of the dioxin receptor in vitro, we have recently observed that ligand (such as dioxin) is necessary but not sufficient to activate the latent, hsp90-associated dioxin receptor complex. In addition, a cellular factor is required to dissociate hsp90 in vitro and to unmask functional activity (McGuire et al, 1994). Moreover, this effect is mediated by the bHLH motif of the receptor. As we interpret these results, dioxin induces the receptor into a potentiated state from which it can be converted into a functional state by a factor that induces release of hsp90. Biochemical analysis and fractionation experi-ments indicate that this cellular factor may be Arnt itself or an Arnt-associated cofactor (McGuire et al, 1994; Pongratz, et al, 1994). As discussed in closer detail below, this observation suggests that the intracellular concentration of Arnt may be an important determinant of the dioxin-responsiveness of a target cell. It will therefore be important to investigate whether, in the most extreme case, overexpression of Arnt can totally by-pass ligand-dependency for induction of dioxin receptor func-tion. Alternatively, Arnt function (and thereby possibly indirectly dioxin receptor function) may be closely controlled by ubiquitous or cell type-restricted novel and as yet unidentified dimerization partners. Interaction with such partner factors may in certain cells limit the pool of Arnt available for dimerization with the ligand-activated dioxin receptor, or it may alter the DNA binding specificity of the resulting heteromeric protein complexes, thus recruiting Arnt into alternative gene regulatory networks.

Functional Architecture of the Dioxin Receptor and Arnt

Fusion of different functional domains of the dioxin receptor and Arnt to heterologous DNA binding domains has permitted us to identify func-tional domains of these proteins. These studies have demonstrated that the ligand binding domain of the dioxin receptor confers conditional regulation on heterologous transcription factors (Whitelaw et al, 1993a), reminiscent of the mode of regulation by the ligand binding domain of the glucocorticoid receptor (Picard et al, 1988). Importantly, fusion of this domain of the dioxin receptor to a heterologous DNA binding motif has uncoupled dioxin receptor function from Arnt. Consequently, we have recently observed that Arnt is not required for dioxin regulation in Arnt-deficient cells (Whitelaw et al, 1993a). The minimal ligand binding domain of the dioxin receptor is located within the carboxyterminal half of the PAS domain, as examined by noncovalent and covalent ligand binding assays (Dolwick et al, 1993b; Whitelaw et al, 1993a). In contrast, the PAS region of Arnt does not generate any detectable complexes with hsp90 in co-immunoprecipitation experiments (McGuire et al, 1994). It is not yet known whether the PAS domain of either the receptor or Arnt is important for stabilization of the Arnt-dioxin receptor heterodimer, as suggested by its role in dimerization processes of the *Drosophila* factor Per (Huang et al, 1993). In any case, deletion of the minimal bHLH motif abrogates physical Arnt-dioxin receptor interaction in vitro (Whitelaw et al, 1993b; Mason et al, 1994) and functional Arnt-receptor interaction in vivo (Whitelaw et al, 1993b), demonstrating that this very motif is critical for dimer formation. A preliminary map of the functional domains of both the dioxin receptor and Arnt is presented in Figure 6.8.

As schematically shown in Figure 6.8, both the dioxin receptor and Arnt harbor glutamine-rich sequence motifs in their carboxytermini. Similar motifs constitute transactivation domains in a number of transcription factors, e.g. Sp1 (Mitchell and Tjian, 1989), and homo-polymeric stretches of glutamine can activate transcription when fused to the DNA binding domain of the Gal4 factor (Gerber et al, 1994).

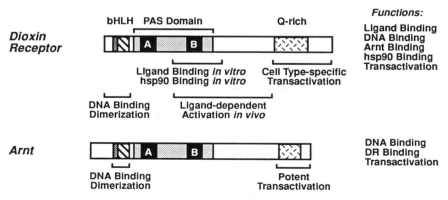

Figure 6.8 Model summarizing the functional architecture of the dioxin receptor and its bHLH partner factor Arnt. A glutamine-rich (Q-rich) region in both proteins is indicated.

Moreover, many developmentally regulated proteins in *Drosophila* such as engrailed, bithorax and Notch contain glutamine stretches termed M repeats (McGinnins et al, 1984) or opa repeats (Wharton et al, 1985). These sequence motifs have the general structure (CAX) whereby X is G or A, and the triplets CAG and CAA code for glutamine in a correct reading frame. In our preliminary analyses (Whitelaw et al, 1993b; Whitelaw et al, 1994) transactivating regions within both the dioxin receptor and Arnt, respectively, largely coincide with the carboxyterminal glutamine-rich sequence motifs. However, the receptor appears to be a rather poor transactivator in cell transfection assays (Whitelaw et al, 1993a). In contrast, Arnt confers potent transactivation on most target promoters (ML Whitelaw et al, 1994), arguing that transcriptional regulation, in addition to determining DNA binding specificity of the dioxin receptor, may be an important functional property of Arnt. When expressed together in transient transfection assays in mammalian cells, full length dioxin receptor and Arnt show strong synergistic transcriptional activation (Mason et al, 1994), indicating that the receptor and Arnt may have very specialized and distinct functional roles in the dioxin signalling pathway, reminiscent of the distinct roles of the p65 versus the p50 subunits in transactivation by NF-κB (Schmitz and Baeuerle, 1991).

Crosscoupling of Dioxin Receptor- and Protein Kinase C-mediated Signal Transduction Pathways

In human keratinocytes the induction process of cytochrome P-450IA1 gene expression is modulated both by extracellular Ca^{2+} and serum (Berghard et al, 1990). Interestingly, treatment of the keratinocytes with the phorbolester 12-O-tetradecanoylphorbol-13-acetate (TPA) at doses and time points which down-regulate protein kinase C (PKC) activity in the cells inhibits both the dioxin induction response and the DNA binding activity of the receptor. This effect is also achieved by treating the cells with a number of different PKC inhibitors, most notably the very specific inhibitor calphostin (Berghard et al, 1993). Dioxin receptor function appears also to be regulated by phorbol ester in cells other than keratinocytes (Carrier et al, 1992; Okino et al, 1992). Taken together, these data indicate that protein kinase C-mediated phosphorylation processes may control dioxin receptor function. Similarly, the bHLH factor myogenin is negatively regulated by protein kinase C-mediated phosphorylation of a threonine residue in the center of the basic DNA binding region (Li et al, 1992). In vitro, the DNA binding activity of the ligand-activated dioxin receptor is inhibited by phosphatase treatment

(Pongratz et al, 1991; Carrier et al, 1992; Berghard et al, 1993). Moreover, we have recently demonstrated that the dioxin receptor is a phosphoprotein in vivo (Berghard et al, 1993). Dephosphorylation experiments have indicated that not only the DNA binding activity of the ligand-activated, heterodimeric receptor-Arnt complex but, in fact, the dimerization process itself between the receptor and Arnt may be regulated by phosphorylation processes (Berghard et al, 1993). As outlined in the model in Figure 6.9 it is therefore conceivable that signal transduction by dioxin from the cytoplasm to the nucleus of target cells may require protein kinase C-dependent phosphorylation of either the receptor, Arnt or both subunits. Finally, it is possible to restore the DNA binding activity of the dephosphorylated dioxin receptor form in vitro by a cytosolic catalytic activity that is sensitive to calphostin (Berghard et al, 1993). We are now attempting to further characterize and purify this catalytic activity. In particular, it will be interesting to test the hypothesis whether this activity represents a protein kinase C isozyme and whether the receptor is the direct target of protein kinase C-catalyzed phosphorylation processes, and, if this is the case, whether amino acids in the basic region are targeted for regulation.

Distinct Roles of hsp90 in Modulation of Dioxin Receptor Function

Although the precise role(s) of hsp90 in modulating dioxin receptor function remains largely unclear, it appears that hsp90 both blocks receptor-Arnt dimerization (Whitelaw et al, 1993b), resulting in repression of receptor function, and chaperones a high affinity ligand binding conformation of the receptor (Pongratz et al, 1992). As discussed above, ligand-induced receptor activation involves release of hsp90 and concomitant unmasking of its dimerization and DNA binding activities (Wilhelmsson et al, 1990; Pongratz et al, 1992; Whitelaw et al, 1993b). As summarized in Figure 6.10, glucocorticoid receptor function appears to be modulated by hsp90 by a similar regulatory strategy. In further similarity to the dioxin receptor system, hsp90-glucocorticoid receptor interaction is mediated by the ligand binding domain (Pratt, 1993; Smith and Toft, 1993).

Interestingly, recent observations indicate that hsp90 may modulate the function of the bHLH factors MyoD and E12. This model is based on the observation that bacterially expressed MyoD exhibits low levels of DNA binding activity. In line with these results, a cellular factor has been reported to stimulate the DNA binding activity of MyoD (Thayer and Weintraub, 1993). Reconstitution experiments indicate that hsp90 may

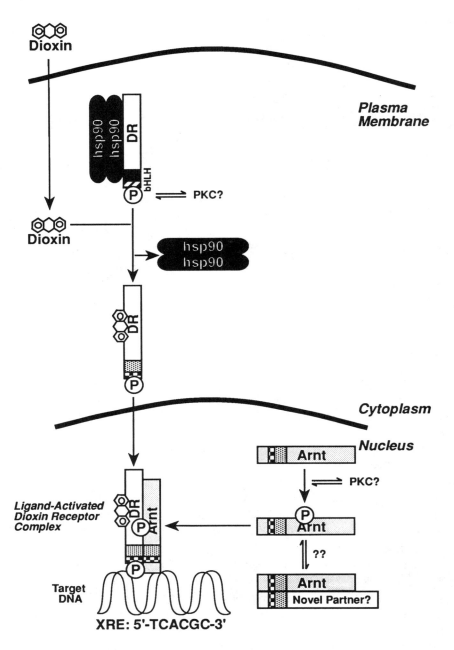

Figure 6.9 Model for signal transduction of dioxin between cytoplasm and nucleus. Possible regulation mechanisms by protein kinase C and dimerization with as yet unidentified partner factors are indicated. See text for discussion and details.

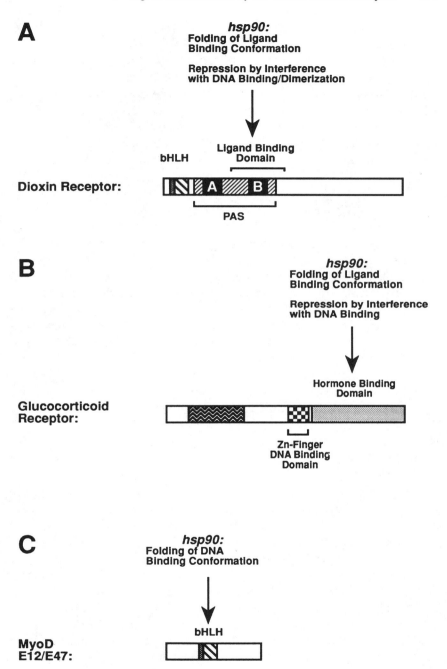

Figure 6.10 Summary of the different postulated roles of hsp90 in modulating functional activities of the dioxin receptor, glucocorticoid receptor bHLH factors MyoD and E12/E47; the bHLH/PAS dioxin receptor and the glucocorticoid receptor.

fold inactive fractions of bacterially expressed MyoD and E12 bHLH domains into DNA binding conformations (Shaknovich et al, 1992; Shue and Kohtz, 1994). However, the interaction between the bHLH domain of MyoD and E12 appears to be weak and transient. In contrast to experiments with the dioxin receptor, it has not been possible to detect any interaction between hsp90 and MyoD or E12 in co-immunoprecipitation experiments (Shaknovich et al, 1992; Shue and Kohtz, 1994). Thus, as schematically indicated in Figure 6.10, hsp90 appears to play distinct roles in modulation of function of different classes of bHLH factors.

Is there a Physiological Ligand of the Dioxin Receptor?

Dioxin exemplifies the prototypical ligand for the dioxin receptor. Like dioxin the vast majority of compounds that have been demonstrated to bind to the receptor are environmental contaminants of mainly industrial origin belonging either to the class of halogenated aromatic hydrocarbons (e.g. polychlorinated biphenyls, dibenzo-p-dioxins or dibenzofurans) or polycyclic aromatic hydrocarbons (e.g. benzo(a)pyrene and methylcholanthrene (Poland and Knutson, 1982; Safe, 1990). In view of the great number of mechanistic similarities between the dioxin and steroid hormone receptor systems, it is conceivable that the physiological ligand for the dioxin receptor is an as yet unidentified hormone. Moreover, given the background that dioxin in certain cells can modulate differentiation processes (Poland and Knutson, 1982; Whitlock 1993), it is also possible that the endogenous dioxin receptor ligand may represent a previously unknown morphogen. In striking contradiction of these hypotheses, it has so far not been possible to identify any truly endogenous or physiological ligand for the receptor. For instance, the dioxin receptor does not bind any known steroid hormone, nor does it exhibit any detectable affinity and specificity for thyroid hormones or retinoic acid (Poellinger et al, 1992). At present it can therefore not be excluded that natural ligands of the dioxin receptor are of xenobiotic nature. However, several lines of evidence indicate that high affinity dioxin receptor ligands (or ligand precursor molecules) occur in certain plants, suggesting that endogenous receptor ligands may be found in the diet. Most notably, certain indole derivatives such as indolo[3,2-b]carbazole (Gillner et al, 1985; Bjeldanes et al, 1991) (Figure 6.1) are at least as potent agonists for both the murine and human dioxin receptor as dioxin (TCDD) itself (Kleman et al, 1994). Moreover, photolysis of tryptophan and tryptamine yields products which bind to the dioxin receptor with high affinity (Rannug et al, 1987), and certain rutaecarpine alkaloids which can be chemically derived from tryptamine bind to the dioxin receptor with a relatively high affinity (Gillner et al, 1989). Finally, certain food-borne heterocyclic amines generated during cooking processes appear to be ligands of the dioxin receptor and induce receptor-dependent DNA binding activity in in vitro assays (Kleman et al, 1992). Thus, these heterocyclic compounds represent a new class of dioxin receptor ligands which are distinct from the two previously known (i.e. halogenated aromatic hydrocarbons and polycyclic aromatic hydrocarbons), and which to date constitute our best candidates for a physiological receptor ligand.

In this context it is noteworthy that Arnt can promote derepression of the dioxin receptor by inducing release of hsp90 via the bHLH-mediated dimerization process with the ligand-activated dioxin receptor form (McGuire et al, 1994; Pongratz et al, 1994). These results suggest the testable model that regulation of receptor function by ligand binding may be by-passed if the receptor is exposed to high intracellular levels of the Arnt partner factor. So far there is a paucity of data with regard to cellular concentrations of Arnt in rodent and human tissues. In preliminary experiments Arnt appears to be expressed in certain cells at levels significantly exceeding those of the dioxin receptor (Poellinger L, 199?). It is not yet known whether Arnt dimerizes with other as yet unidentified bfHLH or non-bHLH partner factors (see below), and if such putative dimerization mechanisms will modulate dioxin receptor function by regulating the concentration of the pool of Arnt available to dimerize with the receptor. Given the apparently relatively high concentrations of Arnt in certain cells, the presence of alternative dimerization partner factors for Arnt, possibly dominant negative HLH factors, would present an attractive model for regulation of dioxin receptor function. This model further implies that, under certain conditions, receptor function may be separated from ligand-dependent control mechanisms. Finally, alternative signal transduction pathways, e.g. phosphorylation cascades, may also modulate dioxin receptor function in certain target cells, possibly resulting in activation of the dioxin receptor even in the absence of ligand.

Conclusions

In view of the very complex regulatory networks of other bHLH factors, in particular of members of the MyoD family of factors (Jan and Jan, 1983; Weintraub, 1993; Olson and Klein, 1994), it is an interesting possibility that the dioxin receptor and/or Arnt interact with additional ubiquitous or cell type-specific dimerization partner factors to modulate receptor function. For instance, the composite dioxin response element of the glutathione *S*-transferase gene creates the stage for interesting positive or negative functional interactions between the dioxin receptor and the leucine zipper factor C/EBP (Pimental et al, 1993), increasing the potential diversity of dioxin-induced responses. Perhaps more importantly, the structural relatedness of the dioxin receptor with the *Drosophila* neural regulators Per and Sim implies that putative partner factors for the dioxin receptor and/or Arnt (see above) may be found in developmental regulatory pathways or, in particular, in the developing and/or adult central or peripheral nervous systems. Given the absence of the bHLH motif in Per, such novel putative partner factors for the receptor or Arnt could very well prove to be either bHLH proteins or Per-like PAS factors lacking the bHLH domain.

If mice are viable following disruption of the dioxin receptor, Arnt or both genes by homologous recombination in embryonal stem cells, we should soon have an answer to the question whether a physiological role of the dioxin receptor and/or its partner factor is to be found in developmental processes. Given the homology to the *Drosophila* factors Per and Sim, such regulatory processes may include as diverse events as neuronal development and circadian rhythm regulation. Moreover, receptor- or Arnt-deficient mice will facilitate studies on the involvement of the receptor in the various pleiotropic toxic responses observed upon exposure to dioxin, e.g. lymphotoxicity, liver damage, and the dramatic so called wasting syndrome (see above). It will also be possible to directly address the question whether the dioxin receptor and/or Arnt are mediating the carcinogenic (i.e. tumor promoting) effects of dioxin and related environmental pollutants. Importantly, studies on human populations may clarify whether genetic polymorphisms in the receptor and/or Arnt genes will affect the susceptibility to certain cancers.

It appears likely that there exist novel partner factors to either Arnt or the dioxin receptor. Given the fact that the basic region of Arnt contains the Arg, His, and Glu residues that have been shown to recognize specific bases in the E box target sequence for other bHLH factors, it is plausible that heterodimerization of Arnt with novel partner factors will dictate a DNA binding specificity of Arnt that is more related to the E box motifs that XRE sequences. Thus, there may very well exist target genes for either the dioxin receptor or Arnt that are not recognized by the heterodimeric dioxin receptor-Arnt complex but by the receptor and Arnt in association with other partner molecules. In addition, it will now also be important to select optimal recognition motifs for both homodimeric receptor and Arnt complexes, and to examine the specificity of these complexes versus that of the heterodimeric complex.

Finally, as outlined above novel partner factors may provide the basis for alternative pathways that may derepress the dioxin receptor in the absence of ligand stimulation and that may therefore give us information with regard to a possible physiological function of the receptor. To my knowledge the dioxin receptor system provides a unique example of signal-controlled bHLH factors and may therefore be a valuable model to study regulatory strategies which modulate the function of the two highly interesting classes of bHLH/PAS and PAS gene regulatory molecules.

Acknowledgments

Research in my laboratory was supported by grants from the Swedish Cancer Society. I am grateful to all members of my laboratory, particularly Murray Whitelaw, who has contributed scientifically and conceptually to the topics discussed in this review. I also thank Anders Berkenstam for stimulating discussions.

References

Axelson O (1993): Seveso: disentangling the dioxin enigma? *Epidemiology* 4: 389–392
Bailar JP (1991): How dangerous is dioxin? *New Engl J Med* 324: 260–262
Baker RE, Masison DC (1990): Isolation of the gene encoding the Saccharomyces cerevisiae centromere binding protein CP1. *Mol Cell Biol* 10: 2458–2467
Beckman H, Su L-K, Kadesh T (1990): TFE3: a helix-loop-helix protein that activates transcription through the immunoglobulin enhancer μE3 motif. *Genes Dev* 4: 167–179
Benezra R, David RL, Lockshon D, Weintraub H (1990): The protein Id, a negative regulator of helix-loop-helix proteins. *Cell* 61: 49–59
Berghard A, Gradin K, Pongratz I, Whitelaw ML, Poellinger L (1993): Cross-coupling of signal transduction pathways: the dioxin receptor mediates induction of cytochrome P-450IA1 expression via a protein kinase C-dependent mechanism. *Mol Cell Biol* 13: 677–689
Berghard A, Gradin K, Toftgård R (1990): Serum and extracellular calcium modulate induction of cytochrome P-450Ia1 in human keratinocytes. *J Biol Chem* 265: 21086–21090
Bjeldanes LF, Kim JY, Grose KR, Bartholomew JC, Bradfield CA (1991): Aromatic hydrocarbon responsiveness — receptor agonists generated from indole-3-carbinol in vitro and in vivo: comparisons with 2,3,7,8-tetrachlorodibenzo-p-dioxin. *Proc Natl Acad Sci USA* 88: 9543–9547
Blackwood EM, Eisenman RN (1991): Max: a helix-loop-helix zipper protein that forms a sequence-specific DNA binding complex with Myc. *Science* 251: 1211–1217
Bohen SP, Yamamoto KR (1993): Isolation of hsp90 mutants by screening for decreased steroid receptor function *Proc Natl Acad Sci USA* 90: 11424–11428

Bresnick EH, Dalman FC, Sanchez ER, Pratt WB (1989): Evidence that the 90-kDa heat shock protein is necessary for the steroid binding conformation of the L cell glucocorticoid receptor. *J Biol Chem* 264: 4992–4997

Burbach KM, Poland A, Bradfield CA (1992): Cloning of the Ah receptor cDNA reveals a distinctive ligand-activated transcription factor. *Proc Natl Acad Sci USA* 89: 8185–8189

Cai M, Davis RW (1990): Yeast centromere binding protein CBF1, of the helix-loop-helix protein family, is required for chromosome stability and methionine prototrophy. *Cell* 61: 437–446

Carrier F, Owens IA, Nebert DW, Puga A (1992): Dioxin-dependent activation of murine CypIa-1 gene transcription requires protein kinase C-dependent phosphorylation. *Mol Cell Biol* 12: 1856–1863

Cuthill S, Wilhelmsson A, Poellinger L (1991): Role of the ligand in intracellular receptor function: receptor affinity determines activation in vitro of the latent dioxin receptor to a DNA-binding form. *Mol Cell Biol* 11: 401–411

Denis M, Cuthill S, Wikström A-C, Poellinger L, Gustafsson J-Å (1988a): Association of the dioxin receptor with mr 90,000 heat shock protein: a structural kinship with the glucocorticoid receptor. *Biochem Biophys Res Commun* 155: 801–807

Denis M, Poellinger L, Wikström A-C, Poellinger L, Gustafsson J-Å (1988b): Requirement of hormone for thermal conversion of the glucocorticoid receptor to a DNA-binding state. *Nature* 333: 686–688

Denis M, Wikström A-C, Gustafsson J-Å (1987): The molybdate-stabilized non-activated glucocorticoid receptor contains a dimer of Mr 90,000 non-hormone binding protein. *J Biol Chem* 262: 11803–11806

Denison MS, Fisher JM, Whitlock JPJr (1988): Inducible, receptor-dependent protein-DNA interactions at a dioxin-responsive transcriptional enhancer. *Proc Natl Acad Sci USA* 85: 2528–2532

Dolwick KM, Schmidt JV, Carver LA, Swanson HI, Bradfield CA (1993a): Cloning and expression of a human Ah receptor cDNA. *Mol Pharmacol* 44: 911–917

Dolwick KM, Swanson H, Bradfield CA (1993b): In vitro analysis of Ah receptor domains involved in ligand-activated DNA recognition. *Proc Natl Acad Sci USA* 90: 8566–8570

Edmondson DG, Olson EN (1993): Helix-loop-helix proteins as regulators of muscle-specific transcription. *J Biol Chem* 268: 755–758

Ema M, Sogawa K, Watanabe Y, Chujoh Y, Matsushita N, Gotoh O, Funae Y, Fujii-Kuriyama Y (1992): cDNA cloning and structure of mouse putative Ah receptor. *Biochem Biophys Res Commun* 184: 246–253

Favreau LV, Pickett CB (1991): Transcriptional regulation of the rat NAD(P)H:quinone oxidoreductase gene: identification of regulatory elements controlling basal expression and inducible expression by planar aromatic compounds and phenolic antioxidants. *J Biol Chem* 266: 4556-4561

Ferré-D'Amaré AR, Pognonec P, Roeder RG, Burley SK (1994): Structure and function of the b/HLH/Z domain of USF. *EMBO J* 13: 180–189

Ferré-D'Amaré AR, Prendergast GC, Ziff EB, Burley SK (1993): Recognition by Max of its cognate DNA through a dimeric b/HLH/Z domain. *Nature* 363: 38–45

Fischer DE, Parent LA, Sharp PA (1993): High affinity DNA binding Myc analogs: recognition by an α helix. *Cell* 72: 467–476

Fujii-Kuriyama Y, Imataka H, Sogawa K, Yasumoto K-I, Kiguchi Y (1992): Regulation of Cyp1A1 expression. *FASEB J* 6: 706–710

Fujisawa-Sehara A, Sogawa K, Yamane M, Fujii-Kuriyama Y (1987): Characterization of xenobiotic response elements upstream from the drug-metabolizing cutochrome P-450c gene: a similarity to glucocorticoid response elements. *Nucl Acids Res* 15: 4179–4191

Fujisawa-Sehara A, Yamane M, Fujii-Kuriyama Y (1988): A DNA-binding factor specific for xenobiotic responsive elements of P-450c gene exists as a cryptic form in cytoplasm: its possible translocation to nucleus. *Proc Natl Acad Sci USA* 85: 5859–5863

Gallo MA, Scheuplein RJ, Van der Heiden KA (1991): Biological basis for risk assessment of dioxins and related compounds. *Banbury Report 35*. Cold Spring Harbor, New York: Cold Spring Harbor Laboratory Press

Gerber H-P, Seipel K, Georgiev O, Höfferer M, Hug M, Rusconi S, Schaffner W (1994): Transcriptional activation modulated by homopolymeric glutamine and proline stretches. *Science* 263: 808–811

Gillner M, Bergman J, Cambilleau C, Fernström B, Gustafsson J-Å (1985): Interactions of indoles with specific binding sites for 2,3,7,8-tetrachlorodibenzo-p-dioxin in rat liver. *Mol Pharmacol* 28: 357–363

Gillner M, Bergman J, Cambilleau C, Gustafsson J-Å (1989): Interactions of rutaecarpine alkaloids with specific binding sites for 2,3,7,8-tetrachlorodibenzo-p-dioxin in rat liver. *Carcinogenesis* 10: 651–654

Gradin K, Wilhelmsson A, Poellinger L, Berghard A (1993): Nonresponsiveness of normal human fibroblasts to dioxin correlates with the presence of a constitutive xenobiotic response element binding factor. *J Biol Chem* 268: 4061–4068

Gregor P, Sawadogo M, Roeder RG (1990): The adenovirus major late transcription factor USF is a member of the helix-loop-helix group of regulatory proteins and binds to DNA as a dimer. *Genes Dev* 4: 1730–1740

Gudas JM, Hankinson O (1986): Intracellular location of the Ah receptor. *J Cell Physiol* 128: 441-448

Guillemot F, Lo L-C, Johnson JE, Auerbach A, Anderson DJ, Joyner AL (1993): Mammalian *achaete-scute* homolog 1 is required for the early development of olfactory and autonomic neurons. *Cell* 75: 463–476

Hankinson O (1983): Dominant and recessive aryl hydrocarbon hydroxylase-deficient mutants of the mouse hepatoma cell line, Hepa 1, and assignment of the recessive mutants to three complementation groups. *Somatic Cell Genet* 9: 497–514

Hapgood J, Cuthill S, Denis M, Poellinger L, Gustafsson J-Å (1989): Specific protein-DNA interactions at a xenobiotic-responsive element: copurification of dioxin receptor and DNA-binding activity. *Proc Natl Acad Sci USA* 86: 60–64

Hoffman EC, Reyes H, Chu FF, Sander F, Conley LH, Brooks BA, Hankinson O (1991): Cloning of a factor required for activity of the Ah (dioxin) receptor. *Science* 252: 954–958

Hu YF, Luescher B, Admon A, Mermod N, Tijian R (1990): Transcription factor AP-4 contains multiple dimerization domains that regulate dimer specificity. *Genes Dev* 4: 1741–1752

Huang ZJ, Edery I, Rosbash M (1993): PAS is a dimerization domain common to Drosophila Period and several transcription factors. *Nature* 364: 259–262

Itoh S, Kamataki T (1993): Human Ah receptor cDNA: analysis for highly conserved sequences. *Nucl Acids Res* 21: 3578

Jan YN, Jan LY (1993): HLH proteins, fly neurogenesis, and vertebrate myogenesis. *Cell* 75: 827–830

Kadesh T (1993): Consequences of heteromeric interactions among helix-loop-helix proteins. *Cell Growth Differentiation* 4: 49–55

Kleman M, Övervik E, Mason GGF, Gustafsson J-Å (1992): In vitro activation of the dioxin receptor by food-borne heterocyclic amines. *Carcinogenesis* 13: 1619–1624

Kleman M, Poellinger L, Gustafsson J-Å (1994): Regulation of human dioxin receptor function by indolocarbazoles, receptor ligands of dietary origin. *J Biol Chem* 269: 5137–5144

Landers JP, Bunce NJ (1991): The Ah receptor and the mechanism of dioxin toxicity. *Biochem J* 276: 273–287

Lassar AB, Buskin JN, Lockshon D, Davis RL, Apone S, Haupschka SD, Weintraub H (1989): MyoD is a sequence-specific DNA binding protein requiring a region of myc homology to bind to the muscle creatine kinase enhancer. *Cell* 58: 823–831

Legraverend C, Hannah RR, Eisen HJ, Owens IS, Nebert DW, Hankinson O (1982): Regulatory gene product of the Ah locus: characterization of receptor mutants among mouse hepatoma clones. *J Biol Chem* 257: 6402–6407

Li L, Zhou J, James G, Heller-Harrison R, Czech M, Olson EN (1992): FGF inactivates myogenic helix-loop-helix proteins through phosphorylation of a conserved protein kinase C site in their DNA binding domains. *Cell* 71: 1181–1194

Lindquist S, Craig EA (1988): The heat shock proteins. *Annu Rev Genet* 22: 631–677

Mason GGF, Witte A-M, Whitelaw ML, Antonsson C, McGuire J, Wilhelmsson A, Poellinger L, Gustafsson J-Å (1994): Purification of the DNA binding form of dioxin receptor: role of the Arnt cofactor in regulation of dioxin receptor function. *J Biol Chem* 269: 4438–4449

Matsushita N, Sogawa K, Ema M, Yoshida A, Fujii-Kuriyama Y (1993): A factor binding to the xenobiotic responsive element (XRE) of P-450IA1 gene consists of at least two helix-loop-helix proteins, Ah receptor and Arnt. *J Biol Chem* 268: 21002–21006

McGinnis W, Levine MS, Hafen E, Kuroiwa A, Gehring WJ (1984): A conserved DNA sequence in homeotic genes of the Drosophila Antennapedia and bithorax complexes. *Nature* 308: 428–433

McGuire J, Whitelaw ML, Pongratz I, Gustafsson J-Å, Poellinger L (1994): A cellular factor stimulates ligand-dependent release of hsp90 from the basic helix-loop-helix dioxin receptor. *Mol Cell Biol* 14: 2438–2446

Mitchell PJ, Tjian R (1989): Transcriptional regulation in mammalian cells by sequence-specific DNA binding proteins. *Science* 245: 371–378

Miyata Y, Yahara I (1992): The 90 kDa heat shock protein, hsp90, binds and protects casein kinase II from self aggregation and enhances its kinase activity. *J Biol Chem* 267: 7042–7047

Nambu JR, Lewis JO, Wharton KA Jr, Crews ST (1991): The drosophila single-minded gene encodes a helix-loop-helix protein that acts as a master regulator of CNS midline development. *Cell* 67: 1157–1167

Nebert DW, Gonzales FJ (1987): P-450 genes: structure, evolution and regulation. *Annu Rev Biochem* 56: 945–993

Nemoto T, Mason GGF, Wilhelmsson A, Cuthill S, Hapgood J, Gustafsson J-Å, Poellinger L (1990a): Activation of the dioxin and glucocorticoid receptors to a DNA binding state under cell-free conditions. *J Biol Chem* 265: 2269–2277

Nemoto T, Ohara-Nemoto Y, Denis M, Gustafsson J-Å (1990b): The transformed glucocorticoid receptor has a lower steroid binding affinity than the nontransformed receptor. *Biochemistry* 29: 1880–1886

Neuhold LA, Shirayoshi Y, Ozato K, Jones JE, Nebert DW (1989): Regulation of mouse CYP1A1 gene expression by dioxin: requirement of two cis-acting elements during induction. *Mol Cell Biol* 9: 2378–2386

Okino ST, Pendurthi UR, Tukey RH (1992): Phorbol esters inhibit the dioxin receptor-mediated transcriptional activation of mice nonresponsive to induction of the mouse Cyp1a1 AND Cyp1a2 genes by 2,3,7,8-tetrachlorodibenzo-p-dioxin. *J Biol Chem* 267: 6991–6998

Olson EN, Klein WH (1994): bHLH factors in muscle development: dead ends and commitments, what to leave in and what to leave out. *Genes Dev* 8: 1–8

Paulson KE, Darnell J Jr, Rushmore T, Pickett CB (1990): Analysis of the upstream elements of the xenobiotic compound-inducible and positionally regulated glutathione S-transferase Ya gene. *Mol Cell Biol* 10: 1841-1852

Perdew GH (1988): Association of the Ah receptor with the 90 kD heat shock protein. *J Biol Chem* 263: 13802-13805

Perdew GH (1991): Comparison of cytosolic and nuclear forms of the Ah receptor from Hepa 1c1c7 cells: charge heterogeneity and ATP binding properties. *Arch Biochem Biophys* 291: 284–290

Perdew GH, Hollenback CE (1990): Analysis of photoaffinity-labeled aryl hydrocarbon receptor heterogeneity by two-dimensional gel electrophoresis. *Biochemistry* 29: 6210–6214

Picard D, Khursheed B, Garabedian MJ, Fortin MG, Lindquist S, Yamamoto KR (1990): Reduced levels of hsp90 compromise steroid receptor action in vivo. *Nature* 348: 166–168

Picard D, Salser SJ, Yamamoto KR (1988): A movable and regulable inactivation function within the steroid binding domain of the glucocorticoid receptor. *Cell* 54: 1073–1080

Pimental RA, Liang B, Yee GK, Wilhelmsson A, Poellinger L, Paulson KE (1993): Dioxin receptor and C/EBP regulate the function of the glutathione S-transferase Ya gene xenobiotic response element. *Mol Cell Biol* 13: 4365–4373

Poellinger L (1994): unpublished observation

Poellinger L, Göttlicher M, Gustafsson J-Å (1992): The dioxin and peroxisome proliferator-activated receptors: nuclear receptors in search of endogenous ligands. *Trends Pharm Sci* 13: 241–245

Poland A, Knutson JC (1982): 2,3,7,8-tetrachlorodibenzo-p-dioxin and related halogenated aromatic hydrocarbons: examination of the mechanism of toxicity. *Annu Rev Pharmacol Toxicol* 22: 517–554

Poland A, Glover E, Ebetino FH, Kende AS (1986): Photoaffinity labeling of the Ah receptor. *J Biol Chem* 261: 6352–6365

Poland A, Glover E, Bradfield CA (1991): Characterization of polyclonal antibodies to the Ah receptor prepared by immunization with a synthetic peptide hapten. *Mol Pharmacol* 39: 20–26

Pollenz RS, Sattler CA, Poland A (1994): The aryl hydrocarbon receptor and aryl hydrocarbon receptor nuclear translocator protein show distinct subcellular localizations in Hepa1c1c7 cells by immunofluorescence microscopy. *Mol Pharmacol* 45: 428–438

Pongratz I, Mason GGF, Poellinger L (1992): Dual roles of the 90 kDa heat shock protein in modulating functional activities of the dioxin receptor. *J Biol Chem* 267: 13728–13734

Pongratz I, Strömstedt P-E, Poellinger L (1991): Inhibition of the specific DNA binding activity of the dioxin receptor by phosphatase treatment. *J Biol Chem* 266: 16813–16817

Pongratz I, Whitelaw ML, Poellinger L (1994): unpublished observation

Pratt WB (1993): The role of heat shock proteins in regulating the function, folding, and trafficking of the glucocorticoid receptor. *J Biol Chem* 268: 21455–21458

Pratt WB, Hutchinson KA, Scherrer LC (1992): Steroid receptor folding by heat-shock proteins and composition of the receptor heterocomplex. *Trends Endocrinol Metab* 3: 326–333

Prendergast GC, Ziff EB (1992): A new bind for myc. *Trends Genet* 8: 91–96

Prendergast GC, Lawe D, Ziff EB (1991): Association of myn, the murine homolog of Max, with c-Myc stimulates methylation-sensitive DNA binding and ras cotransfection. *Cell* 65: 395–407

Probst MR, Reisz-Porszasz S, Agbunag RV, Ong MS, Hankinson O (1993): Role of the aryl hydrocarbon receptor nuclear translocator protein in aryl hydrocarbon (dioxin) receptor function. *Mol Pharmacol* 44: 511–518

Rannug A, Rannug U, Rosenkrantz HS, Winqvist L, Westerholm R, Agurell E, Grafström A-K (1987): Certain photooxidized derivatives of tryptophan bind with very high affinity to the Ah receptor and are likely to be endogenous signal substances. *J Biol Chem* 262: 15422–15427

Reyes H, Reiz-Porszasz S, Hankinson O (1992): Identification of the Ah receptor nuclear translocator protein (Arnt) as a component of the DNA binding form of the Ah receptor. *Science* 256: 1193–1195

Safe S (1986): Comparative toxicology and mechanism of action of polychlorinated dibenzo-p-dioxins and dibenzofurans. *Annu Rev Pharamcol Toxicol* 26: 371–399

Safe S (1990): Polychlorinated biphenyls (PCBFs), dibenzo-p-dioxins (PCDDs), dibenzofurans (PCDFs) and related compounds: environmental and mechanistic considerations which support the development of toxic equivalency factors (TEFs). *Crit Rev Toxicol* 21: 51–88

Schmitz ML, Baeuerle PA (1991): The p65 subunit is responsible for the strong transcription activation potential of NF-κB. *EMBO J* 10:3805–3817

Shaknovich R, Shue G, Kohtz DS (1992): Conformational activation of a basic helix-loop-helix protein (MyoD) by the C-terminal region of murine hsp90 (hsp84). *Mol Cell Biol* 12: 5059-5068

Shen ES, Whitlock JPJr (1992): Protein-DNA interactions at a dioxin-responsive enhancer: mutational analysis of the DNA binding site for the liganded Ah receptor. *J Biol Chem* 267: 6815–6819

Shue G, Kohtz DS (1994): Structural and functional aspects of basic helix-loop-helix protein folding by heat shock protein 90. *J Biol Chem* 269: 2702–2711

Smith DF, Toft DO (1993): Steroid receptors and their associated proteins. *Mol Endocrinol* 7: 4–11

Suskind RR (1985): Chloracne, the "hallmark of dioxin intoxication". *Scand J Work Environ Health* 165: 165–171

Sutter TR, Guzman K, Dold KM, Greenlee WF (1991): Targets for dioxin: genes for plasminogen activator inhibitor-2 and interleukin-1β. *Science* 258: 238–240

Takahashi JS (1992): Circadian clock genes are ticking. *Science* 258: 238–240

Thayer MT, Weintraub H (1993): A cellular factor stimulates the DNA binding activity of MyoD and E47. *Proc Natl Acad Sci USA* 90: 6483–6487

Watson AJ, Hankinson O (1992): Dioxin- and Ah receptor-dependent protein binding to xenobiotic response elements and G-rich DNA studies by in vivo footprinting. *J Biol Chem* 267: 6874–6878

Weintraub H (1993): The MyoD family and myogenesis: redundancy, networks, and thresholds. *Cell* 75: 1241–1244

Wharton KA, Yedvobnick B, Finnerty KA, Artavanis-Tsakonas S (1985): opa: a novel family of transcribed repeats shared by the notch locus and other developmentally regulated lock in Drosophila melanogaster. *Cell* 40: 55–62

Whitelaw ML, Göttlicher M, Gustafsson J-Å, Poellinger L (1993a): Definition of a novel ligand binding domain of a nuclear bHLH receptor: co-localization of ligand and hsp90 binding activities within the regulable inactivation domain of the dioxin receptor. *EMBO J* 12: 4169–4179

Whitelaw ML, Gustafsson JÅ, Poellinger, L (1994): unpublished observations

Whitelaw ML, Pongratz I, Wilhelmsson A, Gustafsson J-Å, Poellinger L (1993b): Ligand-dependent recruitment of the Arnt coregulator determines DNA recognition by the dioxin receptor. *Mol Cell Biol* 13: 2504–2514

Whitlock JPJr (1993): Mechanistic aspects of dioxin action. *Chem Res Toxicol* 6: 754–763

Wiech H, Buchner J, Zimmermann R, Jakob U (1992): Hsp90 chaperones protein folding in vitro. *Nature* 358: 169–170

Wilhelmsson A, Cuthill S, Denis M, Wikström A-C, Gustafsson J-Å, Poellinger L (1990): The specific DNA binding activity of the dioxin receptor is modulated by the 90 kD heat shock protein. *EMBO J* 9: 69–76

Wilhelmsson A, Wikström A-C, Poellinger L (1986): Polyanionic binding properties of the receptor for 2,3,7,8-tetrachlorodibenzo-p-dioxin: a comparison with the glucocorticoid receptor. *J Biol Chem* 261: 13456–13463

Wu L, Whitlock JPJr (1993): Mechanism of dioxin action: receptor-enhancer interactions in intact cells. *Nucl Acids Res* 21: 119–125

7

Transcriptional Regulation by Heavy Metals, Exemplified at the Metallothionein Genes

RAINER HEUCHEL, FREDDY RADTKE, AND WALTER SCHAFFNER

Introduction

Seventeen of the thirty elements known to be essential for life are metals (Cotton and Wilkinson, 1980). They can function as structural or catalytic components of bioorganic molecules or even as signal transducers. (Lippard, 1993). The so-called transition metals are found in the groups IIIB to IIB of the periodic system. Of these, zinc (Group IIB) is the most widely used in living systems. In 1869 it was discovered that zinc is an essential trace element for higher organisms, and in 1940, it was the first trace element to be recognized as a component of an enzyme, namely carbonic anhydrase (Raulin, 1869; Keilin and Mann, 1940). To date, there are more than 300 enzymes known to require zinc for proper functioning (Vallee and Auld, 1990). Pathological zinc deficiency, due to greatly reduced intestinal zinc uptake as in the recessive, autosomal disorder Acrodermatitis enteropathica, leads to death unless treated by high oral zinc doses (Vallee and Falchuk, 1993). Among the zinc dependent enzymes several are involved in nucleic acid metabolism such as the prokaryotic and eukaryotic RNA polymerases (Vallee and Falchuk, 1993). It has been discovered only recently that zinc is also an integral constituent of proteins that regulate the activity of eukaryotic RNA polymerases. These factors, termed zinc finger transcription factors use zinc ions as structural components of those protein subdomains that bind to regulatory DNA sequences. The first representative which was found of this class of proteins is the *Xenopus laevis* RNA polymerase III transcription factor TFIIIA, which binds to the internal 5S RNA gene promoter and can also bind to the 5S RNA gene product itself (Hanas et al, 1983; Miller et al, 1985; Theunissen et al, 1992). Since then, dozens of proteins containing structures reminiscent of zinc fingers or other zinc-binding structures,

INDUCIBLE GENE EXPRESSION, VOLUME 1
P.A. Baeuerle, Editor
© 1995 Birkhäuser Boston

termed zinc clusters or zinc twists, have been found (Kaptain, 1991; Vallee et al, 1991). Other metals essential for life include cobalt (Co^{2+}), nickel (Ni^{2+}), copper ($Cu^{1/2+}$) and iron (Fe^{3+}). Nature has developed at least two ways, to provide for cellular availability of these important components, namely, specific import systems and unspecific cotransport systems. Especially in the latter case, cells need mechanisms to ensure that concentrations of otherwise essential metals do not become too high and that generally toxic metals, taken up fortuitously, are removed from the cell. In prokaryotes this is mainly achieved by specific efflux systems or sequestration of the compounds in question within the cell wall. In eukaryotes the best known mechanism is the intracellular sequestration of essential and toxic metals by a group of proteins called metallothioneins. In a few selected cases the control loops of effector and regulator molecules are reasonably well understood. This review will present our current knowledge regarding the transcriptional regulation of genes involved in heavy metal homeostasis and heavy metal detoxification with a main emphasis on metallothionein genes.

Metallothionein, a Protein Meant to Bind Heavy Metals

Sometime ago a protein responsible for the natural accumulation of cadmium in equine kidney cortex was described (Margoshes and Vallee, 1957). Due to its remarkably high content in sulfur, in the form of cysteine, and its ability to bind heavy metal it was named metallothionein (MT). Since then, it has been shown that metallothioneins comprise a class of highly conserved isoproteins found in organisms as different as fungi and man (Figure 7.1) (Kaegi and Kojima, 1987). For example, the *Neurospora crassa* MT has its cysteine residues at exactly the same positions as

Mouse	MT-I	Ac-MDPNCSCSTGGSCTCTSSCACKNCKCTSCKKSCCSCCPVGCSKCAQGCVCKGAADKCTCCA
Mouse	MT-II	Ac-MDPNCSCASDGSCSCAGACKCKQCKCTSCKKSCCSCCPVGCAKCSQGCICKQASDKCSCCA
Rat	MT-I	X-MDPNCSCSTGGSCTCSSSCGCKNCKCTSCKKSCCSCCPVGCSKCAQGCVCKGASDKCTCCA
Rabbit	MT-I	Ac-MDPNCSCAABGSCTCATSCRCKECKCTSCKKSCCSCCPAGCTKCAQGCICKGASDKCSCCA
Monkey	MT-I	MDPNCSCATGVSCTCADSCKCKECKCTSCKKSCCSCCPVGCAKCAQGCVCKGASEKCNCCA
Human	MT-Iᴀ	MDPNCSCATGGSCTCTGSCKCKECKCNSCKKSCCSCCPMSCAKCAQGCICKGASEKCSCCA
N.Crassa	MT	MGDCGCSGASSCNCGSGCSCSNCGSK

Figure 7.1 Amino acid sequences of class I metallothioneins (mouse, rat, rabbit, monkey, human and *Neurospora crassa*). MT-I and MT-II designate two closely related isoforms of the class I metallothionein proteins which can be readily distinguished by reversed phase HPLC, due to the presence of an acidic amino acid residue in position 10 or 11 of the standard sequence of MT-II compared to the neutral residue found in MT-I isoforms (Kaegi and Kojima, 1987). The cysteines of the characteristic Cys-Xaa-Cys and Cys-Xaa-Xaa-Cys motifs (Xaa = any amino acid except cysteine) are in bold. X indicates an undetermined blocked aminoterminus, Ac indicates an acetylated aminoterminus.

mammalian metallothioneins, however, it is only half the size of a mammalian metallothionein, and thus corresponds to their N-terminal β-domain (described below) (Münger et al, 1985). In the mouse, there are four metallothionein isogenes (MT-I to MT-IV) clustered within some 50 kb on chromosome 8, and in human there is one MT II gene and a cluster of closely linked MT I genes on chromosome 16 (Searle et al, 1984; West et al, 1990; Quaife et al, 1994). Among the human metallothionein genes there are also several pseudogenes.

Mammalian metallothioneins generally contain 61 amino acids, 20 of which are cysteines. These cysteines are organized in characteristic Cys-Xaa-Cys or Cys-Xaa-Xaa-Cys motifs (where Xaa is any amino acid except Cys) at conserved positions within the metallothionein (see Figure 7.1). Generally, metallothioneins do not contain aromatic amino acids or histidine. All cysteines are involved in the binding of seven equivalents of bivalent transition metal ions, which in most cells are predominantly zinc, copper and cadmium (Table 1).

The metal ions are exclusively bound via thiolate clusters in the alpha-domain and beta-domain of metallothionein (Figure 7.2 A, B) (Andrews, 1990; Hamer, 1986). Interestingly, the highly toxic cadmium is bound with a 10,000-fold higher avidity than zinc, underlining the possible role of metallothionein in heavy metal detoxification (Durnam and Palmiter, 1987). Indeed, it has been shown recently that organisms deficient for their metal-inducible metallothionein genes are much more sensitive to heavy metals than their wild-type counterparts (Hamer et al, 1985; Ecker et al, 1986; Michalska and Choo 1993; Masters et al, 1994). Other

Table 1. Occurrence and Metal Composition of Metallothionein

Species	Organ	Metal composition			
		Zn	Cd	Cu	Hg
Man	Liver	+ + + + + +	+/−	+/−	
	Fetal liver	+ + + +		+ +	
	Neonatal liver	+ + + +		+ +	
	Kidney	+ + +	+ + +	+	+/−
Horse	Liver	+ + + + + +	+	+/−	
	Kidney	+ + +	+ + +	+/−	
	Intestine	+ + + +	+ +	+/−	
Rat	Neonatal liver	+ + + + +		+	
	Neonatal kidney	+ + + + +			
	Adult kidney	+ +		+ + + +	
	Adult testis	+ + + + +		+	

All data refer to metallothioneins obtained from organisms not subjected to experimental pretreatment with metals (Reprinted with permission of Birkhäuser Verlag, from Kaegi and Kojima, 1987).

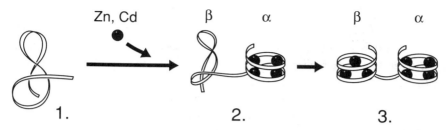

Figure 7.2A Model for binding of heavy metals to the metal-free apometallothionein. Apometallothionein exists as a random coil (1) which binds metal ions shown in black spheres in a sequential and ordered fashion. It first forms a carboxyterminal alpha-domain (2), containing four equivalents of a divalent metal ion, and then an amino-terminal beta-domain (3), containing three equivalents of a divalent metal ion (Pande et al, 1985; Stillman et al, 1987).

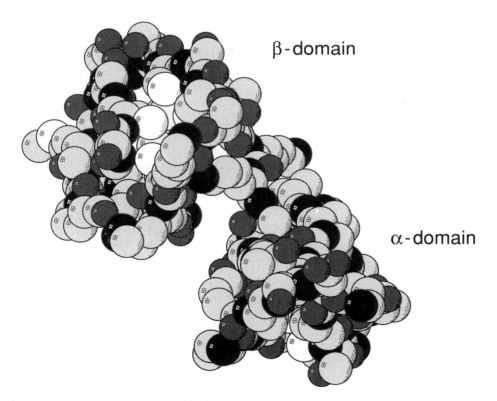

β-domain

α-domain

Figure 7.2B Space filling model of Zn_2Cd_5-metallothionein. The beta-domain contains a cluster of three metal ions, respectively. White spheres denote sulfur atoms; the white spheres appearing in a vertical line from the bottom to top represent cysteines 13, 7 and 5 of the beta-cluster. Stippled spheres, carbon; grey spheres,-oxygen; black spheres, nitrogen atoms. (Reprinted with permission of Academic Press LTD from Robbins et al, 1991.)

possible functions discussed for metallothioneins I and II are homeostasis of essential metals, i.e. zinc and copper, in vivo (Bremner and Beatti, 1990), and generalized cellular stress responses as deduced from their inducibility by such diverse stimuli as heavy metals, different forms of irradiation, high oxygen tension, hormones, interleukins, tumor promoters, infection, inflammation and many more (Table 2).

In marked contrast to the ubiquitously expressed metallothionein-I and -II genes (Hamer, 1986), there are the cell type- and developmental

Table 2. Factors that induce metallothionein synthesis in cultured cells or in vivo

Heavy metal ions	Antibiotics
Cd, Zn, Cu, Au, Ag, Co,	Streptozotocin
Ni, Bi	Cycloheximide
Hormones and second messengers	Mitomycin
Glucocorticoids	Cytotoxic agents
Progesterone	Hydrocarbons
Estrogen	Ethanol
	Isopropanol
Catecholamines	Formaldehyde
Glucagon	Fatty acids
Angiotensin II	Butyrate
Arg-Vasopressin	Chloroform
Adenosine	Carbon tetrachloride
	Bromobenzene
cAMP	Iodoacetate
Diacylglycerol	Urethane
Calcium	Ethionine
Growth factors	Di(2-ethylhexyl)phthalate
Serum factors	α-Mercapto-β-(furyl)acrylate
Insulin	6-Mercaptopurine
IGF-1	Diethyldithiocarbamate
EGF	Penicillamine
Inflammatory agents and cytokines	2,3-Dimercaptopropanol
Lipopolysaccharide (LPS)	2,3-Dimercaptosuccinate
Carrageenan	EDTA
Dextran	5-Azacytidine
Endotoxin	Acetaminophen
	Indomethacin
Interleukin-1	Stress-producing conditions
Interleukin-6	Starvation
Interferon-γ	Inflammation
Tumor necrosis factor	Laparotomy
Tumor promoters and oncogenes	Physical stress
Phorbol esters	X-irradiation
ras	O_2 tension
Vitamins	Ultraviolet radiation
Ascorbic acid	
Retinoate	
1α,25-Dihydroxyvitamin D_3	

(Reprinted with permission of Academic Press, from Kaegi, 1991)

stage-specific metallothionein-III and -IV genes. Human metallothionein-III, about 70 % homologous to human metallothionein-IIA, is expressed exclusively in the brain and has been reported to be reduced in patients with Alzheimer's disease. In cell culture, the addition of purified metal-lothionein-III reduces the growth of neurons, and it is speculated that the lack of metallothionein-III contributes to the increased regenerative processes that accompany the extensive degeneration of hippocampal and cortical brain structures of Alzheimer patients (Uchida et al, 1991). Metallothionein-IV is specifically expressed in stratified squamous epithelia associated with several organs such as oral epithelia and footpads (Quaife et al, 1994).

Although all four metallothionein isoproteins can confer elevated cadmium resistance when overexpressed in tissue culture, only the metallothionein-I and -II are inducible by heavy metal (Palmiter et al, 1992; Quaife et al, 1994). Therefore we will restrict our discussion to the metallothionein-I and -II, unless otherwise mentioned.

Transcriptional Regulation of the Metallothioneins

The cis Elements

The regulation of metallothionein is mostly exerted at the transcriptional level, since first, the relative rates of synthesis of rat liver metallothionein-I and -II directly correlate with the amounts of metallothionein mRNAs in these tissues and second, the induction of metallothionein mRNA synthesis is independent of the protein biosynthesis inhibitor cyclohex-imide (Karin et al, 1980; Durnam and Palmiter, 1981).

Initial investigations of the mouse metallothionein-I promoter including deletion and linker scanning mutation analyses lead to the conclusion that a set of similar short sequence motifs present within the first 200 bp upstream of the transcription start site are responsible for induction by heavy metals. Hence, these sequences were called MREs, for metal responsive elements (Stuart et al, 1984; Carter et al, 1984). Palmiter and colleagues have shown that each single MRE of the mouse metallothionein-I promoter can confer metal-inducible transcription to a reporter gene when cloned as tandemly repeated sequences upstream of the reporter gene's TATA box. In this assay they further note that different MREs also have a different activation potential, with MREd being the strongest inducible element (Stuart et al, 1985). By comparing all known MRE sequences and performing detailed analyses of specific point mutation-MREs, a 15 bp consensus sequence containing a mini-

m M T - I	a	-54	CTTTGCGCCCGGACT	-40
	b	-56	GTTTGCACCCAGCAG	-70
	f	-94	CTATGCGTGGGCTGG	-80
	c	-132	AAGTGCGCTCGGCTC	-118
	d	-150	CTCTGCACTCCGCCC	-136
	e	-175	CTGTGCACACTGGCG	-161

CONSENSUS   CTN<u>TGCRC</u>NCGGCCG

Figure 7.3 MRE sequences of the mouse metallothionein I promoter. Numbers denote nucleotide positions relative to the transcription start site. The consensus sequence shown below is derived from a comparison of MREs present in the mouse metallothionein I promoter. The core region, containing the five virtually invariant bases is underlined. The MREs a to e were originally defined by mutational analyses, whereas MREf was detected later by in vivo footprinting studies (Stuart et al, 1985, Mueller et al, 1988).

mal core of 7 bp has been established to be necessary for functional integrity as a metal regulatory *cis* element (Figure 7.3) (Searle et al, 1987; Culotta and Hamer, 1989; Imbert et al, 1990). Additional interesting features of MREs are that they can be found, in either orientation, upstream of all heavy metal-inducible metallothionein genes analyzed to date (Karin et al, 1984; Otto et al, 1987; Harlow et al, 1989; Andersen et al, 1986; Zafarullah et al, 1988), and that both the mouse metallothionein-I promoter or a synthetic 8xMREd element can confer metal-inducible transcription to a heterologous gene from a remote position, i.e. work as inducible enhancers (Serfling et al, 1985; Westin and Schaffner, 1988a). There are other known *cis*-acting transcriptional activator sequences in metallothionein promoters, e.g. binding sites for the transcription factors Sp1, AP1, AP2, MLTF and GR, some of which have been shown to activate transcription of metallothionein promoters in vitro (Lee et al, 1987a; Lee et al, 1987b; Mitchell et al, 1987) or in vivo (Figure 7.4) (Yagle and Palmiter, 1985; Karin et al, 1984). However, metal-inducible transcription can only be mediated by MREs. This general observation has been confirmed by in vivo footprinting, a technique that uses either chemical or enzymatic modification of DNA to analyze the interaction of DNA-binding proteins and their target sites in situ (Mueller et al, 1988). In the case of the mouse metallothionein-I promoter it has been shown that from the MRE sites, only MREd is protected to some extent by a bound protein under non-inducing conditions. After the addition of zinc however, a marked increase of protection is seen over MREd and most notably over the other 5 MRE sites. The protection pattern over the Sp1 and MLTF binding sites shows constitutive protein binding, i.e. independent of metal treatment of the cells (Mueller et al, 1988).

Mouse metallothionein MT-I gene

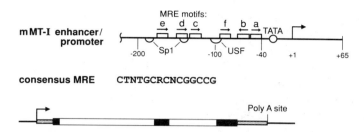

consensus MRE   CTNTGCRCNCGGCCG

amino acid sequence

MDPNCSCSTGGSCTCTSSCACKNCKCTSCKKSCCSCCPVGCSKCAQGCVCKGAADKCTCCA

Drosophila metallothionein

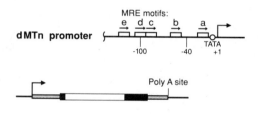

amino acid sequence

MPCPCGSGCKCASQATKGSCNCGSDCKCGGDKKSACGCSE

Yeast (S. cerevisiae) copper metallothionein (CUP1)

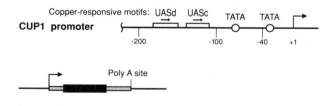

amino acid sequence

MFSELINFQNEGHECQCQCGSCKNNEQCQKSCSCPTGCNSDDKCPCGNKSEETKKSCCSGK

Figure 7.4 Promoter sequences from the genes of mouse metallothionein I (mMT-I), the *D. melanogaster* metallothionein (Mtn), and the yeast *S. cerevisiae* metallothionein gene (CUP1) are shown together with their respective gene structure and amino acid sequences. MRE, metal responsive element; UAS, upstream activator sequence; upstream/downstream untranslated sequences are represented as stippled boxes in the gene schema; black boxes and open boxes in the gene schema designate exon and intron sequences, respectively.

The Hunt for the Metal Inducibility Conferring Principle

After the detailed analysis of the metal-inducible promoter of the metal-lothionein genes, different laboratories tried to identify and ultimately clone and characterize factors interacting with the corresponding DNA sequences. First results were obtained by bandshift analyses (Westin and Schaffner, 1988a; Searle, 1990; Koizumi et al, 1992), in vitro and in vivo footprints (Mueller et al, 1988; Séguin, 1991), UV-crosslinking experiments (Andersen et al, 1990), and Southwestern blot analyses (Séguin and Prévost, 1988; Czupryn et al, 1992). Westin and Schaffner detected a specific protein-DNA interaction using the so-called bandshift or gel retardation assay. They incubated nuclear HeLa cell extracts and radioactively labelled MREd oligonucleotides from the mouse metallothionein-I promoter. These reaction mixtures were then resolved on a native (nondenaturing) polyacrylamide gel (PAGE). Labelled MREd oligonucleotides which had been specifically bound by protein showed a retarded migration (shift) compared to the free labeled DNA. Depending on the conditions for the initial binding reaction, they detected differently retarded bands. Using nuclear extracts without adding zinc to the binding reaction, only the constitutively active transcription factor Sp1 binds to MREd. Upon addition of zinc however another protein bound to MREd, resulting in a slightly faster migrating band. This DNA binding-activity has been termed MTF-1 (MRE-binding transcription factor) (Westin and Schaffner, 1988a).

Using methylation interference analyses, it has been shown that Sp1 and MTF-1 have overlapping but not identical binding sites. This in vitro technique allows the determination of individual bases that interfere with sequence specific binding of proteins due to chemical modification of the DNA prior to the binding reaction. Based on these results a model has been suggested in which elevated intracellular zinc concentrations trigger the binding of a preexisting zinc-dependent factor(s) to the MREs, resulting in metal-induced transcription. This model is also consistent with earlier experiments showing that zinc-induced metallothionein transcription in HeLa cells occurs even in the presence of protein synthesis inhibitors (Karin et al, 1980). The obvious zinc-dependence of MTF-1 for DNA-binding lead Westin and Schaffner (1988a) to propose that MTF-1 will bind to DNA with so-called zinc finger motifs as defined earlier for other transcription factors (Miller et al, 1985).

MTF-1 is a Zinc Finger Protein

MTF-1 has been cloned in our laboratory using a specifically designed MRE oligonucleotide to screen a mouse cDNA expression library of B-cell origin (Radtke et al, 1993). This oligonucleotide has the advantage of binding very strongly to MTF-1, but unlike the original MREd oligonucleotide, it is unable to bind Sp1.

The cloned cDNA sequence of MTF-1 contains an open reading frame of 675 amino acids with a calculated molecular weight of 72.6 kDa. The amino-terminal half harbors six zinc fingers similar to the type found in the RNA polymerase III transcription factor TFIIIA (Cys_2His_2) (Brown et al, 1985; Miller et al, 1985). These structures are followed by three regions reminiscent of transcriptional activator domains, with high densities of acidic amino acids, proline and serine/threonine (Mitchell and Tjian, 1989; Seipel et al, 1992). From the three putative activation domains, the acidic one was shown to be active when fused to the GAL4 DNA binding domain (Xu et al, 1994).

Recombinant MTF-1 is Identical to the Endogenous MRE-binding Activity

Mouse recombinant MTF-1 which has been overexpressed in monkey COS cells, and the endogenous activity from mouse 3T6 cells both display identical migration behavior and binding activities in bandshift analyses. In addition, no difference in sensitivity to chelator treatment or partial proteolysis, or binding specificity and affinity to a set of mutant MRE oligonucleotide can be detected (Radtke et al, 1993).

MTF-1 is a Transcriptional Activator Protein

To test the biological activity of recombinant mouse MTF-1, human HeLa cells were cotransfected with an MTF-1 expression vector plus either natural or synthetic MRE-containing promoter/reporter gene plasmids. Recombinant MTF-1 strongly activated transcription of such reporter genes, but surprisingly, it did so even without zinc treatment of the transfected cells. These observations were not due to testing a mouse factor in human cells, since transfection of several mouse cell lines yielded the same result. There always was a clear dose-dependent relationship between the amount of transfected MTF-1 and the evoked basal, i.e. uninduced, transcriptional response. At the same time, the metal-induced transcription levels of MTF-1 transfected cells usually did not exceed the ones of cells without extra MTF-1 (Radtke et al, 1993). Therefore, some doubts remained regarding the role of MTF-1 in metallothionein gene regulation, despite the facts that recombinant MTF-1 bound to an MRE oligonucleotide in the same zinc-dependent manner as the endogenous MRE-binding activity and that MTF-1 was the only detectable MRE-binding activity. Also, it was comforting to see that human MTF-1, recently cloned in our group, showed a pronounced zinc response in transfected cells (Brugnera et al, 1994).

Zinc Response in Higher Eukaryotes : The Role of MTF-1

To find out unambiguously whether MTF-1 is involved in metal regulated transcription of the metallothionein genes, a murine null mutant embryonic stem (ES) cell line ($-/-$) that lacks a functional MTF-1 gene was generated (Heuchel et al, 1994). Targeting vectors for homologous recombination were constructed in order to replace most of the first zinc finger exon with either the neomycin phosphotransferase gene or the hygromycin gene. These two replacement vectors were consecutively electroporated into ES cells. Positive clones were tested for homologous recombination by PCR and confirmed by Southern blot analysis (Figure 7.5).

In bandshift assays it has been demonstrated that nuclear extracts from $-/-$ ES cells still contain the ubiquitous transcription factor Sp1, but no MTF-1 activity, irrespective of whether the nuclear extract is prepared

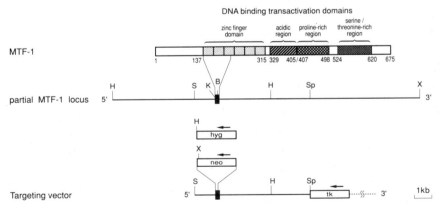

Figure 7.5 Disruption of the mouse MTF-1 locus in embryonic stem (ES) cells. A schematic diagram of the MTF-1 protein is shown together with the part of the MTF-1 gene locus containing the first zinc finger exon of 238 bp. The targeting vectors include 6.7 kb of genomic sequence. Two-thirds of the first zinc finger exon were replaced by either the neomycin cassette (neo) or hygromycin cassette (hyg) via homologous recombination. The neomycin and hygromycin genes were used for positive selection, whereas the herpes simplex virus thymidine kinase gene (tk) was used for negative selection. Sites for restriction enzymes: B, *BamHI*; H, *HindIII*; K, *KpnI*; S, *SacI*; Sp, *SpeI* (not all sites shown); X, *XbaI*; thin horizontal lines, intron sequences; black rectangle, first zinc finger exon; dotted line, pBluescript; arrows above positive and negative selection marker cassettes denote direction of their transcription (Heuchel et al, 1994).

from uninduced or zinc-induced cells. $+/+$ ES control cells (wild-type for the MTF-1 locus but neomycin resistant due to fortuitous, nonhomologous vector integration) however, contain Sp1 and zinc-dependent MTF-1 activity.

To investigate the role of MTF-1 in metallothionein gene regulation, mRNA levels of the endogenous metallothionein-I and -II genes were measured. $+/+$ ES cells contain MTF-1 mRNA whose level was only marginally, if at all, changed by zinc treatment, which makes an autoregulatory loop for MTF-1 transcription rather unlikely. However, as expected, the levels of metallothionein-I/-II transcripts were significantly induced upon zinc treatment. In marked contrast, the $-/$ $-$ ES cells did not contain detectable amounts of MTF-1 transcripts or of metallothionein-I/-II mRNA, either before or after treatment of the cells with zinc. Similar results were obtained with other well known inducers of metallothionein genes, namely cadmium, copper, nickel, or lead (Figure 7.6). Results supporting the influence of MTF-1 on metallothionein expression came also from antisense experiments, where inducibility by a number of bivalent metals to stably integrated reporter genes driven by a 5xMREd promoter was found to be reduced (Palmiter, 1994).

In an attempt to restore metallothionein transcription by expression of additional MTF-1, we have transfected $+/+$ and $-/-$ ES cells with reporter genes under the control of either 4 copies of the strong metal-responsive element MREd (4xMREd OVEC), or the complete mouse metallothionein-I promoter (MT-I OVEC). Treatment of $+/+$ ES cells with $400\,\mu M$ zinc resulted in a 10-fold increase of transcription from a transfected 4xMREd reporter gene. By contrast, in the $-/-$ ES cell line, reporter gene expression was barely detectable either with or without zinc treatment. After cotransfection of the cloned MTF-1 gene, transcription was restored to the same levels as observed with MTF-1 cotransfected $+/$ $+$ ES cells. These results show that the metal-inducibility of natural and synthetic metal-responsive promoters is lost upon disruption of the MTF-1 gene and can be restored to a large extent by cotransfection of the MTF-1 expression vector (Heuchel et al, 1994).

Models for Heavy Metal Regulated Transcription of Metallothionein Genes

The experiments done by Heuchel et al demonstrate that normal mouse MT-I/II gene regulation is dependent on the presence of MTF-1. Interestingly, even the complete metallothionein-I/II enhancer/promo-

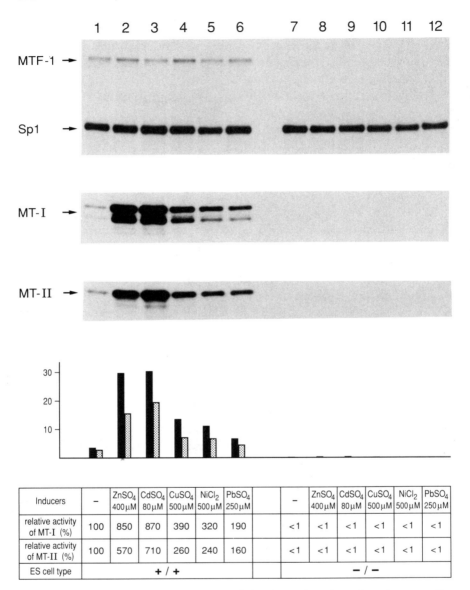

Figure 7.6 Loss of metallothionein gene regulation in MTF-1 $-/-$ embryonic stem cells. Transcript levels for MTF-1, metallothionein-I and metallothionein-II were determined in MTF-1 $+/+$ (lanes 1 to 6) and MTF-1 $-/-$ ES cells (lanes 7 to 12). Sp1 transcript levels were used as internal controls for RNA loading. Before harvesting, cells were treated with different metal salts as indicated. In the presence of MTF-1, a several-fold induction of both the metallothionein-I and -II genes can be observed upon challenging $+/+$ ES cells with different heavy metals (lanes 1 to 6). The transcript levels of Sp1 and MTF-1 itself are not influenced by this treatment. However, neither basal nor heavy metal-induced transcripts of both metallothionein genes can be detected in $-/-$ ES cells which lack MTF-1, whereas Sp1 transcript levels are unchanged as expected (lanes 7 to 12) (Heuchel et al, 1994).

ter region was not activated to any appreciable extent in the absence of MTF-1. This means that MTF-1 is not only necessary for metal-induced but also for basal transcription of the metallothionein-I and -II genes. This is surprising, since it has been shown that the binding sites for the ubiquitous transcription factors Sp1 and MLTF/USF within the mouse metallothionein-I promoter are occupied in vivo, even without heavy metal challenge, and one might thus have expected them to be responsible for basal transcription (Mueller et al, 1988). These factors may nevertheless have some auxiliary role in concert with MTF-1. Based on (1) the absolute dependence on MTF-1 for metallothionein transcription, (2) the independence of de novo protein synthesis for transcriptional induction and (3) the zinc-dependent DNA binding of MTF-1 in vivo and in vitro, several models for metal induction can be envisaged.

In the uninduced case, i.e. without heavy metal challenge, only a small percentage of MTF-1 protein is able to bind to its recognition sites, with MREd being the site with the highest binding affinity. There are several explanations for this finding. It is conceivable that the binding of nuclear MTF-1 to DNA is very sensitive to changes in intracellular zinc concentrations. Indeed, Radtke et al noticed a four-fold increase in MTF-1 binding activity in vitro after challenging the cells for four hours with zinc (Figure 7.7) (Radtke et al, 1993). At low zinc concentrations, it might be that only a fraction of the whole nuclear MTF-1 population is competent for DNA binding or that only a fraction of the six zinc fingers necessary for DNA binding are saturated with zinc. Alternatively, the nuclear factor concentration could be subcritical at low zinc conditions because, for example,

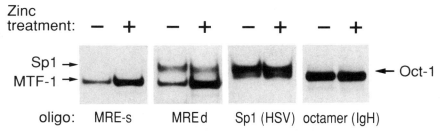

Figure 7.7 Bandshift analysis using nuclear extracts from uninduced (−) and zinc-induced (+) mouse 3T6 cells. For induction, cells were treated with 100 μM ZnSo$_4$ for 4 hr before harvesting. The positions of the protein-DNA interactions are indicated as Sp1, MTF-1 or Oct-1. MRE-s contains a single binding site for MTF-1, whereas MREd contains overlapping binding sites for both MTF-1 and Sp1. In marked contrast to the MTF-1 signal intensity, which increases about four fold upon zinc induction, the signal intensities for Sp1 and Oct-1 remain unchanged (Reprinted with permission of Oxford University Press from Radtke et al, 1993).

MTF-1 may be sequestered in the cytoplasm by (1) an RNA as in the case of the zinc finger factor TFIIIA, which can bind to the 5S RNA gene internal control region and to 5S RNA itself (Picard and Wegnez, 1979; Theunissen et al, 1992) or (2) as speculated by R.D. Palmiter, by a cytoplasmic anchoring factor as for example seen with NFκBF and IκB (Henkel et al, 1993; Palmiter, 1994). We have shown that a nuclear extract from zinc-treated cells has always a higher MTF-1 binding activity than nuclear extracts from untreated cells even though saturating amounts of zinc were added to the in vitro binding reaction (Figure 7.8), which is compatible with several possibilities.

If the intracellular zinc concentration is elevated, it could be that all six zinc fingers become saturated with zinc and bind, here in the case of the mouse metallothionein-I promoter, to all MRE sites thereby cooperating to bring about a high transcription rate (Figure 7.9A), or MTF-1 might be released from its interaction with some cytoplasmic component for transport into the nucleus (Figure 7.9B). It is also conceivable that there is a modification system that modulate the transcriptional competence of MTF-1 according to intracellular changes in the zinc concentrations. For example, the transcription factor c-Jun is differently phosphorylated upon different stimuli which modulates its transcriptional competence (Hunter and Karin, 1992). Another possibility would be the existence of a repressor which, in the absence of zinc, keeps the metallothionein promoter in a closed, inaccessible chromatin state (Figure 7.9C), or there might even be a specific coactivator involved as illustrated in

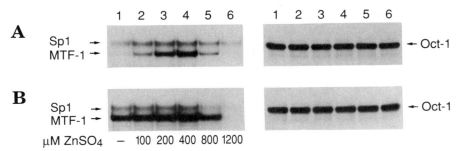

Figure 7.8 Zinc-induced DNA binding of MTF-1 from untreated and zinc-treated cells. Nuclear extracts were prepared from untreated cells (A) and cells treated with 100 μM zinc sulfate for 4 hr prior to harvest and extract preparation (B). Lanes 1-6, increasing amounts of ZnSO$_4$ as indicated were added to the binding buffer before the DNA-protein binding reaction and gel electrophoresis. The lefthand side shows bandshifts with the MREd oligonucleotide, which binds both Sp1 and MTF-1. The righthand side shows bandshifts using an octamer site as a control for the amount of protein loaded, since the Oct-1 binding activity is known to be insensitive to zinc treatment (Westin and Schaffner, 1988a). MTF-1 binding in nuclear extracts from zinc-pretreated cells is always higher than from untreated cells, even if saturating amounts of zinc are added to the binding reaction.

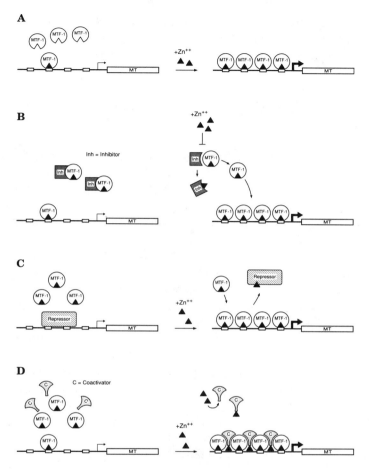

Figure 7.9 Models for metal-induced transcription of metallothionein genes by MTF-1 (A) Allosteric zinc finger model. Transcriptional induction of the metallothionein gene is solely dependent on promoter occupancy by MTF-1. Zinc acts as a coinducer in that it transforms the loose zinc finger structures of MTF-1 into a DNA binding-competent form. This model proposed for mammalian MTF-1 has been shown independently to be correct for the yeast copper metallothionein systems (Westin and Schaffner, 1988; Fuerst et al, 1988). (B) Protein/ MTF-1 inhibitor model. Under normal conditions most of the MTF-1 is bound by an inhibitor that is released by intracellular increase in the zinc concentration. (C) DNA repressor model. The metallothionein promoter is kept in an inactive state by a repressor bound to the DNA. Upon an increase in the intracellular zinc concentration the repressor, which itself may have an affinity for zinc is exchanged for high affinity binding MTF-1. However, this scenario is rather unlikely in the light of the in vivo footprinting data by Mueller et al (1988). They noted that only MREd among all MREs of the mouse metallothionein-I promoter is bound by protein in untreated cells. Treating the cells with $ZnSO_4$ only increases the general intensity of the footprint over MREd, but there is no qualitative change in any of the protected guanosine bases. From this one still cannot exclude the possibility of a repressor with binding properties similar to MTF-1. (D) Coactivator model. In this model, a specific coactivator binds zinc upon increase of the intracellular zinc concentration and interacts with MTF-1 proteins to fully induce transcription of the metallothionein genes. A combination of model B, C or D with model A is possible.

Figure 7.9D. Finally, it is also possible that the heavy metal regulated transcription of the metallothionein genes is in fact a mixture of all possibilities mentioned above.

MerR, a Mercury Regulated Repressor/activator of Prokaryotic Transcription

While exciting problems remain to be solved in heavy metal-inducible gene transcription of mammals, more is known about such regulation processes in micro-organisms. Interestingly, bacteria, and yeasts, have evolved their own systems specifically tailored to cope with heavy metal load. In prokaryotes metal ions are taken up either by specific and regulated transport systems as in the case of nickel, or they are coimported by constitutive Mg^{2+} transport systems. Due to the broad specificity of the ion uptake systems, nonessential or even toxic metals such as cadmium (Cd^{2+}) can also enter the cell. In addition, even essential metals can accumulate to toxic levels within a bacterial cell (Silver and Walderhaug, 1992; Nies, 1992). Therefore resistance mechanisms, mostly encoded on plasmids, have evolved which either actively export metal ions themselves, inactivate and remove metal ions by sequestration, or reduce the ions to metallic form which can passively leave the cell. The latter is found for mercury. Resistance towards mercury is widespread in gram-negative and gram-positive bacteria (Helmann et al, 1990; Misra, 1992; O'Halloran, 1993). This complex system, encoded by several genes within the *mer* operon is a means for many bacteria to clear their microenvironment of toxic mercury. The operon comprises genes for mercury transport designated *merT* and *merP*, mercury metabolism (*merA merB*) and for the transcriptional regulation (*merR*) of the operon itself. The key enzyme in the detoxification process is the mercuric ion reductase (*merA*). This enzyme catalyses the reduction of Hg(II) to the volatile and lipophilic Hg(0), which then passively diffuses from the cell. Many *mer* operons also contain another mercury specific enzyme, organomercurit lyase (*merB*), which breaks the C-Hg bond, thereby converting a highly toxic compound into the less toxic Hg(II) which can then be metabolized by MerA. The *mer* operon is divergently expressed with the structural genes *merT, P, (C), A,* and *D* transcribed into a single polycistronic mRNA encoded by one strand and the overall regulator protein *merR* encoded by the other strand of the DNA molecule. The *merR* gene encodes a transcriptional repressor/ activator of the classical helix-turn-helix protein class (Helmann, 1989). It binds to its operator sequence as a homodimer between the two hexanucleotide polymerase recognition elements at the positions -35 and -10 of the P_T promoter. Independently of the presence of Hg, repressor binding introduces a slight bend into the operator DNA (Ansari and O'Halloran, 1992). In the absence of Hg(II), MerR represses the

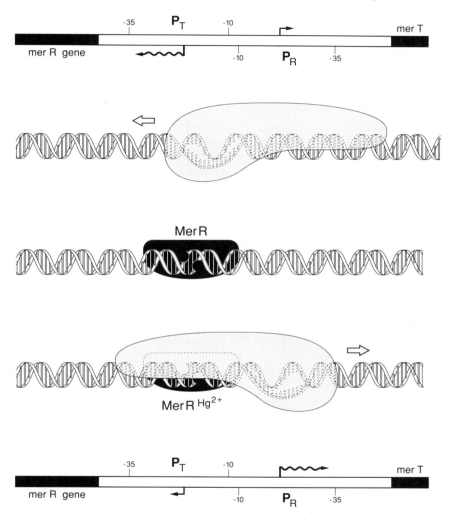

Figure 7.10 Model for the regulation of the divergently arranged promoters of the *mer* operon. Based on footprinting results with σ^{70}RNA polymerase, MerR and the *mer* promoters (P_R and P_T), the following scenario can be envisaged: in the absence of Mer R, polymerase binds to the P_R promoter and expresses *mer* R. The repressor MerR binds between the -35 and -10 RNA polymerase recognition elements of P_T, thereby sterically hindering binding of RNA polymerase to P_R. Instead, RNA polymerase binds loosely to MerR-bound P_T. In this form RNA polymerase is unable to form an open transcription initiation complex, which is only possible if MerR binds mercury. This way, MerR is transformed from a repressor to an activator protein. Adapted with permission fromO'Halloran et al (1989).

structural gene promoter P_T by keeping it a low affinity site for RNA polymerase, and it also represses its own promoter P_R by steric hindrance (Figure 7.10). In the presence of mercury, however, bound MerR homodimer binds one Hg(II) and by an allosteric mechanism induces an additional unwinding of its DNA recognition site of about 30° when compared to the mercury-free form (Ansari and O'Halloran, 1993). Thereby the -10 and -35 regions of P_T, which are suboptimally phased by an unusually large spacing of 19 base pairs (bp) instead of the optimal 17 bp for *E.coli* promoters (Figure 7.11A) (Harley and Reynolds, 1987; Hawley and McClure, 1983) are twisted to achieve a perfect architecture resulting in a high affinity promoter for RNA polymerase (Figure 7.11B, C) (Ansari et al, 1992). Thus MerR fulfills two tasks at the same time. It represses its own transcription independent of the presence of Hg(II) as long as the repressor concentration is high enough, and it activates the genes for Hg-metabolism/detoxification only when the specific ligand is present.

Heavy Metal Resistance in Lower Eukaryotes Conferred by Class II and Class III Metallothioneins

The class I metallothioneins of higher eukaryotes are characterized by the specific arrangement of cysteines closely related to the first characterized prototype of metallothioneins, from horse kidney. Recently, groups of clearly distinct metallothioneins have been detected, termed class II and class III metallothioneins (Fowler et al, 1987). The class II metallothioneins are characterized by an arrangement of cysteine-rich motifs which are only distantly related to those in horse metallothionein. Representative of this group were found in the cyanobacterium *Synechococcus spec.* (Olafson et al, 1988; Shi et al, 1992), in the yeasts *S. cerevisiae* and *C. glabrata* (Winge et al, 1985; Thiele, 1992), the worm *Caenorhabditis elegans* (Slice et al, 1990; Imagawa et al, 1990) and a higher plant (Kawashima et al, 1992). The atypical class III metallothioneins were isolated first from the fission yeast *S. pombe*, here called cadystins, (Murasugi et al, 1981; Kondo et al, 1984) or from plants where they are called phytochelatins (Grill et al, 1985; Grill et al, 1991; Robinson et al, 1993). Chemically, the class III metallothioneins are not proteins or peptides encoded by a specific gene but rather γ-glutamyl isopeptides (γ-glutamylcysteinyl-glycine; Figure 7.12), enzymatically synthesized from glutathione and range in M_T from 2000 to 10,000 (Figure 7.11) (Rauser, 1990; Steffens, 1990). In plants the phytochelatins are mainly involved in binding of copper and cadmium (Grill E, 1987; Robinson et al, 1987). An

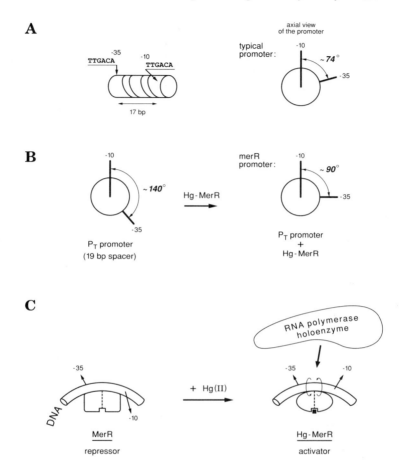

Figure 7.11 Change of promoter geometry allows transcriptional activation of the *mer* promoter P$_T$. (A) The relative positions of the -35 and -10 σ^{70}RNA polymerase recognition elements are schematically shown on an *E.coli* consensus promoter, here depicted as a cylinder. If we look down the helix axis, the DNA appears as a circle and the bars that are placed at the center of the -10 and the -35 regions are offset by a dihedral angle of 74°. (B) Between the -35 and -10 elements of the P$_T$ promoter, there is a 19 bp spacing sequence. As a result of this unusual spacing, the dihedral angle is offset 140° , and consequently P$_T$ is only a weak promoter. The underwinding introduced by binding of merR and Hg-MerR would face the -35 and -10 promoter elements such that they would fit quite closely to the dihedral angle typically seen in consensus *E. coli* promoters. (C) Local DNA distortion model for allosteric activation of the *mer* T promoter. Independently of the presence of mercury, homodimeric repressor MerR binds to the *mer* operator/promoter DNA, shown as a cylinder. This binding introduces a slight bending in the target DNA. The arrows projecting from the major groove of the DNA double helix indicate the relative positions of the -10 (projecting into the plane of the paper) and -35 (projecting out of the plane of the paper) σ^{70}RNA polymerase recognition elements. Upon binding of one mercury ion, Hg(II)-MerR twists the DNA in between the repressor monomer hands of the dimer-operator DNA complex, thereby underwinding the DNA and phasing the -10 and -35 regions for optimal interaction with the RNA polymerase (to initiate transcription). Adapted with permission from Ansari and O'Halloran (1994).

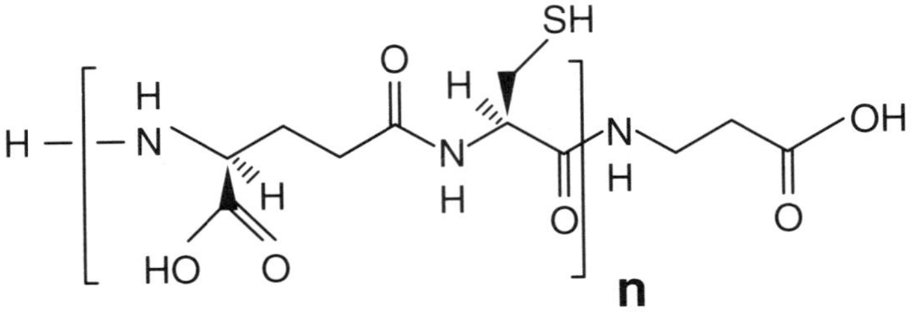

Figure 7.12 General formula of phytochelatins, the so-called class III metallothioneins. In plants the main compound to sequester cadmium ions is a group of peptides called γ-glutamyl isopeptides. The most common ones have the structure (γ-Glu-Cys)$_n$-Gly, where $n = 2$ to 11, depending on the organism. In the bean *Phaseolus spec.* (order Fabales), a slightly different variant is found. In the example shown here glycine has been replaced by β-alanine (Grill et al, 1986).

interesting aspect in the regulation of the phytochelatins is that their expression is stimulated by cadmium. In keeping with this notion, the constitutively expressed enzyme, γ-glutamylcysteine dipeptidyl transferase (phytochelatin synthetase), which synthesizes phytochelatins, requires cadmium for catalytic activity (Grill et al, 1989).

Copper Resistance in Lower Eukaryotes

There are two yeasts, namely the baker's yeast *Saccharomyces cerevisiae* and the opportunistic pathogenic yeast *Candida glabrata*, which have well studied copper-inducible metallothionein genes (Thiele, 1992). Both systems have evolved from a common ancestor, but the one of *C. glabrata* is far more sophisticated, both with respect to the number of metallothionein genes and to regulation of the regulatory factor itself.

The Regulation of Metallothionein in Saccharomyces cerevisiae

S. cerevisiae has a single class II metallothionein gene, designated CUP1, which confers copper resistance on yeast cells (Brenes-Pomales et al, 1955; Butt and Ecker, 1987). CUP1 codes for a 61 amino acid long protein that has been shown to bind eight copper molecules per polypeptide, thereby preventing toxic effects of this metal (Karin et al, 1984; Butt et al, 1984; Winge et al, 1985). CUP1 gene transcription is inducible by copper and, to a lesser extent, by its electrochemical analog silver (Fuerst et al, 1988). This metal induction is mediated in *cis* by so-called upstream activator sequences (UAS$_{CUP1}$) within the CUP1 promoter. These confer metal-inducible transcription when fused to a heterologous reporter gene and tested in yeast (Thiele and Hamer, 1986). However the MRE sequences regulating class I metallothioneins in higher eukaryotes do not show any sequence similarity to the yeast UAS_{cup1} sequences (Thiele, 1992). The fact that Cup1 confers copper-resistance in yeast was exploited by D. Thiele in an elegant series of experiments, applying classical yeast genetics to clone the responsible regulating factor. Towards this end he chemically mutagenized the copper-resistant yeast strain BR10 with EMS (ethylmethane sulfonate) to select for copper-sensitive survivors, which no longer accumulated CUP1 mRNA. He termed the resulting string ace1-1 for activation of CUP1 expression and used it to clone the responsible ACE1 gene by complementation (Thiele, 1988). Shortly thereafter these results were confirmed by the cloning of CUP2 by others, a gene which was later shown to be identical to ACE1 (Welch et al, 1989; Buchman et al, 1990). The transcriptional activator protein ACE1 is 225 amino acids long and its amino-terminal half exhibits striking similarity to CUP1 itself by the presence of the characteristic metallothionein Cys-Xaa-Cys and Cys-Xaa-Xaa-Cys motifs. Eleven of the twelve cysteine residues are crucial for copper dependent binding to the upstream activator sequences of the CUP1 promoter (Fuerst et al, 1988; Thiele, 1988; Huibregste et al, 1989; Buchman et al, 1990; Evans et al, 1990; Hu et al, 1990). In the absence of copper this combined metal and DNA binding domain does not have an ordered structural motif. Upon copper binding the polypeptide adopts a so-called copper fist structure, which is able to bind to the upstream activating sequences within the CUP1 promoter (Figure 7.13A). The carboxyterminal half is very rich in acidic amino acids, reminiscent of other yeast transcriptional activation domains such as those of GCN4 or GAL4 (Hope and Struhl, 1986; Ma and Ptashne, 1987). ACE1 is, however, not only required for metallothionein gene expression, but also regulates other cellular genes. It activates transcription of the yeast copper/zinc superoxide dismutase gene (Cu/Zn-SOD1), whose gene product protects the cell from oxygen toxicity (Gralla et al, 1991). Interestingly however, the ACE1 gene is not essential for the viability of *S. cerevisiae*, at least not under standard laboratory conditions (Thiele, 1988; Butler and Thiele, 1991).

The Regulation of Metallothioneins in the Yeast Candida glabrata

Candida glabrata has, in contrast to *S. cerevisiae*, two classes of metallothionein genes, a single MT-I gene and two distinct MT-II genes. The MT-II genes consist of a tandemly-amplified (3 to 9) MT-IIa

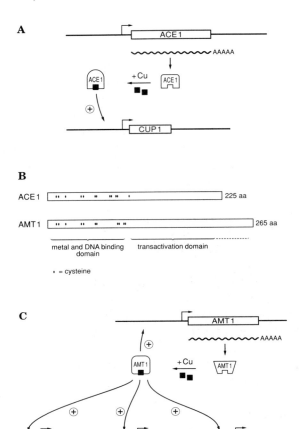

Figure 7.13 Model for the induction of the *S. cerevisiae* copper metallothionein gene CUP1 by ACE1. (A) The metal-regulatory transcription factor ACE1 is constitutively expressed and adopts a random coil structure in the absence of copper. In the presence of inducing amounts of copper the loose amino-terminal part of ACE1 changes into a so-called copper fist structure which is able to bind to the CUP1 upstream activator sequences (UAS_{CUP1}) for full transcriptional activation. (B) Schematic comparison of the yeast metallothionein gene activator proteins ACE1 and AMT1 from *S. cerevisiae* and *C. glabrata*, respectively. Relative locations of the metal and DNA-binding domains and the transactivation domains are indicated. Cysteine residues, indicated by dots in the metal and DNA binding domain, are arranged in Cys-Xaa-Cys motifs and Cys-Xaa-Xaa-Cys motifs characteristic for heavy metal binding proteins. Adapted with permission from Jungmann et al, 1993. Curiously, there are no cysteines whatsoever in the carboxyterminal transactivating portion of these factors.(C) Model for the induction of the *C. glabrata* copper metallothionein genes. Although the *C. glabrata* metallothionein system in principle functions like that of *S. cerevisiae*, namely via a copper-inducible transcriptional activator protein, there are fundamental differences. First, there are different metallothionein genes coding for isoproteins, reminiscent of the class I metallothionein gene families in vertebrates. Second, AMT1 which plays the role of the *S. cerevisiae* ACE1 in *C. glabrata*, not only induces the MT-I and MT-II genes, but also induces its own expression in a copper-dependent, autoregulatory fashion.

gene and an unlinked single copy metallothionein-IIb gene. The transcription of both classes of MT genes is activated by copper and silver but not by cadmium, unlike the class I metallothioneins of higher eukaryotes (Mehra et al, 1989; Mehra et al, 1990; Mehra et al, 1992). Again it was the group of D. Thiele and colleagues who cloned the ACE1 analog from *C. glabrata*. This time they selected for the ability to rescue a copper-sensitive *S. cerevisiae* host strain by transfecting a *C. glabrata* cDNA library which contained a *C. glabrata* MT-I cDNA. The factor responsible for the metal-induced activation was designated AMT1. As with ACE1, AMT1 acts as a copper sensor and transcriptional activator. Both factors show a high degree of structural and functional homology, an aminoterminal metallothionein-like copper and DNA binding domain, and a carboxyterminal acidic domain for transcriptional activation (Figure 7.13B) (Zhou and Thiele, 1991; Zhou et al, 1992). A significant and highly interesting difference between these proteins is, that the expression of ACE1 is constitutive, i.e. not influenced by the copper status of the cell, whereas the expression of AMT1 is more sophisticated in that it is induced by copper in an autoregulatory fashion (Figure 7.13C) (Szczypka and Thiele, 1989; Zhou and Thiele, 1993). As one would expect for a preexisting, inducible factor, AMT1 exhibits very fast activation kinetics in activating the MT-I and -II promoter as well as its own promotor within minutes (Zhou and Thiele, 1993).

Physiological Functions of Metallothioneins : Facts and Speculations

Originally, metallothionein was found as a mammalian protein responsible for the natural accumulation of cadmium, and to bind cadmium much more avidly than zinc. For this reason it has been assumed that metallothionein could have a function in heavy metal detoxification (Kaegi and Vallee, 1960; Piscator, 1964). This idea is supported by several findings: (1) a correlation has been found between the expression rate of metallothionein genes and a concomitantly increased resistance to heavy metals. This is achieved by either stable transformation of MT genes in cell culture or by selection for heavy metal-resistent cell lines which are found to have undergone amplification of the endogenous MT genes (Beach and Palmiter, 1981; Compere and Palmiter, 1981; Gick and McCarty, 1982; Karin et al, 1983; Schmidt et al, 1985); (2) a mutant strain of yeast *Saccharomyces cerevisiae* containing a functionally inert CUP1 gene, is much more sensitive to copper poisoning than the wild-type strain (Brenes-Pomales et al, 1955; Fogel and Welch, 1982; Hamer et al, 1985; Ecker et al, 1986); (3) mouse strains carrying a homozygous mutation for the metallothionein-I and -II genes are much more sensitive to cadmium toxicity than wild-type mice (Michalska and Choo, 1993; Masters et al, 1994). For unknown reasons, there is apparently a sex-specific difference in that female homozygous mutant mice are slightly more resistant to cadmium treatment than male homozygous mutant mice (Masters et al, 1994). Based on the many different ways metallothionein expression can be stimulated, a few additional possible functions for the metallothionein protein have been proposed, such as homeostatic control of zinc and copper, free radical scavenging, or as a general stress response protein.

The metallothionein of *Neurospora crassa*, which, as previously mentioned, is half the size of mammalian metallothioneins, functions as a copper storage and transfer protein (see Figure 7.1 for amino acid sequence). The copper enzyme tyrosinase is produced exclusively during sexual differentiation in *N. crassa*. Tyrosinase is a key enzyme involved in the synthesis of melanin, which gives the fruiting body its typical dark appearance. While the mycelium is growing under the surface, the fruiting body protrudes into the open, and melanin thus is needed to protect its cells from sunlight damage. There is good evidence from a combination of in vitro and in vivo studies that copper is stored during the vegetative growth phase in the form of Cu-metallothionein, which in turn can transfer copper by an as yet unknown mechanism to apotyrosinase at the time of fruiting body formation. Tyrosinase gene expression itself is independent of copper, whereas the catalytic activity of the enzyme is completely dependent on copper, as is shown when *N. crassa* is grown in copper-free medium (Lerch, 1980; Beltramini and Lerch, 1982; Huber and Lerch, 1987).

These findings argue for a general function of metallothionein in cellular metal homeostasis, ensuring that a sufficiently high intracellular concentration of essential metals are available at any particular time. However, since the metallothioneins bind their heavy metal ions with a very high affinity one can envisage several mechanisms for a redistribution of heavy metals into recipient molecules: (1) heavy metal-transfer molecules may serve as go-betweens to link metallothionein and a metal-free apoprotein; (2) (active) degradation of metallothionein releases metal that is then bound by apoproteins; (3) on the basis of the extremely high exchange rate for these metals, metallothionein may share metal ions with other proteins (Vasák and Kaegi, 1983; Nettesheim et al, 1985; Petering et al, 1987; Otvos et al, 1987; Schmid et al, 1990).

However, there are also data in support of the opposite process, namely active removal of metal from target proteins by metallothionein whereby these target proteins would be downregulated or inactivated. In collaboration with the group of J.H.R. Kaegi and his colleagues, we have compared the activity of the zinc-dependent zinc finger transcription factor Sp1 and the zinc-independent homeo-domain transcription factor Oct-1 in HeLa cell nuclear extracts in the presence or absence of added apothionein (i.e. metal-free metallothionein). In vitro transcription studies showed that in the presence of added apothionein, only the reporter gene driven by a promoter containing binding sites for the octamer factor but not for Sp1 is transcribed. The reason for this behavior is explained by bandshift assays. Only the homeo-domain factor Oct-1, but not the zinc finger factor Sp1 is able to bind to its respective DNA recognition sequence in the presence of apothionein in the binding reaction. Similar results have been obtained for the RNA polymerase transcription factor TFIIIA (Zeng et al, 1991). These results are interesting in the light of the fact that RNA polymerases are also zinc dependent enzymes. This means that metallothionein may modulate the activity of certain metal-dependent proteins, whereas others like the vital RNA polymerases would not be affected. At first glance it seems quite unlikely that metallothionein is used for downregulation of some but not other classes of zinc-binding proteins. If a protein like Sp1, which has binding sites in the promoters of most housekeeping genes could be inhibited this way, vital functions would be affected. Zinc deficiency is rather detrimental to life, with those cells being the most sensitive to zinc deprivation that have a high proliferation rate (Vallee and Falchuk, 1993). One should also keep in mind that the expression of metallothionein is completely dependent on MTF-1, whose DNA-binding activity seems to be much more sensitive to the zinc concentration than the DNA-binding activity of Sp1 (Westin and Schaffner, 1988a; Heuchel et al, 1994). Therefore it is difficult, if not impossible, to produce enough metallothionein for a serious zinc depletion of the cell unless there would be an as yet unknown mechanism for producing metallothionein at low intracellular zinc concentration. At present, we favour a model in which MTF-1 senses the intracellular zinc concentration as follows. Under normal conditions, i.e. sufficient environmental zinc, metallothionein is only moderately expressed. If environmental zinc drops under a certain threshold level, MTF-1 is unable to bind to the MRE sequences in the metallothionein promoters and as a consequence metallothionein synthesis ceases. Metal transfer from metallothionein to a hypothetical heavy metal transfer-protein, or the decay, or active degradation of metallothionein might ensure zinc-dependent functions by releasing the last zinc reserves. Upon increase in environmental zinc, or cytotoxic metals such as cadmium, metal-lothionein expression will be boosted via activation of MTF-1 for metal sequestration and/or detoxification.

Conclusions

In this review we have compared four different metal inducible gene systems. Even though the task in all of them, taken at face value, is to induce transcription of specific genes as a result of heavy metal load, in each of them the problem is solved in a specific way. In bacteria, the mercury response is best studied, MerR factor binds constitutively to DNA, but only after mercury binding twists the promoter such that it can be recognized by RNA polymerase. Like several known bacterial transcription regulators, the MerR protein has activator as well as repressor properties. In the yeast *S. cerevisiae*, ACE-1 is a copper dependent DNA binding transcription factor which activates the copper metallothionein gene. In another yeast, *C. glabrata*, a similar metallothionein regulator (AMT-1) activates not one but a multitude of metallothionein genes. In addition, AMT-1 regulates itself by positive feedback upon metal treatment. In mammals finally, both man and mouse induce metallothionein gene transcription via the zinc finger factor MTF-1. This factor can reversibly bind to DNA as a consequence of the presence or absence of zinc in the zinc fingers. Therefore, these zinc fingers are likely to have a metal sensory function in vivo. Given the amazing complexity of the mammalian transcription apparatus in general, it is to be expected that MTF-1 does not exert its effect directly on RNA polymerase II but rather in concern with cofactors. These cofactor(s) would help to activate and/or inhibit transcription in presence or absence of heavy metals, respectively. While MTF-1 is highly conserved among mammals, the greater multitude of MT genes in human as compared to mouse suggests a more complex role for metallothioneins. In spite of all these differences, in each of the systems described here, metal induced genes are activated via one key factor which binds to specific upstream sequence elements.

Of the systems described the mammalian one, due to its complexity, may yield many surprises in future studies. With the isolation and characterization of MTF-1 the first crucial player in this system has been identified. It would be interesting, for example, to find out why MTF-1 contains a proline-rich and a serine-threonine-rich domain in addition to the acidic activation domain. Of course it will be important to elucidate the signal transduction cascade for heavy metal-induced transcription, and also to find out how nonmetals induce metallothionein gene transcription. Naturally, this will raise a question about the interrelatedness of the metal induction system with other stress inducible gene systems, such as the heat shock response or the oxidative stress (NF-κB) systems. Do these systems share cofactors? Does the phenomenon of the ready-to-go, or poised RNA polymerase II, which is binding to the promoter but not released for elongation in absence of heat shock, also exist for metal induction?

References

Andersen RD, Birren BW, Taplitz SJ, Herschman HR (1986): Rat metallothionein-I structural gene and three pseudogenes, one of which contains 5'-regulatory sequences. *Mol Cell Biol* 6: 302–314

Andersen RD, Taplitz SJ, Oberbauer AM, Calame KL, Herschman HR (1990): Metal-dependent binding of a nuclear factor to the rat metallothionein-I promoter. *Nucleic Acids Res* 18: 6049–6055

Ansari AZ, O'Halloran TV (1994): An emerging role for allosteric modulation of DNA structure in transcription. In: *Transcription Mechanisms and Regulation*, Raven Press

Ansari AZ, Chael ML, O'Halloran TV (1992): Allosteric underwinding of DNA is a critical step in positive control of transcription by Hg-MerR. *Nature* 355: 87–89

Beach LR, P, RD (1981): Amplification of the metallothionein-I gene in cadmium-resistant mouse cells. *Proc Natl Acad Sci USA* 78: 2110–2114

Beltramini M, Lerch K (1982): Copper transfer between Neurospora copper metallothionein and type 3 copper apoproteins. *Febs Lett* 142: 219–222

Bremner I, Beattie JH (1990): metallothionein and the trace minerals. *Annu Rev Nutr* 10: 63–83

Brenes-Pomales A, Lindegren G, Lindegren CC (1955): Gene control of copper-sensitivity in *Saccharomyces Nature* 176: 841–842

Brown RS, Sander C, Argos P (1985): The primary structure of transcription factor TFIIIA has 12 consecutive repeats. *FEBS Lett* 186: 271–274

Brugnera E, Georgiev O, Radtke F, Heuchel R, Baker E, Sutherland GR, Schaffner W (1994): Cloning, chromosomal mapping and characterization of the human metal-regulatory transcription factor MTF-1. *Nucl Acids Res* 22: 3167–3173

Buchman C, Skroch P, Dixon W, Tullius TD, Karin M (1990): A single amino acid change in CUP2 alters its mode of DNA binding. *Mol Cell Biol* 10: 4778–4787

Butler G, Thiele DJ (1991): ACE2, an activator of yeast metallothionein expression which is homologous to SW15. *Mol Cell Biol* 11: 476–485

Butt TR, Ecker DJ (1987): Yeast metallothionein and applications in biotechnology. *Microbiol Rev* 51: 351–364

Butt TR, Sternberg EJ, Gorman JA, Clark P, Hamer D, Rosenberg M, Crooke ST (1984): Copper metallothionein of yeast, structure of the gene, and regulation of expression. *Proc Natl Acad Sci USA* 81: 3332–3336

Carter AD, Felber BK, Walling MJ, Jubier MF, Schmidt CJ, Hamer DH (1984): Duplicated heavy metal control sequences of the mouse metallothionein-I gene. *Proc Natl Acad Sci USA* 81: 7392–7396

Compere SJ, Palmiter RD (1981): DNA methylation controls the inducibility of the mouse metallothionein-I gene in lymphoid cells. *Cell* 25: 233–240

Cotton FA, Wilkinson G (1980): *Advanced Inorganic Chemistry, A Comprehensive Text* New York: John Wiley and Sons

Culotta VC, Hamer DH (1989): Fine mapping of a mouse metallothionein gene metal response element. *Mol Cell Biol* 9: 1376–1380

Czupryn M, Brown WE, Vallee BL (1992): Zinc rapidly induces a metal response element-binding factor. *Proc Natl Acad Sci USA* 89: 10395–10399

Durnam DM, Palmiter RD (1981): Transcriptional regulation of the mouse metallothionein-I gene by heavy metals. *J Biol Chem* 256: 5712–5716

Durnam DM, Palmiter RD (1987): Analysis of the detoxification of heavy metal ions by mouse metallothionein. *Experientia Suppl*, 457–463

Ecker DJ, Butt TR, Sternberg EJ, Neeper MP, Debouck C, Gormon JA, Crooke ST (1986): Yeast metallothionein function in metal ion detoxification. *J Biol Chem* 261: 16895–16900

Evans CF, Engelke DR, Thiele DJ (1990): ACE1 transcription factor produced in Escherichia coli binds multiple regions within yeast metallothionein upstream activation sequences. *Mol Cell Biol* 10: 426–429

Fogel S, Welch JS (1982): Tandem gene amplification mediates copper resistance in yeast. *Proc Natl Acad Sci USA* 79: 5342–5346

Fowler BA, Hildebrand CE, Kojima Y, Webb M (1987): Nomenclature of metallothionein. *Experientia Suppl*, 19-22

Furst P, Hu S, Hackett R, Hamer D (1988): Copper activates metallothionein gene transcription by altering the conformation of a specific DNA binding protein [published erratum appears in Cell 1989 Jan 27;56(2):following 321]. *Cell* 55: 705–717

Gick GG, McCarty KSr (1982): Amplification of the metallothionein-I gene in cadmium- and zinc-resistant Chinese hamster ovary cells. *J Biol Chem* 257: 9049–9053

Gralla EB, Thiele DJ, Silar P, Valentine JS (1991): ACE1, a copper-dependent transcription factor, activates expression of the yeast copper, zinc superoxide dismutase gene. *Proc Natl Acad Sci USA* 88: 8558–8562

Grill E (1987): Phytochelatins, the heavy metal binding peptides of plants: characterization and sequence determination. *Experientia Suppl*, 317–322

Grill E, Loffler S, Winnacker EL, Zenk MH (1989): Phytochelatins, the heavy-metal-binding peptides of plants, are synthesized from glutathione by a specific gamma-glatmylcysteine dipeptidyl transpeptidase (phytochelatin synthetase). *Proc Natl Acad Sci USA* 86: 6838–6842

Grill E, Winnacker EL, Zenk MH (1985): Phytochelatins: The principal heavy-metal complexing peptides of higher plants. *Science* 230: 4726.

Grill E, Winnacker EL, Zenk MH (1986): Homo-phytochelatins are heavy metal-binding peptides of homo-glutathione containing *Fabales*. *FEBS Lett* 205: 47–50

Grill E, Winnacker EL, Zenk MH (1991): Phytochelatins. In: *Methods Enzymol*, New York: Academic Press

Hamer DH (1986): metallothionein. *Annu Rev Biochem* 55: 913–951

Hamer DH, Thiele DJ, Lemontt JE (1985): Function and autoregulation of yeast coppertionein. *Science* 228: 685–690

Hanas JS, Hazuda DJ, Bogenhagen DF, Wu FY, Wu CW (1983): Xenopus transcription factor A requires zinc for binding to the 5S RNA gene. *J Biol Chem* 258:14120–14125

Harley CB, Reynolds RP (1983): Analysis of *E. coli* promoter sequences. *Nucleic Acids Research* 15: 2343–2361

Harlow P, Watkins E, Thornton RD, Nemer M (1989): Structure of an ectodermally expressed sea urchin metallothionein gene and characterization of its metal-responsive region. *Mol Cell Biol* 9: 5445–5455

Hawley DK, McClure WR (1983): Compilation and analysis of Escherichia coli promoter DNA sequences. *Nucleic Acids Res* 11: 2237–2255

Helman JD, Shewchuk LM, Walsh CT (1990): *Metal-Ion Induced Regulation of Gene Expression*, New York: Elsevier

Helmann JD, Wang Y, Mahler I, Walsh CT (1989): Homologous metalloregulatory proteins from both gram-positive and gram-negative bacteria control transcription of mercury resistance operons. *J Bacteriol* 171: 222–229

Henkel T, Machleidt T, Alkalay I, Kronke M, Ben-Neriah Y, Baeuerle PA (1993): Rapid proteolysis of I kappa B-alpha is necessary for activation of transcription factor NF-kappa B. *Nature* 365: 182–185

Heuchel R, Radtke F, Georgiev O, Stark G, Aguet M, Schaffner W (1994): The transcription factor MTF-1 is essential for basal and heavy metal-induced metallothionein gene expression. *EMBO J* 13: 2870–2875

Hope IA, Struhl K (1986): Functional dissection of a eukaryotic transcriptional activator protein, GCN4 of yeast. *Cell* 46: 885–894

Hu S, Furst P, Hamer D (1990): The DNA and Cu binding functions of ACE1 are interdigitated within a single domain. *New Biol* 2: 544–555

Huber M, Lerch K (1987): The influence of copper on the induction of tyrosinase and laccase in Neurospora crassa. *FEBS Lett* 219: 335–338

Hulbregtse JM, Engelke DR, Thiele DJ (1989): Copper-induced binding of cellular factors to yeast metallothionein upstream activation sequences. *Proc Natl Acad Sci USA* 86: 65–69

Hunter T, Karin M (1992): The regulation of transcription by phosphorylation. *Cell* 70: 375–387

Imagawa M, Onozawa T, Okumura K, Osada S, Nishihara T, Kondo M (1990): Characterization of metallothionein cDNAs induced by cadmium in the nematode Caenorhabditis elegans. *Biochem J* 268: 237–240

Imbert J, Fürst P, Gedamu P, Hamer D (1990): Regulation of metallothionein gene transcription by metals. *Adv Inorg Biochem* 8: 139–164

Jungmann J, Reins H-A, Lee J, Romeo A, Hassett R, Kosman D, Jentsch S (1993): MAC1, a nuclear regulator protein related to Cu-dependent transcription factors is involved in Cu/Fe utilization and stress resistance in yeast. *EMBO J* 12: 5051–5056

Kadonaga JT, Carner KR, Masiarz FR, Tijian R (1987): Isolation of cDNA encoding transcription factor Sp1 and functional analysis of the DNA binding domain. *Cell* 51: 1079–1090

Kaegi JHR (1991): Overview of metallothionein. In: *Methods Enzymol*, New York: Academic Press

Kaegi JHR, Kojima Y (1987): Chemistry and biochemistry of metallothionein. In: *Experientia Suppl*, 25–61

Kaegi JH, Schaffer A (1988): Biochemistry of metallothionein. *Biochemistry* 27: 8509–8515

Kaegi JHR, Vallee B (1960): metallothionein: a cadmium- and zinc-containing protein from equine renal cortex. *J Biol Chem* 235: 3460–3465

Kaptain R (1991): Zinc-finger structures. *Curr Opin Struct Biol* 2: 109–115

Karin M, Andersen RD, Slater E, Smith K, Herschman HR (1980): metallothionein mRNA induction in HeLa cells in response to zinc or dexamethasone is a primary induction response. *Nature* 286:

Karin M, Cathala G, Nguyen-Huu MC (1983): Expression and regulation of a human metallothionein gene carried on an autonomously replicating shuttle vector. *Proc Natl Acad Sci USA* 80: 4040–4044

Karin M, Haslinger A, Holtgreve H, Richards RI, Krauter P, Westphal HM, Beato M (1984): Characterization of DNA sequences through which cadmium and glucocorticoid hormones induce human metallothionein-IIA gene. *Nature* 308: 513–519

Karin M, Najarian R, Haslinger A, Valenzuela P, Welch J, Fogel S (1984): Primary structure and transcription of an amplified genetic locus: the CUP1 locus of yeast. *Proc Natl Acad Sci USA* 81: 337–341

Kawashima I, Kennedy TD, Chino M, Lane BG (1992): Wheat Ec metallothionein genes. Like mammalian Zn2+ metallothionein genes, wheat Zn2+ metallothionein genes are conspicuously expressed during embryogenesis. *Eur J Biochem* 209: 971–976

Keilin D, Mann T (1940): Carbonic anhydrase. Purification and nature of the enzyme. *Biochem J* 34: 1163–1176

Koizumi S, Suzuki K, Otsuka F (1992): A nuclear factor that recognizes the metal-responsive elements of human metallothionein IIA gene. *J Biol Chem* 267: 18659–18664

Kondo N, Imai K, Isobe M, Goto T, Murasugi A, Wada-Nakagawa C, Hayashi Y (1984): Cadystin A and B, major unit peptides comprising cadmium binding peptides induced in a fission yeast—Separation, revision of structures and synthesis. *Tetrahedron Lett* 25: 3869–3872

Lee W, Haslinger A, Karin M, Tjian R (1987a): Activation of transcription by two factors that bind promoter and enhancer sequences of the human metallothionein gene and SV40. *Nature* 325: 368–372

Lee W, Mitchell P, Tjian R (1987b): Purified transcription factor AP-1 interacts with TPA-inducible enhancer elements. *Cell* 49: 741–752

Lerch K (1980): Copper metallothionein, a copper-binding protein from *Neurospora crassa*. *Nature* 284: 368–370

Lippard SJ (1993): Bioinorganic chemistry: a maturing frontier [comment]. *Science* 261: 699–700

Ma J, Ptashne M (1987): Deletion analysis of GAL4 defines two transcriptional activating segments. *Cell* 48: 847–853

Mansour SL, Thomas KR, Capecchi MR (1988): Disruption of the proto-oncogene int-2 in mouse embryo-derived stem cells: a general strategy for targeting mutations to non-selectable genes. *Nature* 336: 348–352

Margoshes M, Vallee BL (1957): A cadmium protein from equine kidney cortex. *J Am Chem Soc* 79: 4813–4814

Masters BA, Kelly EJ, Quaife CJ, Brinster RL, Palmiter RD (1994): Targeted disruption of metallothionein I and II genes increases sensitivity to cadmium. *Proc Natl Acad Sci USA* 91: 584–588

Mehra RK, Garey JR, Butt TR, Gray WR, Winge DR (1989): Candida glabrata metallothioneins. Cloning and sequence of the genes and characterization of proteins. *J Biol Chem* 264: 19747–19753

Mehra RK, Garey JR, Winge DR (1990): Selective and tandem amplification of a member of the metallothionein gene family in Candida glabrata. *J Biol Chem* 265: 6369–6375

Mehra RK, Thorvaldsen JL, Macreadie IG, Winge DR (1992): Disruption analysis of metallothionein-encoding genes in Candida glabrata. *Gene* 114: 75–80

Michalska AE, Choo KH (1993): Targeting and germ-line transmission of a null mutation at the metallothionein I and II loci in mouse. *Proc Natl Acad Sci USA* 90: 8088–8092

Miller J, McLachlan AD, Klug A (1985): Repetitive zinc-binding domains in the protein transcription factor IIIA from Xenopus oocytes. *EMBO J* 4: 1609–1614

Misra TK (1992): Bacterial resistances to inorganic mercury salts and organomercurials. *Plasmid* 27: 4–16

Mitchell PJ, Tjian R (1989): Transcriptional regulation in mammalian cells by sequence-specific DNA binding proteins. *Science* 245: 371–378

Mitchell PJ, Wang C, Tjian R (1987): Positive and negative regulation of transcription in vitro: enhancer-binding protein AP-2 is inhibited by SV40 T antigen. *Cell* 50: 847–861

Mueller PR, Salser SJ, Wold B (1988): Constitutive and metal-inducible protein:DNA interactions at the mouse metallothionein I promoter examined by in vivo and in vitro footprinting. *Genes Dev* 2: 412–427

Munger K, Germann UA, Lerch K (1985): Isolation and structural organization of the Neurospora crassa copper metallothionein gene. *EMBO J* 4: 2665–2668

Murasugi A, Wada C, Hayashi Y (1981): Purification and unique properties in UV and CD spectra of Cd-binding peptide 1 from *Schizosaccharomyces pombe*. *Biochem Biophys Res Commun* 103: 1021-1028

Nettesheim DG, Engeseth HR, Otvos JD (1985): Products of metal exchange reactions of metallothionein. *Biochemistry* 24: 6744–6751

Nies DH (1992): Resistance to cadmium, cobalt, zinc, and nickel in microbes. *Plasmid* 56: 17–28

O'Halloran TV (1993): Transition metals in control of gene expression [see comments]. *Science* 261: 715–725

O'Halloran TV et al (1989): The MerR heavy metal receptor mediates positive activation in a topologically novel transcription complex. *Cell* 56: 119–129

Olafson RW, McCubbin WD, Kay CM (1988): Primary- and secondary-structural analysis of a unique prokaryotic metallothionein from a Synechococcus sp. cyanobacterium. *Biochem J* 251: 691–699

Otto E, Allen JM, Young JE, Palmiter RD, Maroni G (1987): A DNA segment controlling metal-regulated expression of the Drosophila melanogaster metallothionein gene Mtn. *Mol Cell Biol* 7: 1710–1715

Otvos JD, Engeseth HR, Nettesheim DG, Hilt CR (1987): Interprotein metal exchange reactions of metallothioneins. *Experientia Suppl*, 171–178

Palmiter RD (1994): Regulation of metallothionein genes by heavy metals appears to be mediated by a zinc-sensitive inhibitor that interacts with a constitutively active transcription factor, MTF-1. *Proc Natl Acad Sci USA* 91: 1219–1223

Palmiter RD, Findley SD, Whitmore TE, Durnam DM (1992): MT-III, a brain-specific member of the metallothionein gene family. *Proc Natl Acad Sci USA* 89: 6333–6337

Pande J, Vasak M, Kagi JH (1985): Interaction of lysine residues with the metal thiolate clusters in metallothionein. *Biochemistry* 24: 6717–6722

Petering DH, Krezoski S, Villalobos J, Shaw CF, Otvos JD (1987): Cadmium-zinc interactions in the Ehrlich cell: metallothionein and other sites. In: *Experientia Suppl*, 573–580

Picard B, Wegnez M (1979): Isolation of a 7S particle from Xenopus laevis oocytes: A 5S RNA/protein complex. *Proc Natl Acad Sci USA* 76: 241–245

Piscator M (1964): *Nord Hyg Tidskr* 48: 76–82

Quaife CJ, Findley SD, Erickson GJ, Froelick GJ, Kelly EJ, Zambrowicz BP, Palmiter RD (1994): Induction of a new metallothionein isoform (MT–IV) occurs during differentiation of stratified squamous epithelia. *Biochemistry* 33: 7250–7259

Quaife CJ, Findley SD, Erickson GJ, Kelly EJ, Zambrowicz BW, Palmiter RD (1994): personal communication

Radtke F, Heuchel R, Georgiev O, Hergersberg M, Gariglio M, Dembic Z, Schaffner W (1993): Cloned transcription factor MTF-1 activates the mouse metallothionein I promoter. *EMBO J* 12: 1355–1362

Raulin J (1969): Etudes Cliniques sur la vegetation. *Ann Sci Nat Bot Biol Veg* 11: 93–299

Rauser WE (1990): Phytochelatins. *Annu Rev Biochem* 59: 61–86

Robbins AH, McRee DE, Williamson M, Collett SA, Xuong NH, Furey WF, Wang BC, Stout CD (1991): Refined crystal structure of Cd, Zn metallothionein at 2.0 A resolution. *J Mol Biol* 221: 1269–1293

Robinson JN, Barton K, Naranjo CM, Sillerud LO, Trewhella J, Watt K, Jackson PJ (1987): Characterization of metal binding peptides from cadmium resistent plant cells. *Experientia Suppl*, 323–327

Robinson JN, Tommey AM, Kuske C, Jackson P (1993): Plant metallothioneins. *Biochem J* 295: 1–10

Schmid R, Zeng J, Schäffer A (1990): *Experientia* 46: A36

Schmidt CJ, Jubier MF, Hamer DH (1985): Structure and expression of two human metallothionein-I isoform genes and a related pseudogene. *J Biol Chem* 260: 7731–7737

Schreiber E, Matthias P, Muller MM, Schaffner W (1988): Identification of a novel lymphoid specific octamer binding protein (OTF- 2B) by proteolytic clipping bandshift assay (PCBA). *EMBO J* 7: 4221–4229

Searle PF (1990): Zinc dependent binding of a liver nuclear factor to metal response element MRE-a of the mouse metallothionein-I gene and variant sequences. *Nucleic Acids Res* 18: 4683–4690

Searl PF, Davison BL, Stuart GW, Wilkie TM, Norstedt G, Palmiter RD (1984): Regulation, linkage and sequence of mouse metallothionein I and II genes. *Mol Cell Biol* 4: 1221–1230

Searl PF, Stuart GW, Palmiter RD (1987): Metal regulatory elements of the mouse metallothionein-I gene. *Experientia Suppl*, 407–414

Seipel K, Georgiev O, Schaffner W (1992): Different activation domains stimulate transcription from remote ('enhancer') and proximal ('promoter') positions. *EMBO J* 11: 4961–4968

Serfling E, Lubbe A, Dorsch-Hasler K, Schaffner W (1985): Metal-dependent SV40 viruses containing inducible enhancers from the upstream region of metallothionein genes. *EMBO J* 4: 3851–3859

Séguin C (1991): A nuclear factor requires Zn2 + to bind a regulatory MRE element of the mouse gene encoding metallothionein-I. *Gene* 97: 295–300

Séguin C, Prevost J (1988): Detection of a nuclear protein that interacts with a metal regulatory element of the mouse metallothionein I gene. *Nucleic Acids Res* 16: 10547–10560

Shi J, Lindsay WP, Huckle JW, Morby AP, Robinson NJ (1992): Cyanobacterial metallothionein gene expressed in Escherichia coli. Metal- binding properties of the expressed protein. *FEBS Lett* 303: 159–163

Silver S, Walderhaug M (1992): Gene regulation of plasmid- and chromosome-determined inorganic ion transport in bacteria. *Microbiol Rev* 56: 195–228

Slice LW, Freedman JH, Rubin CS (1990): Purification, characterization, and cDNA cloning of a novel metallothionein- like, cadmium-binding protein from Caenorhabditis elegans. *J Biol Chem* 265: 256–263

Steffens JC (1990): *Ann Rev Plant Physiol Plant Mol Biol* 533–575

Stillman MJ, Cai W, Zelazowski AJ (1987): Cadmium binding to metallothioneins. Domain specificity in reactions of alpha and beta fragments, apometallothionein, and zinc metallothionein with Cd2 + . *J Biol Chem* 262: 4538–4548

Stuart GW, Searl PF, Chen HY, Brinster RL, Palmiter RD (1984): A 12-base-pair DNA motif that is repeated several times in metallothionein gene promoters confers metal regulation to a heterologous gene. *Proc Natl Acad Sci USA* 81: 7318–7322

Stuart GW, Searle PF, Palmiter RD (1985): Identification of multiple metal regulatory elements in mouse metallothionein-I promoter by assaying synthetic sequences. *Nature* 317: 828–831

Sczypka MS, Thiele DJ (1989): A cysteine-rich nuclear protein activates yeast metallothionein gene transcription. *Mol Cell Biol* 9: 421–429

Theunissen O, Rudt F, Guddat U, Mentzel H, Pieler T (1992): RNA and DNA binding zinc fingers in Xenopus TFIIIA. *Cell* 71: 679–690

Thiele DJ, Hamer DH (1986): Tandemly duplicated upstream control sequences mediate copper induced transcription of saccharomyces cerevisiae copper-metallothionein gene. *Mol Cell Biol* 6: 1158–1163

Thiele DJ (1988): ACE1 regulates expression of the Saccharomyces cerevisiae metallothionein gene. *Mol Cell Biol* 8: 2745–2752

Thiele DJ (1992): Metal-regulated transcription in eukaryotes. *Nucleic Acids Res* 20: 1183–1191

Uchida Y, Takio K, Titani K, Ihara Y, Tomonaga M (1991): The growth inhibitory factor that is deficient in the Alzheimer's disease brain is a 68 amino acid metallothionein-like protein. *Neuron* 7: 337–347

Vallee BL, Auld DS (1990): Zinc coordination, function, and structure of zinc enzymes and other proteins. *Biochemistry* 29: 5647–5659

Vallee BL, Falchuk KH (1993): The biochemical basis of zinc physiology. *Physiol Rev* 73: 79–118

Vallee BL, Coleman JE, Auld DS (1991): Zinc fingers, zinc clusters, and zinc twists in DNA-binding protein domains. *Proc Natl Acad Sci USA* 88: 999–1003

Vasák M, Kaegi JHR (1983): *Metal Ions In Biological Systems*, Sigel -, ed. New York: Marcel Dekker

Welch J, Fogel S, Buchman C, Karin M (1989): The CUP2 gene product regulates the expression of the CUP1 gene, coding for yeast metallothionein. *Embo J* 8: 255–260

West AK, Hildebrand CE, Karin M, Richards RI (1990): Human metallothionein genes: Structure of the functional locus at 16q13. *Genomics* 8: 513–518

Westin G, Schaffner W (1988a): A zinc-responsive factor interacts with a metal-regulated enhancer element (MRE) of the mouse metallothionein-I gene. *EMBO J* 7: 3763-3770

Westin G, Schaffner W (1988b): Heavy metal ions in transcription factors from HeLa cells: Sp1, but not octamer transcription factor requires zinc for DNA binding and for activator function. *Nucleic Acids Res* 16: 5771–5781

Winge DR, Nielson KB, Gray WR, Hamer DH (1985): Yeast metallothionein. Sequence and metal-binding properties. *J Biol Chem* 260: 14464–14470

Xu L, Rungger D, Georgiev O, Seipel K, Schaffner W (1994): Different potential of cellular and viral activators of transcription revealed in oocytes and early embryos of *Xenopus laevis*. *Biol Chem Hoppe-Seyler* 375: 105–112

Yagle MK, Palmiter RD (1985): Coordinate regulation of mouse metallothionein I and II genes by heavy metals and glucocorticoids. *Mol Cell Biol* 5: 291–294

Zafarullah M, Bonham K, Gedamu L (1988): Structure of the rainbow trout metallothionein B gene and characterization of its metal-responsive region. *Mol Cell Biol* 8: 4469–4476

Zeng J, Heuchel R, Schaffner W, Kagi JH (1991): Thionein (apometallothionein) can modulate DNA binding and transcription activation by zinc finger containing factor Sp1. *FEBS Lett* 279: 310–312

Zeng J, Vallee BL, Kagi JH (1991): Zinc transfer from transcription factor IIIA fingers to thionein clusters. *Proc Natl Acad Sci USA* 88: 9984–9988

Zhou P, Szczypka MS, Sosinowski T, Thiele DJ (1992): Expression of a yeast metallothionein gene family is activated by a single metalloregulatory transcription factor. *Mol Cell Biol* 12: 3766–3775

Zhou P, Thiele DJ (1993): Rapid transcriptional autoregulation of a yeast metalloregulatory transcription factor is essential for high-level copper detoxification. *Genes Dev* 7: 1824–1835

Zhou P, Thiele DJ (1991): Isolation of a metal-activated transcription factor gene from Candida glabrata by complementation in *Saccharomyces cerevisiae*. *Proc Natl Acad Sci USA* 88: 6112–6116

8

Post-Transcriptional Regulation of Gene Expression by Iron

MATTHIAS W. HENTZE

Heavy metals play an ambivalent role in biology: their toxicity threatens cellular integrity, but they are required as cofactors for many biological reactions. This situation necessitates the regulation of heavy metal acquisition, storage and utilization in response to supply and demand. A common safeguard system, metallothionein, binds and detoxifies most heavy metals and is transcriptionally induced by cellular exposure to these (see Chapter 7). In contrast, cells have evolved exclusive regulatory networks for the second most common heavy metal, iron. The task of coordinating iron uptake, storage and utilization has been solved differently by bacteria, yeast and multicellular eukaryotic organisms. In *E. coli*, the transcription of genes involved in iron metabolism, including those for a secreted iron chelator (a siderophore) and a siderophore receptor, is regulated by the iron-containing repressor protein FUR (Braun et al, 1991). In *S. cerevisiae*, a ferric reductase/ferrous iron transporter system localized on the cell surface mediates iron acquisition. Its expression is also transcriptionally regulated by iron (Dancis et al, 1992). The regulation of iron storage and utilization in *Escherichia coli* and *Saccharomyces cerevisiae* is less well understood than its uptake.

Multicellular organisms control their iron metabolism both at the systemic and the cellular level. In the human body, iron homeostasis is achieved by regulation of iron absorption from the gut (Skikne and Baynes, 1994). Once iron has passed into the circulation, the majority binds to the serum protein transferrin. Transferrin-bound iron can be taken up by the various cells and tissues in the body, but no physiological mechanisms exist for its excretion from the circulation. At the cellular level, an elegant post-transcriptional regulatory circuit has evolved which coordinates iron uptake, storage and utilization. In contrast to the other regulatory systems described in this book, this iron control circuit

INDUCIBLE GENE EXPRESSION, VOLUME 1
P.A. Baeuerle, Editor
© 1995 Birkhäuser Boston

operates almost exclusively extra-nuclear, and it involves regulatory interactions between cytoplasmic proteins and mature, fully processed mRNAs.

Proteins and Pathways Involved in the Regulation of Cellular Iron Metabolism

Transferrin-bound iron enters cells by endocytosis through a specific plasma membrane receptor, the transferrin receptor (TfR). Although other mechanisms of iron uptake exist, the TfR pathway is the major route of iron entry into cells under physiological conditions (Aisen and Listowski, 1990). The number of TfRs on the cell surface directly correlates with and limits the amount of iron taken up (Klausner et al, 1983). Following endocytosis and acidification of the endosome, iron is released from transferrin. The apotransferrin/TfR complex recycles to the cell surface, while iron leaves the endosome by as yet poorly defined mechanisms.

Conceptually, the distribution of cytoplasmic iron can be subdivided into storage, regulation and utilization pools. Intracellular iron storage occurs within a shell consisting of 24 subunits of ferritin (heavy and light) chains. The intracellular level of ferritin correlates with the fraction of iron which is taken up and stored in ferritin. When ferritin levels are high, a higher percentage of the incoming iron is sequestered into the ferritin core, whereas lower ferritin levels leave a bigger fraction unsequestered and available for metabolic functions (Mattia et al, 1986). To what extent ferritin iron can be mobilized for utilization within the cell is still a controversial question (Halliday et al, 1994).

Non-ferritin iron is required for the synthesis of heme and hemoproteins, iron-sulfur (Fe-S) proteins as well as a variety of non-heme, non-Fe-S proteins, and frequently participates in electron transfer reactions. Overall, the synthesis of heme in erythroid cells constitutes the major iron utilization pathway in the human body, and hemoglobin synthesis and degradation account for $> 80\%$ of the total body iron turnover (Bothwell et al, 1983). The expression of the enzyme that catalyzes the first step in heme biosynthesis, 5-aminolevulinate synthase, is increased when erythroid cells (MEL cells) are treated with iron and decreases following treatment with an iron chelator (Melefors et al, 1993). This regulation in erythroid cells probably helps to adjust the activity of the major iron utilization pathway to iron availability.

Cellular iron levels are buffered against harmful increases or decreases by adjusting the expression of transferrin receptors (TfRs) and ferritin to the supply and demand. As one would expect, low iron levels trigger increased TfR synthesis to augment iron uptake and reduce the expression of the storage protein ferritin to increase the fraction of free non-ferritin iron. Conversely, exposure of cells to a high iron load reduces TfR expression while raising the levels of ferritin (Melefors and Hentze, 1993).

Post-Transcriptional Regulation of Iron Proteins by Two Different Mechanisms: Role of Iron-Responsive Elements (IREs)

Iron regulates the expression of transferrin receptor (TfR), ferritin and erythroid 5-aminolevulinate synthase (eALAS) largely at the post-transcriptional level, although quantitatively minor transcriptional effects of iron on the TfR (Casey et al, 1988a), and ferritin (White and Munro, 1988) genes have been described. Iron stimulates the translation of ferritin H- and L-chain as well as eALAS mRNAs, while it reduces the expression of the TfR by destabilization of its mRNA. In all four cases, similar cis-regulatory elements (referred to as iron-responsive elements, IREs) have been identified within the untranslated regions (UTRs) of the mRNAs. Single IREs in the 5′ UTRs of ferritin and eALAS mRNAs regulate translation, whereas five IREs are located within the 3′ UTR of TfR mRNA which is responsible for the regulation of TfR mRNA stability.

When the IREs from different mRNAs and species are compared to one another, the homology between ferritin IREs from different species is higher than the similarity amongst the IREs found in human ferritin, TfR and eALAS mRNAs (Kühn and Hentze, 1992). A consensus IRE derived from phylogenetic comparison of all naturally occurring IREs can be defined (Hentze et al, 1988) (Figure 8.1): IREs are RNA motifs of ≈30 nucleotides, which are characterized by conserved structural features and nucleotide sequences. The double-stranded helical structure of an IRE is terminated with a six nucleotide loop. The sequence of this loop (5′ CAGUGN 3′, N = any nucleotide except G) is conserved, as is a bulged C-residue that precedes the loop by five nucleotides. This phylogenetic consensus IRE has been confirmed by mutational analyses (Barton et al, 1990; Leibold et al, 1990; Jaffrey et al, 1993).

IREs are Binding Sites for Iron Regulatory Protein (IRP)

Gel retardation assays with a radioactively labelled ferritin IRE and cytoplasmic extracts from different cells and tissues were used to identify proteins that specifically bind to the IRE probe (Leibold and Munro,

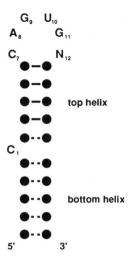

Figure 8.1 Definition of a consensus iron-responsive element (IRE) by phylogenetic comparison of cloned ferritin, transferrin receptor and eALAS IREs. The IRE is composed of conserved sequence and structure determinants. It is not known whether all conserved features of IREs are necessary for high affinity IRP-binding. Deletion of C_7 strongly diminishes IRP-binding and causes loss of function in vivo and in vitro.

1988). With extracts from human cell lines, a single IRE/protein complex was identified (Rouault et al, 1988; Müllner et al, 1989). Analysis of rodent cell extracts yielded two IRE/protein complexes, with the slower migrating one corresponding to the human protein (Leibold and Munro, 1988; Dandekar et al, 1991; Henderson et al, 1993). UV-crosslinking experiments suggested a molecular weight of 90 to 100 kDa for this protein, which is now referred to as iron regulatory protein (IRP). Former names include iron regulatory factor (IRF), IRE-binding protein (IRE-BP), ferritin repressor protein (FRP) and p90. IRP occurs in all mammalian cells that have been examined for its presence, and has been conserved during evolution. IRE-binding activity is found in chicken, frog, fish, fly and worm, but not in extracts from plants, fission and budding yeast, or bacteria (Rothenberger et al, 1990). Cross-competition experiments demonstrated that cellular and recombinant human IRP also bind to the eALAS and the five TfR IREs (Koeller et al, 1989; Müllner et al, 1989; Cox et al, 1991; Dandekar et al, 1991; Emery-Goodman et al, 1993; Gray et al, 1993), suggesting that IRP coordinates the post-transcriptional regulation of ferritin, TfR and eALAS mRNAs.

IRP has been purified from rabbit liver by conventional biochemical techniques (Walden et al, 1989), and from human tissues by exploiting its specific binding to IREs by affinity chromatography (Rouault et al, 1989; Neupert et al, 1990). Purified IRP displays essentially the same IRE-binding characteristics as it does in cellular extracts, indicating that no additional proteins are required for IRE-binding. Complementary DNAs for IRP have been cloned from human (Rouault et al, 1990; Hirling et al, 1992), mouse (Philpott et al, 1991), rabbit (Patino and Walden, 1992), and rat (Yu et al, 1992) libraries. The sequences show remarkable conservation with 93% to 98% identity and predict a protein of ≈ 98 kDa, suggesting that IRP is not extensively modified post-translationally.

Gel retardation and UV-crosslinking experiments with extracts from rodent cells have identified a second protein that specifically binds to IREs (referred to as IRF_B) (Henderson et al, 1993). On native gels, the IRE/IRF_B complex migrates faster than IRE/IRP complexes, and the molecular weight of the immunologically distinct IRF_B protein has been estimated to be around 105 kDa (Henderson et al, 1993). The tissue distribution of IRP (most abundant in liver, intestine and kidney) and IRF_B (most abundant in intestine and brain) differs, although most rodent tissues express both proteins. The function of IRF_B and the question of whether a human homologue exists are currently unresolved. However, a cDNA for a protein with 57% identity and 75% similarity with human IRP has been cloned from a human T-cell library (referred to as clone 10.1) (Rouault et al, 1990). There is no functional information about the encoded protein, but the corresponding gene has been localized to human chromosome 15 (Rouault et al, 1990), distinct from the IRP gene which is located on chromosome 9 (Hentze et al, 1989a).

How Iron and Other Cellular Signals Regulate IRP

Changes in the IRE-binding activity of IRP can be demonstrated by gel retardation assays in extracts from cells treated with iron salts or hemin as iron donors or with the iron chelator desferrioxamine (Leibold and Munro, 1988; Rouault et al, 1988). When compared to extracts from untreated cells, iron starvation increases IRE-binding, whereas iron administration reduces the RNA-binding activity of IRP. These changes are mediated post-translationally. First, iron perturbations do not affect IRP mRNA or protein levels (Patino and Walden, 1992; Tang et al, 1992). Second, treatment of cellular extracts with high concentrations of reductants (2% 2-mercaptoethanol) has little effect on the high IRE-binding activity found in preparations from iron-starved cells, but increases the low IRE-binding activity in extracts from iron replete cells to comparably high levels (Hentze et al, 1989b; Haile et al, 1989; Rothenberger et al, 1990). Third, the increase in IRE-binding following treatment of human RD4 or murine B6 cells with iron chelators is not blocked by inhibitors of protein synthesis (Hentze et al, 1989b; Tang et al, 1992), although conflicting results were reported for murine L cells (Müllner et al, 1989). Whether or not cell type-dependent differences exist will require further analysis. Thus, it appears as if dormant IRP can be post-translationally activated, at least in some cells, by iron starvation and by reducing agents in vitro.

How do cellular iron levels affect IRP? Is this a direct effect of some form of free iron, or are second messengers involved in the transduction of the iron signal? It has been postulated that alternations in the level of free iron induce corresponding changes in a regulatory heme pool, and heme has been suggested to serve as a second messenger to IRP (Goessling et al, 1992). In support of this hypothesis, it has been shown that heme can be crosslinked to IRP in vitro (Lin et al, 1991) and that incubation of IRP with heme negatively affects its binding to ferritin mRNA (Lin et al, 1990). Immunoprecipitation of metabolically pulse-labelled IRP shows that incubation of rabbit RAB-9 cells with hemin rapidly ($<30\,min$) shifts the 98 kDa protein into larger ($\approx 200\,kDa$) complexes, followed by their disappearance. These data form the basis of a model with heme serving as a second messenger for the iron signal and triggering the degradation of IRP (Goessling et al, 1992). The general validity of this model has been challenged for several reasons (Haile et al, 1990; Eisenstein et al, 1991; Tang et al, 1992), including its failure to account for the strong increase in IRE-binding in extracts from hemin-treated cells by incubation with 2-mercaptoethanol (see above).

Following the cloning of IRP cDNAs, similarities between its deduced primary amino acid sequence and the mitochondrial protein aconitase have been noted (Hentze and Argos, 1991; Rouault et al, 1991). Over their entire lengths (98 kDa and 83 kDa, respectively), the two proteins display 57% conservation with 30% amino acid identity. Even more remarkable is the 100% identity of the 20 amino acids which form the catalytic core of mitochondrial aconitase (Robbins and Stout, 1989a; Robbins and Stout, 1989b) and corresponding positions in IRP. The relevance of this similarity becomes evident from the mechanism by which aconitase catalyzes the conversion of its substrate citrate to isocitrate: citrate directly interacts with one of the four iron atoms of a 4Fe-4S cluster of aconitase (Beinert, 1990). Three of these four iron atoms are liganded to cysteines, while the fourth iron interacts with citrate. Therefore, loss of the complete iron sulfur cluster, or only of this fourth iron atom, results in inactivity of the enzyme. Based on the homology between the two proteins, IRP has been suggested to be an iron sulfur protein itself (Hentze and Argos, 1991; Rouault et al, 1991). Cellular iron levels have been hypothesized to affect the iron sulfur cluster which, in turn, changes the IRE-binding activity of IRP (Constable et al, 1992).

Subsequent experiments have established that IRE-binding by IRP is specifically inhibited by incubation of the purified or recombinant protein with iron salts under conditions that reconstitute the 4Fe-4S cluster in mitochondrial aconitase (Constable et al, 1992; Haile et al, 1992a; Emery-Goodman et al, 1993; Gray et al, 1993). Moreover, IRP displays aconitase activity under these conditions, and the enzymatic activity of IRP matches that of mitochondrial aconitase (Kaptain et al, 1991; Haile et al, 1992a; Emery-Goodman et al, 1993; Gray et al, 1993). Analysis of IRP from cells treated with an iron donor or an iron chelator shows that the apoprotein form of IRP predominates in iron-starved cells and binds to iron-responsive elements, whereas the 4Fe-4S form prevails in iron-replete cells and acts as a cytoplasmic aconitase (Kennedy et al, 1992; Haile et al, 1992b). Taken together, the data demonstrate that IRP is a bifunctional protein which responds to changes in cellular iron availability by alterations in the state of its iron sulfur cluster (Figure 8.2).

When the three cysteines that have been predicted to coordinate the Fe-S cluster (C437, C503 and C506) are mutated to serines, each individual substitution abolishes aconitase activity and renders IRP constitutive for IRE-binding (Philpott et al, 1993; Hirling et al, 1994). Combinations of cysteine mutations suggest that C437 can form a disulfide bridge with C503 or C506 in the absence of an Fe-S cluster. Alkylation of apoIRP with N-ethylmaleimide at C437 (but not the other two cysteines) prevents

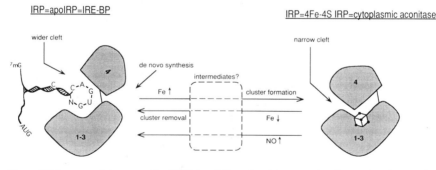

Figure 8.2 Iron regulatory protein (IRP) is a bifunctional iron-regulated cytoplasmic protein. IRP is depicted as a four domain protein with a hinge-linker connecting the C-terminal fourth with the N-terminal three domains. This structural representation is derived from the three dimensional structure of the homologous mitochondrial aconitase (Robbins and Stout, 1989a; Robbins and Stout, 1989b). In iron replete cells (right), IRP is predominantly found in the 4Fe-4S form with a cubane Fe-S cluster. As a cytoplasmic aconitase, the cleft between the fourth domain and the rest of the protein is probably narrow, allowing access of citrate, but not of an IRE. In iron starved cells (and probably in cells exposed to nitric oxide) (left), IRP exists mainly as an Fe-S free apoprotein. The cleft is wider and allows access of IREs to the (still largely undefined) RNA-binding region of the protein. The possibility of conversions between the two forms, which may involve intermediates, is discussed in the text.

IRE-binding, while alkylation of C437 with the less bulky compound iodoacetamide has no such negative effect (Philpott et al, 1993; Hirling et al, 1994). These findings indicate that C437 is in close proximity to the IRE-binding site in the three dimensional structure of IRP, but not directly part of it. This interpretation is consistent with the UV cross-linking of an IRE to the region of amino acids 121–130 (Basilion et al, 1994). Indirect evidence suggests that the IRE-binding site is quite complex, because deletions of 99 amino acids from the N-terminus or 132 amino acids from the C-terminus of the 889 amino acid protein both render IRP unable to bind IREs (Rouault et al, 1990; Hirling et al, 1992).

The crystallographic analysis of mitochondrial aconitase reveals that this enzyme consists of four domains. The N-terminal first three domains are connected with the fourth domain by a hinge-linker (schematically illustrated in Figure 8.2) (Robbins and Stout, 1989a; Robbins and Stout, 1989b). By analogy, a relatively narrow cleft between the first three and the fourth domain of the 4Fe-4S (aconitase) form of IRP may permit access of the substrate citrate, but hide the IRE-binding site. In apoIRP, the cleft is envisioned to be wide enough to accommodate the IRE (Figure 8.2) (Klausner et al, 1993; Melefors and Hentze, 1993).

Which form of iron is used to assemble the 4Fe-4S cluster from apoIRP in vivo remains an open question. In vitro, the reaction can occur spontaneously at physiological pH in the presence of reducing agents and inorganic iron and sulfur (Constable et al, 1992; Haile et al, 1992a; Emery-Goodman et al, 1993). Likewise, it is not entirely clear under which conditions the aconitase form of IRP is converted into the apoprotein in vivo. Results obtained in RD4 and B6 cells treated with protein synthesis inhibitors strongly suggest that generation of the apoprotein has no obligatory requirement for de novo synthesis (Hentze et al, 1989b; Tang et al, 1992). On the other hand, Müllner et al, have reported that the protein synthesis inhibitor cycloheximide delayed the increase in IRE-binding following treatment of mouse L cells with an iron chelator (Müllner et al, 1989). Interestingly, cells respond to iron administration and iron chelation with different kinetics. Iron administration reduces the IRE-binding activity and increases ferritin translation fairly rapidly, whereas the increase in IRE-binding and the repression of ferritin translation display slower kinetics (Müllner et al, 1992). This may indicate that the formation of the Fe-S protein from apoIRP is a faster, perhaps spontaneous process in iron loaded cells. In contrast, conversion of the Fe-S protein into apoIRP is a slow process which may not occur in all cell types and possibly involves intermediates and auxiliary factors (Figure 8.2).

The iron sulfur cluster also seems to sensitize IRP for signalling by nitric oxide (NO). NO is a diffusible, short-lived transmitter molecule involved in the regulation of vascular tone, signal transduction in the brain and macrophage-mediated cytotoxicity towards pathogens and tumor cells (Moncada et al, 1991; Lowenstein and Snyder, 1992; Nathan, 1992). A common denominator of many biological roles of NO is its reactivity with iron, a characteristic of NO which is biologically exploited to modulate the activity of NO-responsive iron-containing enzymes (Stamler et al, 1992).

NO is synthesized from L-arginine by specific enzymes, NO synthases. In murine macrophage cell lines and mouse peritoneal macrophages, NO synthase is induced following treatment with gamma-interferon and lipopolysaccharide. This treatment activates IRE-binding by IRP, diminishes cytoplasmic aconitase activity and represses ferritin translation (Weiss et al, 1993; Drapier et al, 1993). These responses require NO synthesis in vivo and NO gas has similar effects on recombinant IRP in vitro (Weiss et al, 1993; Drapier et al, 1993). Thus, NO acts as an additional signal transducer to IRP in vivo and in vitro. While it cannot be concluded that NO regulates the activities of IRP via the Fe-S cluster, the demonstrated effect of NO on the Fe-S cluster of mitochondrial aconitase (Drapier et al, 1991) strongly suggests this explanation. The physiological role of the connection between NO and iron metabolism is not yet clear (Pantopoulos et al, 1994). However, its relevance is supported by the finding that cellular iron levels regulate nitric oxide synthase activity in the murine macrophage cell line J774, probably by transcriptional mechanisms (Weiss et al, 1994). The consequences and implications of this apparent feedback loop between iron and NO requires further investigation.

Finally, serine phosphorylation of IRP by protein kinase C has been demonstrated in vitro and following stimulation of HL60 cells or rat fibroblasts with phorbol esters (Eisenstein et al, 1993). The response to phorbol esters is also accompanied by an increase in the cellular IRE-binding activity without an apparent increase in IRP synthesis. These results raise the possibility that phosphorylation may be an additional means of signal transduction to IRP.

How IRP-Binding to IREs Regulates Translation

The regulation of ferritin expression by iron was shown to be translational by Munro and co-workers (Zähringer et al, 1976), and ferritin H- and L-chain mRNAs were the first to be studied for translational regulation by IREs (Hentze et al, 1987a; Hentze et al, 1987b; Aziz and Munro, 1987). Subsequently, the mRNA encoding the erythroid specific isoform of 5-

aminolevulinate synthase (eALAS), the first enzyme required for heme synthesis, has been found to harbor an IRE (Dierks, 1990; Cox et al, 1991; Dandekar et al, 1991) and demonstrated to be translationally regulated by iron (Melefors et al, 1993). More recently, the IRE in the 5′ UTR of mitochondrial aconitase (Dandekar et al, 1991) has been shown to mediate translational repression by IRP in vitro (Gray and Hentze, 1994b).

The common denominator shared by all of these mRNAs is the presence of an IRE within the 5′ UTR of the transcript. No other sequences or recognizable structural motifs are conserved. The IRE is necessary for iron regulation of ferritin mRNA (Hentze et al, 1987a) and sufficient for regulation of indicator mRNAs in transfected mammalian cells (Hentze et al, 1987a; Hentze et al, 1987b; Aziz and Munro, 1987). Translational control by IRE/IRP interactions has been reconstituted in yeast with an inducible IRP expression system and luciferase reporter transcripts bearing a human ferritin IRE in the 5′ UTR (Oliveira et al, 1993). In vitro, the translation of capped polyadenylated ferritin mRNA is specifically repressed by purified IRP (Walden et al, 1989). In cell free translation systems derived from wheat germ or rabbit reticulocytes, IRE/IRP-controlled translation can be reconstituted with capped, non-polyadeny-lated reporter transcripts and recombinant human IRP from *E. coli* (Gray et al, 1993). All of these experiments show that the IRE is the only cis-regulatory element required for regulation and that binding of IRP suffices to repress translation, even in extracts from cells (wheat germ, yeast) or living cells (yeast) that have not evolved to regulate endogenous IRE-containing mRNAs. Furthermore, the mechanism of translational control has no obligatory requirement for polyadenylation of the mRNA.

A notable feature of ferritin, eALAS and mitochondrial aconitase IREs is the conservation of their position within the 5′ UTR of the mRNAs (Goossen and Hentze, 1992). Experimentally, the distance between the IRE and the initiator codon is functionally irrelevant (Hentze et al, 1987b; Goossen and Hentze, 1992), and it varies from ≈150 nucleotides (in ferritin mRNAs) to zero (the AUG initiator codon is part of the aconitase IRE). In contrast, iron regulation diminishes when the distance of normally 20–40 nucleotides between the IRE and the 5′ cap structure is increased by insertion of spacer RNA sequences (Goossen et al, 1990; Goossen and Hentze, 1992). When a ferritin IRE is placed more than 70 nucleotides downstream from the cap structure, iron regulation is virtually lost, although the binding of IRP is unaffected. The position-dependence of IRE function suggests that the IRE/IRP complex interferes with an early step in the translation initiation pathway which occurs in the cap-proximal region of the mRNA (see below). The nucleotides that flank the IRE in ferritin mRNAs have been suggested to participate in the regulatory process and structural changes in this region following binding of IRP to the IRE have been observed (Harrell et al, 1991). However, there is no direct evidence for a contribution of the IRE-flanking sequences to translational regulation, and deletion or replacement of the ferritin IRE-flanking sequences with unrelated nucleotides yields no qualitative or quantitative differences in several transfection systems or in vitro (Caughman et al, 1988; Goossen and Hentze, 1992; Gray et al, 1993; Oliveira et al, 1993).

How does a cap-proximal IRE/IRP complex control translation initiation? With regard to the interaction of IRP with the translation machinery, two opposing scenarios can be envisioned. First, IRP inhibits initiation by engaging in specific protein/protein interactions with components of the translational apparatus or by enzymatic modification of translation factors. Second, the binding of IRP to an IRE poses a steric barrier preventing the access of the translation apparatus to the mRNA. To distinguish between these two alternatives, the IRE in the 5' UTR of reporter mRNAs has been replaced by binding sites for the spliceosomal protein U1A or the bacteriophage MS2 coat protein. Addition of the recombinant proteins in cell-free translation experiments or co-transfection of yeast and mammalian cells with indicator plasmids and expression vectors for the respective RNA-binding proteins, results in specific translational repression by binding of U1A or MS2 coat protein to the mRNAs (Stripecke and Hentze, 1992; Stripecke et al, 1994). Similar to the situation with IRE/IRP, the inhibitory effect is position-dependent and requires a cap-proximal location of the binding sites (Stripecke and Hentze, 1992). Therefore, RNA-binding proteins with physiological functions unrelated to eukaryotic translational regulation can act as translational repressor proteins, showing that the ability to engage in specific protein/protein interactions or to exert enzymatic activities is a highly improbable requirement for translational repression from cap-proximal binding sites. Rather, high affinity binding of proteins (presumably including IRP) in proximity to the cap structure sterically blocks a sensitive step in the translation initiation pathway.

In Figure 8.3A, the translation initiation pathway is schematically subdivided into three steps (Hershey, 1991). In the first step, a 43S preinitiation complex consisting of the small ribosomal subunit, the ternary complex (comprising eIF2, initiator tRNA and GTP) and associated initiation factors bind to the 5' end of the mRNA. This step also requires the activity of additional initiation factors that are not associated with the preinitiation complex. In the second step, the associated 43S complex moves along the 5' UTR to identify the initiator codon (almost always an AUG). Following selection of the initiator

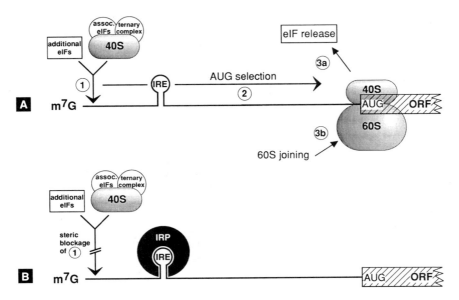

Figure 8.3 A simplified scheme of translation initiation (A) and the mechanism of translational repression of ferritin and eALAS mRNAs by IRP (B). The 5' UTR of an IRE-containing mRNA is depicted with the AUG initiator codon and a truncated open reading frame (ORF). For a discussion and further details, see text.

codon (aided by codon/anticodon recognition with the initiator tRNA), GTP is hydrolyzed, initiation factors are released and the 60S large ribosomal subunit joins to form a translation-competent 80S ribosome in the third step (Figure 8.3). Which of these steps is inhibited by IRP? Using in vitro translation and translation initiation assays, the binding of the small ribosomal subunit to the mRNA has been shown to be blocked by the presence of IRP or steric repressors like U1A (Gray and Hentze, 1994) (Figure 8.3B). As one might expect, binding of the 43S complex is not impaired when the U1A binding site is placed at a distance from the cap (Gray and Hentze, 1994b). Taken together, the mechanism of translational control of the ferritin, eALAS and probably aconitase mRNAs by IRP results from a (sterical) blockage of 43S complex binding (step 1 in Figure 8.3A).

In hepatoma cells, the translation of ferritin mRNA is also stimulated by interleukin-1(IL-1) β (Rogers et al, 1990). This observation is interesting, because ferritin expression is known to increase during the acute phase response, and adjustments in the regulation of iron metabolism are thought to play an important role in inflammatory processes (Brock, 1994). The IL-1β effect is not mediated through IRE/IRP, but it can be conferred to indicator mRNAs by a 60 nucleotide fragment which is located in the 5' UTR of ferritin-H chain mRNA downstream from the

IRE (Rogers, 1992). A similar motif has been detected in ferritin L-chain mRNA and within the mRNAs encoding other acute phase reactant proteins. Little is currently known about transacting factors or the mechanism underlying these findings. However, IL-1β fails to stimulate ferritin translation in iron-starved cells, suggesting that the IRE/IRP block is dominant over the stimulatory IL-1β response (Rogers et al, 1990).

How IRP-Binding to IREs Regulates Transferrin Receptor mRNA Stability

The regulation of transferrin receptor (TfR) mRNA stability by IRE/IRP interactions is mechanistically more complex than the translational regulation of ferritin or eALAS mRNAs, and unfortunately less detailed information is available at the moment. The higher complexity of TfR mRNA regulation includes several aspects. First, TfR mRNA harbors five IREs in its 3' UTR which are involved in iron regulation, but they are neither all necessary nor sufficient for regulation (see below). Second, iron starvation of cells activates IRE-binding of IRP and induces stabilization of the TfR transcript (Casey et al, 1988a; Casey et al, 1988b; Müllner et al, 1989). However, nitric oxide activates IRE-binding and represses ferritin translation in murine macrophages, but stabilization of TfR mRNA cannot be observed under these conditions (Pantopoulos et al, 1994). Likewise, iron starvation increases the IRE-BP activity of IRP in the murine T-cell line B6.1, but TfR mRNA stabilization unexpectedly also requires the presence of interleukin 2 (Seiser et al, 1993). These results indicate that, at least in some cell types, multiple signalling pathways contribute to the post-transcriptional regulation of TfR expression. Third, TfR mRNA levels are controlled by various biological signals through transcriptional and post-transcriptional responses. For example, the iron chelator desferrioxamine induces a $\approx$10-fold stabilization of the TfR mRNA and stimulates TfR transcription $\approx$3-fold (Casey et al, 1988a). Similarly, the responses to interleukin 2 and cellular mitogens are also in part transcriptional (Seiser et al, 1993). These complexities have to be taken into account when considering the biology of transferrin receptor regulation, but the following discussions will focus on the cytoplasmic mechanism by which iron-responsive elements and iron regulatory protein control the stability of the TfR message.

The 3' UTRs of human, rat and chicken TfR mRNAs contain two conserved regions of $\approx$170 nucleotides each which are separated by 220 to 330 nucleotide spacer regions of lower conservation (Koeller et al, 1989;

Chan et al, 1989; Roberts and Griswold, 1990). Transfer of a 678 nucleotide fragment which includes both conserved regions of human TfR mRNA to the 3' UTR of growth hormone or HLA-A2 indicator transcripts suffices to confer iron-dependent mRNA stability to the chimeric transcripts (Müllner and Kühn, 1988; Casey et al, 1988b). Two IRE motifs (A and B) are found in the upstream and three IREs (C, D and E) are located in the downstream conserved region. When IRE_B or IRE_C are cloned into the 5' UTR of reporter mRNAs, they mediate translational regulation (Casey et al, 1988b). This experiment shows that both IREs can bind IRP in vivo and that their function is position and context dependent. When tested in gel retardation assays, all five IREs specifically bind IRP in vitro (Koeller et al, 1989), and at least four of the five IREs can be occupied simultaneously by IRP (Müllner et al, 1992).

Deletions from the regulatory region show that IRE_A and IRE_E can be removed without affecting function. Moreover, the nonconserved region between the two conserved blocks is predicted to form a long loop of 332 nucleotides which can be shortened to 6 nucleotides (Casey et al, 1988b; Müllner and Kühn, 1988; Casey et al, 1989). These deletions have helped to define a synthetic minimal regulatory element of 250 nucleotides (referred to as TRS-1) which contains three IREs and appears to be functionally equivalent to the wild-type regulatory region (Casey et al, 1989).

Deletion of the first C-residue from an IRE (ΔCIRE) prevents the binding of IRP (Hentze et al, 1988). When the three IREs of TRS-1 were converted into ΔCIREs, the resulting mRNA (TRS-4) failed to be iron regulated and appeared to be constitutively unstable (Casey et al, 1989). This experiment shows that IRP-binding is important for stabilization of the mRNA. In addition, it indicates that TRS-4 contains elements which destabilize the message when IRP is not bound. TRS-1 and TRS-4 both contain conserved non-IRE sequences. Small nonoverlapping deletions affecting these sequences (which are separated in human TfR mRNA by more than 400 nucleotides) abolish iron regulation and yield constitutively stable transcripts (Müllner and Kühn, 1988; Casey et al, 1988b). Thus, these mutations disturb the function of instability elements. Taken together, the cis-regulatory region of the TfR mRNA is comprised of IREs and a somewhat ill-defined instability determinant(s). There is no indication that AU-rich sequences, which are involved in the destabilization of several lymphokine and growth factor mRNAs (Shaw and Kamen, 1986), play a role as instability determinants for TfR mRNAs.

IRP-binding stabilizes the TfR transcript (Figure 8.4), but it is not clear whether the mRNA undergoes a structural change before being degraded by the responsible cellular nuclease(s) when IRP is not bound. Concei-

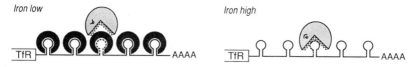

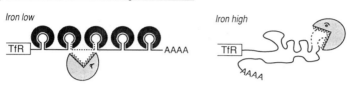

Figure 8.4 Models of possible mechanisms for the regulation of transferrin receptor (TfR) mRNA stability by IRP. The 3′ UTR of TfR mRNA with five IREs is depicted with the 3′ end of the open reading frame and the poly(A)-tail. Divergent and conserved non-IRE regions of the 3′ UTR including the large stem-loop region separating IRE_B from IRE_C (see text) are not depicted. The face-symbol indicates the ribonuclease as an endonuclease, although the possibility of an exonucleolytic mechanism has to be considered. (A) The nuclease is shown to initially attack a region of the mRNA (broken line) which can be **directly** protected by IRP-binding in iron-starved cells. (B) Degradation-prone and protected mRNA are viewed to be folded differently. The equilibrium between the structure required for degradation and the structure displaying IREs is affected by IRP-binding. For further discussion, see text.

vably, a part of the nucleolytic target site could be directly protected by IRP-binding (Figure 8.4A). Alternatively, exposure of the nucleolytic site may require an RNA secondary structure different from that which exposes the IREs. In this scenario, IRP affects the equilibrium between the two alternative secondary structures (Figure 8.4B). The stabilization of the mRNA by distant nonoverlapping deletions indicates that long range interactions within the regulatory region could be required for TfR mRNA degradation, favouring the latter scenario. However, structural analysis of the TRS-1 RNA element in the presence and absence of IRP suggests that IRP-binding does not change the folding of the RNA (Horowitz and Harford, 1992). At present, the characterization of the components and the structure of the cis-regulatory region of TfR mRNA is still incomplete.

Which are the transacting factors that participate in TfR mRNA regulation? As described above, IRP protects the message when bound to (several of?) the IREs. Little information is available concerning the nature of the nuclease(s) involved. Since the binding of IRP is iron-regulated, there is no a priori requirement for iron regulation of the nuclease. As is the case for most other mRNAs whose stability is regulated, intermediates of degradation have not yet been identified. The identification of bona fide intermediates with a direct kinetic relationship to the specific degradation process is difficult, because these intermediates are usually rapidly destroyed by abundant exonucleases. It is also still unclear whether the primary attack on the TfR mRNA is endo- or exonucleolytic, whether the RNase is a protein, a ribozyme or an RNA/protein complex, and whether factors other than IRP bind to the TfR regulatory region to stabilize or destabilize the message. In contrast to the translational regulation by IRE/IRP interactions, the current lack of a suitable cell-free system and the difficulty to reconstitute this pathway in yeast has impeded the elucidation of the underlying molecular mechanism.

At least some pharmacological characteristics of TfR mRNA degradation in iron-loaded cells have been identified. The transcription inhibitor actinomycin D stabilizes TfR mRNA, which may reflect the lack of an RNA or protein component with a short half life. Since all three RNA polymerases are inhibited by actinomycin D, it is not clear whether the missing component is an mRNA or perhaps a small pol III transcript. Furthermore, actinomycin D inhibits transcription by intercalation into the double-stranded DNA; it is conceivable that intercalation into structured regions of the TfR mRNA could be the cause of stabilization by actinomycin D. It has also been investigated whether ribosome association is required for TfR mRNA degradation. This is required for the degradation of several stability-regulated mRNAs including tubulin (Yen et al, 1988), c-fos and c-myc (Schuler and Cole, 1988). Both cycloheximide, a translation inhibitor which stalls ribosomes on the mRNA, and puromycin, an inhibitor of protein synthesis which induces premature release of the mRNA from ribosomes, retard or completely block the degradation of the TfR mRNA (Müllner and Kühn, 1988; Koeller et al, 1991). These results do not allow one to discriminate between a requirement of TfR mRNA to be translated for degradation (a cis effect), and the lack of a necessary component of the nuclease when protein synthesis is blocked (a trans effect). To distinguish between these two possibilities, the translation of TRS-4 mRNA has been selectively perturbed. This transcript cannot be protected by IRP and is rapidly degraded, almost certainly following the same pathway as wild-type TfR mRNA in iron replete cells. Introduction of an IRE into the 5' UTR of TRS-4 mRNA allows selective regulation of the translation of this mRNA. A more than 20-fold difference in translation rate had no effect on stability (Koeller et al, 1991), suggesting that degradation occurs independently from translation.

Conclusions

The investigation of the molecular processes underlying the control of iron metabolism in mammalian cells has led to the identification and subsequent characterization of a cytoplasmic regulatory network. A signal (primarily the cellular iron state) affects the RNA-binding activity of a cytoplasmic protein (IRP), which in turn controls the translation (ferritin, eALAS, aconitase?) and stability (transferrin receptor) of mature, fully spliced and polyadenylated cytoplasmic mRNAs. The current state of knowledge allows to explain key events in the coordination and maintenance of cellular iron homeostasis. The dissection of the components of the regulatory machinery has also yielded fruitful experimental model systems for studying translational control and mRNA stability regulation by RNA/protein interactions in general, and given insight into a novel mechanism by which the nucleic acid-binding activity of a protein can be regulated.

Figure 8.5 summarizes central aspects of the post-transcriptional regulation of gene expression by iron. Iron is taken up into cells by multiple routes, with the uptake of diferric transferrin via the transferrin receptor being the physiologically most relevant one. Following uptake, iron is distributed for storage (in ferritin) or utilization, and participates in regulation. An as yet poorly characterized pool of iron (which can be accessed pharmacologically by desferrioxamine) is sensed, perhaps directly, by iron regulatory protein (IRP). In iron-loaded cells, IRP assembles a 4Fe-4S cluster and functions, as such, as the cytoplasmic enzyme aconitase. In iron-starved cells, IRP remains as (or is converted into, see above) an apoprotein, which functions as an IRE-binding protein (IRE-BP). Binding to iron-responsive elements in the 3' UTR of transferrin receptor mRNA stabilizes the message against degradation and thus allows increased TfR expression. This increase in TfR expression counterbalances iron starvation by increased iron uptake. Binding of IRP to IREs in the 5' UTR of ferritin, eALAS and perhaps aconitase mRNA represses their translation by blocking the binding of the 43S translation preinitiation complex. This response contributes to the homeostatic effect by reducing the storage of available intracellular iron in ferritin and by reducing the expression of the first enzyme in erythroid heme biosynthesis, and thus probably iron consumption by this pathway. The role of reduced synthesis of mitochondrial aconitase, if this occurs in vivo, is less clear (see below). Since the regulation of the target mRNAs occurs post-transcriptionally, and of IRP even post-translationally, in the cytoplasm, the role of nuclear events in these processes is less dynamic and only involves the steady state synthesis of the mature mRNAs (Figure 8.5).

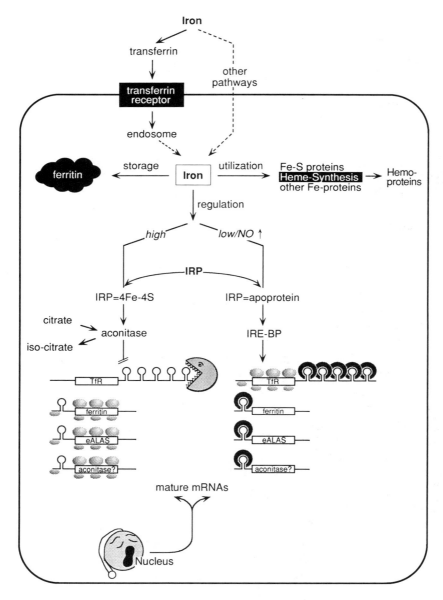

Figure 8.5 Synopsis of iron regulation by the IRE/IRP system. A eukaryotic cell is depicted with the extracellular space, the cell membrane and a nucleus, omitting cellular organelles. IRP is symbolized by a circular structure binding to IREs an iron-starved or NO-exposed cells. Oval structures represent ribosomal subunits engaged with actively translated mRNAs. The primarily cytoplasmic nature of this regulatory network is underscored by the passive appearance of the nucleus releasing the mature mRNAs. The question mark in mitochondrial aconitase mRNA indicates the current lack of direct evidence for regulation by IRP in vivo. Broken arrows represent availability of limited biochemical information. For a detailed discussion, refer to the text.

The above summarizes a framework for explaining the regulation of iron metabolism at the cellular level. However, apart from its implications for the understanding of heme synthesis in erythroid cells, it gives little insight into critical events for the maintenance of iron homeostasis in the whole mammalian organism. In particular, the connections between the IRE/IRP regulatory network and the regulation of iron absorption from the gut need to be identified, as well as the control of iron release from cells, particularly macrophages. In addition to other approaches, the identification of further IRE-containing target mRNAs of IRP may help to uncover connections between the control of systemic and cellular iron metabolism. Information concerning these problems may also provide a more profound understanding of the role of nitric oxide in the control of IRP, as well as the involvement of the IRE/IRP system in human pathology (Melefors and Hentze, 1993).

Several important questions pertaining to the function of the IRE/IRP system at the cellular level are left to be answered. Much remains to be learned about the mechanism by which TfR mRNA is degraded. With regard to IRP, we do not know how the iron sulfur cluster is assembled in iron-loaded or removed in iron-starved cells. Which form of iron is sensed? Are co-factors and enzymes involved? Why has the aconitase function of IRP been conserved, and why does IRP appear to control the translation of mitochondrial aconitase mRNA? Perhaps the modulation of cellular citrate levels in response to iron availability is important, particularly when citrate can bind and perhaps transport iron within cells (Frausto da Silva and Williams, 1991). Finally, how does this regulatory system communicate with cellular surveillance mechanisms for redox state and oxidative stress? Given the chemistry and the biological roles of iron, such communication has to be anticipated. Much has already been learned, and many surprises have been encountered, but it may only be the beginnings of recognizing the cytoplasm as a compartment for gene regulation.

Acknowledgments

I would like to thank the past and present members of our group at the EMBL for their experimental and conceptual contributions, Petra Riedinger for artwork, and the Deutsche Forschungsgemeinschaft for support.

References

Aisen P, Listowski I (1980): Iron transport and storage proteins. *Annu Rev Biochem* 49:357–393

Aziz N, Munro HN (1987): Iron regulates ferritin mRNA translation through a segment of its 5'untranslated region. *Proc Natl Acad Sci USA* 84: 8478–8482

Barton HA, Eisenstein RS, Bomford A, Munro HN (1990): Determinants of the interaction between the iron-responsive element-binding protein and its binding site in rat L-ferritin mRNA. *J Biol Chem* 265: 7000–7008

Basilion JP, Rouault TA, Massinople CM, Klauser RD, Burgess WH (1994): The iron-responsive element-binding protein: localization of the RNA-binding site to the aconitase active-site cleft. *Proc Natl Acad Sci USA* 91: 574–578

Beinert H (1990): Recent developments in the field of iron-sulfur proteins. *FASEB J* 4: 2483–2491

Bothwell TH, Charlton RW, Motulski AG (1983): Idiopathic hemochromatosis. In: *The Metabolic Basis of Inherited Disease*, Stanbury, Wyngaarden, Fredrickson, Goldstein, Brown, eds. New York: McGraw-Hill

Braun V, Günter K, Hantke K (1991): Transport of iron across the outer membrane. *Biol Met* 4: 14–22

Brock JH (1994): Iron in infection, immunity, inflammation and neoplasia. In: *Iron Metabolism in Health & Disease*, Brock JH, Halliday JW, Pippard MJ, Powell LW, eds. London: W.B. Saunders Company Ltd

Casey JL, Di Jeso B, Rao K, Klausner RD, Harford JB (1988a): Two genetic loci participate in the regulation by iron of the gene for the human transferrin receptor. *Proc Natl Acad Sci USA* 85: 1787–1791

Casey JL, Hentze MW, Koeller DM, Caughman SW, Rouault TA, Klausner RD, Harford JB (1988b): Iron-responsive elements: regulatory RNA sequences that control mRNA levels and translation. *Science* 240: 924–928

Casey JL, Koeller DM, Ramin VC, Klausner RD, Harford JB (1989): Iron regulation of transferrin receptor mRNA levels requires iron-responsive elements and a rapid turnover determinant in the 3' untranslated region of the mRNA. *EMBO J* 8: 3693–3699

Caughman SW, Hentze MW, Rouault TA, Harford JB, Klausner RD (1988): The iron-responsive element is the single element responsible for iron-dependent translational regulation of ferritin biosynthesis: evidence for function as the binding site for a translational repressor. *J Biol Chem* 263: 19048–19052

Chan L-NL, Grammatikakis N, Banks JM, Gerhardt EM (1989): Chicken transferrin receptor gene: conservation of 3' noncoding sequences and expression in erythroid cells. *Nucleic Acids Res* 17: 3763–3771

Constable A, Quick S, Gray NK, Hentze MW (1992): Modulation of the RNA-binding activity of a regulatory protein by iron in vitro: switching between enzymatic and genetic function? *Proc Natl Acad Sci USA* 89: 4554–4558

Cox TC, Bawden MJ, Martin A, May BK (1991): Human erythroid 5-aminolevulinate synthase: promoter analysis and identification of an iron-responsive element in the mRNA. *EMBO J* 10: 1891–1902

Dancis A, Roman DG, Anderson GJ, Hinnebusch AG, Klausner RD (1992): Ferric reductase of *Saccharomyces cerevisiae*: molecular characterization, role in iron uptake, and transcriptional control by iron. *Proc Natl Acad Sci USA* 89: 3869–3873

Dandekar T, Stripecke R, Gray NK, Goossen B, Constable A, Johansson HE, Hentze MW (1991): Identification of a novel iron-responsive element in murine and human erythroid δ-aminolevulinic acid synthase mRNA. *EMBO J* 10: 1903–1909

Dierks P (1990): Molecular biology of eukaryotic 5-aminolevulinate synthase. In: *Biosynthesis of Heme and Chlorophylls*, Dailey HA, ed. New York: McGraw-Hill

Drapier JC, Hirling H, Wietzerbin J, Kaldy P, Kühn LC (1993): Biosynthesis of nitric oxide activates iron regulatory factor in macrophages. *EMBO J* 12: 3643–3649

Drapier JC, Pellat C, Yann H (1991): Generation of EPR-detectable nitrosyl-iron complexes in tumor target cells co-cultured with activated macrophages. *J Biol Chem* 266: 10162–10167

Eisenstein RS, Garcia-Mayol D, Pettingell W, Munro HN (1991): Regulation of ferritin and heme oxygenase synthesis in rat fibroblasts by different forms of iron. *Proc Natl Acad Sci USA* 88: 688–692

Eisenstein RS, Tuazon PT, Schalinske KL, Anderson SA, Traugh JA (1993): Iron-responsive element-binding protein. *J Biol Chem* 268: 27363–27370

Emery-Goodman A, Hirling H, Scarpellino L, Henderson B, Kühn LC (1993): Iron regulatory factor expressed from recombinant baculovirus: conversion between the RNA-binding apoprotein and Fe-S cluster containing aconitase. *Nucl Acids Res* 21: 1457–1461

Frausto da Silva JJR, Williams RJP (1991): The inorganic chemistry of life. In: *The Biological Chemistry of the Elements*, Oxford: Clarendon Press

Goessling LS, Daniels-McQueen S, Bhattacharyya-Pakrasi M, Lin J-J, Thach RE (1992): Enhanced degradation of ferritin repressor protein during induction of ferritin messenger RNA translation *Science* 256: 670–673

Goossen B, Caughman SW, Harford JB, Klausner RD, Hentze MW (1990): Translational repression by a complex between the iron-responsive element of ferritin mRNA and its specific cytoplasmic binding protein is position-dependent in vivo. *EMBO J* 9: 4127–4133

Goossen B, Hentze MW (1992): Position is the critical determinant for function of iron-responsive elements as translational regulators. *Mol Cell Biol* 12: 1959–1966

Gray NK, Hentze MW (1994): Iron regulatory protein prevents binding of the 43S translation pre-initiation complex to ferritin and eALAS mRNA. *EMBO J* 13: 3882–3891

Gray NK, Hentze MW (1994b): unpublished observation

Gray NK, Quick S, Goossen B, Constable A, Hirling H, Kühn LC, Hentze MW (1993): Recombinant iron regulatory factor functions as an iron responsive element-binding protein, a translational repressor and an aconitase. A functional assay for translational repression and direct demonstration of the iron switch. *Eur J Biochem* 218: 657–667

Haile DJ, Hentze MW, Rouault TA, Harford JB, Klausner RD (1989): Regulation of interaction of the iron-responsive element binding protein with iron-responsive RNA elements. *Mol Cell Biol* 9: 5055-5061

Haile DJ, Rouault TA, Harford JB, Klausner RD (1990): The inhibition of the iron responsive element RNA-protein interaction by heme does not mimic in vivo iron regulation. *J Biol Chem* 265: 12786–12789

Haile DJ, Rouault TA, Tang CK, Chin J, Harford JB, Klausner RD (1992a): Reciprocal control of RNA-binding and aconitase activity in the regulation of the iron-responsive element binding protein: Role of the iron-sulfur cluster. *Proc Natl Acad Sci USA* 89: 7536–7540

Haile DJ, Rouault TA, Harford JB, Kennedy MC, Blondin GA, Beinert H, Klausner RD (1992b): Cellular regulation of the iron-responsive element binding protein:

Disassembly of the cubane iron-sulfur cluster results in high-affinity RNA binding. *Proc Natl Acad Sci USA* 89: 11735–11739

Halliday JW, Ramm GA, Powell LW (1994): Cellular iron processing and storage: The role of ferritin. In: *Iron Metabolism in Health & Disease*, Brock JH, Halliday JW, Pippard MJ, Powell LW, eds. London: W.B. Saunders.

Harrell CM, McKenzie AR, Patino MM, Walden WE, Theil EC (1991): Ferritin mRNA: Interactions of iron regulatory element with translational regulator protein P-90 and the effect on base-paired flanking regions. *Proc Natl Acad Sci USA* 88: 4166–4170

Henderson BR, Seiser C, Kühn LC (1993): Characterization of a second RNA-binding protein in rodents with specificity for iron-responsive elements. *J Biol Chem* 268: 27327–27334

Hentze MW, Argos P (1991): Homology between IRE-BP, a regulatory RNA-binding protein, aconitase and isopropylmalate isomerase. *Nucl Acids Res* 19: 1739–1740

Hentze MW, Caughman SW, Rouault TA, Barriocanal JG, Dancis A, Harford JB, Klausner RD (1987b): Identification of the iron-responsive element for the translational regulation of human ferritin mRNA. *Science* 238: 1570–1573

Hentze MW, Caughman SW, Casey JL, Koeller DM, Rouault TA, Harford JB, Klausner RD (1988): A model for the structure and function of iron-responsive elements. *Gene* 72: 201–208

Hentze MW, Rouault TA, Caughman SW, Dancis A, Harford JB, Klausner RD (1987a): A cis-acting element is necessary and sufficient for translational regulation of human ferritin expression in response to iron. *Proc Natl Acad Sci USA* 84: 6730–6734

Hentze MW, Rouault TA, Harford JB, Klausner RD (1989b): Oxidation-reduction and the molecular mechanism of a regulated RNA-protein interaction. *Science* 244: 357–359

Hentze MW, Seuanez HN, O'Brien SJ, Harford JB, Klausner RD (1989a): Chromosomal localization of nucleic acid-binding proteins by affinity mapping: assignment of the IRE-binding protein gene to human chromosome 9. *Nucl Acids Res* 17: 6103–6108

Hershey JWB (1991): Translational control in mammalian cells. *Annu Rev Biochem* 60: 717–755

Hirling H, Emery-Goodman A, Thompson N, Neupert B, Seiser C, Kühn LC (1992): Expression of active iron regulatory factor from a full-length human cDNA by in vitro transcription/translation. *Nucl Acids Res* 20: 33–39

Hirling H, Henderson BR, Kühn LC (1994): Mutational analysis of the [4Fe-4S]-cluster converting iron regulatory factory from its RNA-binding form to cytoplasmic aconitase. *EMBO J* 13: 453–461

Horowitz JA, Harford JB (1992): The secondary structure of the regulatory region of the transferrin receptor mRNA deduced by enzymatic cleavage. *New Biol* 4: 330–338

Jaffrey SR, Haile DJ, Klausner RD, Harford JB (1993): The interaction between the iron-responsive element binding protein and its cognate RNA is highly dependent upon both RNA sequence and structure. *Nucl Acids Res* 21: 4627–4631

Kaptain S, Downey WE, Tang C, Philpott C, Haile D, Orloff DG, Harford JB, Rouault TA, Klausner RD (1991): A regulated RNA binding protein also possesses aconitase activity. *Proc Natl Acad Sci USA* 88: 10109–10113

Kennedy MC, Mende-Mueller L, Blondin GA, Beinert H (1992): Purification and characterization of cytosolic aconitase from beef liver and its relationship to the iron-responsive element binding protein. *Proc Natl Acad Sci USA* 89: 11730–11734

Klausner RD, Ashwell G, van Renswoude J, Harford JB, Bridges KR (1983): Binding of apotransferrin to K562 cells: explanation of the transferrin cycle. *Proc Natl Acad Sci USA* 80: 2263–2266

Klausner RD, Rouault TA, Harford JB (1993): Regulating the fate of mRNA: The control of cellular iron metabolism. *Cell* 72: 19–28

Koeller DM, Casey JL, Hentze MW, Gerhardt EM, Chan LN, Klausner RD, Harford JB (1989): A cytosolic protein binds to structural elements within the iron regulatory region of the transferrin receptor mRNA. *Proc Natl Acad Sci USA* 86: 3574–3578

Koeller DM, Horowitz JA, Casey JL, Klausner RD, Harford JB (1991): Translation and the stability of mRNAs encoding the transferrin receptor and c-fos. *Proc Natl Acad Sci USA* 88: 7778–7782

Kühn LC, Hentze MW (1992): Coordination of cellular iron metabolism by post-transcriptional gene regulation. *J Inorgan Biochem* 47: 183–195

Leibold EA, Munro HN (1988): Cytoplasmic protein binds in vitro to a highly conserved sequence in the 5′ untranslated region of ferritin heavy- and light-subunit mRNAs. *Proc Natl Acad Sci USA* 85: 2171–2175

Leibold EA, Laudano A, Yu Y (1990): Structural requirements of iron-responsive elements for binding of the protein involved in both transferrin receptor and ferritin mRNA post-transcriptional regulation. *Nucl Acids Res* 18: 1819–1824

Lin JJ, Daniels-McQueen S, Patino MM, Gaffield L, Walden WE, Thach RE (1990): Derepression of ferritin messenger RNA translation by hemin in vitro. *Science* 247: 74–77

Lin JJ, Patino MM, Gaffield L, Walden WE, Smith A, Thach RE (1991): Crosslinking of hemin to a specific site on the 90-kDa ferritin repressor protein. *Proc Natl Acad Sci USA* 88: 6068–6071

Lowenstein CJ, Snyder SH (1992): Nitric oxide, a novel biologic messenger. *Cell* 70: 705–707

Mattia A, Josic D, Ashwell G, Klausner R, van Renswoude J (1986): Regulation of intracellular iron distribution of K562 human erythroleukemia cells. *J Biol Chem* 261: 4587–4593

Melefors Ö, Hentze MW (1993): Iron regulatory factor — the conductor of cellular iron regulation. *Blood Rev* 7: 251–258

Melefors Ö, Goossen B, Johansson HE, Stripecke R, Gray NK, Hentze MW (1993): Translational control of 5-aminolevulinate synthase mRNA by iron-responsive elements in erythroid cells. *J Biol Chem* 268: 5974–5978

Moncada S, Palmer RMJ, Higgs EA (1991): Nitric oxide: physiology, pathophysiology and pharmacology. *Pharmacol Rev* 43: 109–142

Müllner EW, Kühn LC (1988): A stem-loop in the 3′ untranslated region mediates iron-dependent regulation of transferrin receptor mRNA stability in the cytoplasm. *Cell* 53: 815–825

Müllner EW, Neupert B, Kühn LC (1989): A specific mRNA binding factor regulates the iron-dependent stability of cytoplasmic transferrin receptor mRNA. *Cell* 58: 373–382

Müllner EW, Rothenberger S, Müller AM, Kühn LC (1992): In vivo and in vitro modulation of the mRNA-binding activity of iron-regulatory factor. Tissue distribution and effects of cell proliferation, iron levels and redox state. *Eur J Biochem* 208: 597–605

Nathan C (1992): Nitric oxide as a secretory product of mammalian cells. *FASEB J* 6: 3051-3064

Neupert B, Thompson NA, Meyer C, Kühn LC (1990): A high yield affinity purification method for specific RNA-binding proteins: isolation of the iron regulatory factor from human placenta. *Nucl Acids Res* 18: 51–55

Oliveira CC, Goossen B, Zanchin NIT, McCarthy JEG, Hentze MW, Stripecke R (1993): Translational repression by the human iron-regulatory factor (IRF) in *Saccharomyces cerevisiae*. *Nucl Acids Res* 21: 5316–5322

Pantopoulos K, Weiss G, Hentze MW (1994): Nitric oxide and the post-transcriptional control of cellular iron traffic. *Trends Cell Biol* 4: 82–86

Patino MM, Walden WE (1992): Cloning of a functional cDNA for the rabbit ferritin mRNA repressor protein. *J Biol Chem* 267: 19011–19016

Philpott CC, Haile D, Rouault TA, Klausner RD (1993): Modification of a free Fe-S cluster cysteine residue in the active iron-responsive element-binding protein prevents RNA binding *J Biol Chem* 268: 17655–17658

Philpott CC, Rouault TA, Klausner RD (1991): Sequence and expression of the murine iron-responsive element binding protein. *Nucl Acids Res* 19: 6333

Robbins AH, Stout CD (1989a): The structure of aconitase. *PROTEINS: Structure, Function, and Genetics* 5: 289–312

Robbins AH, Stout CD (1989b): Structure of activated aconitase: Formation of the [4Fe-4S] cluster in the crystal. *Proc Natl Acad Sci USA* 86: 3639–3643

Roberts KP, Griswold MD (1990): Characterization of rat transferrin receptor cDNA: The regulation of transferrin receptor mRNA in testes and in Sertoli cells in culture. *Mol Endocrinol* 4: 521–542

Rogers J (1992): Genetic regulation of the iron transport and storage genes: Links with the acute phase response. In: *Iron and Human Disease*, Lauffer RB, ed. Boca Raton: CRC Press

Rogers JT, Bridges KR, Durmowicz GP, Glass J, Auron PE, Munro HN (1990): Translational control during the acute phase response. *J Biol Chem* 265: 14572–14578

Rothenberger S, Müllner EW, Kühn LC (1990): The mRNA-binding protein which controls ferritin and transferrin receptor expression is conserved during evolution. *Nucl Acids Res* 18: 1175–1179

Rouault TA, Hentze MW, Caughman SW, Harford JB, Klausner RD (1988): Binding of a cytosolic protein to the iron-responsive element of human ferritin messenger RNA. *Science* 241: 1207–1210

Rouault TA, Hentze MW, Haile DJ, Harford JB, Klausner RD (1989): The iron-responsive element binding protein: A method for the affinity purification of a regulatory RNA-binding protein. *Proc Natl Acad Sci USA* 86: 5768–5772

Rouault TA, Stout CD, Kaptain S, Harford JB, Klausner R (1991): Structural relationship between an iron-regulated RNA-binding protein (IRE-BP) and aconitase: Functional implications. *Cell* 64: 881–883

Rouault TA, Tang CK, Kaptain S, Burgess WH, Haile DJ, Samaniego F, McBride OW, Harford JB, Klausner RD (1990): Cloning of the cDNA encoding an RNA regulatory protein-the human iron-responsive element-binding protein. *Proc Natl Acad Sci USA* 88: 7958–7962

Schuler GD, Cole MD (1988): GM-CSF and oncogene mRNA stabilities are independently regulated in *trans* in a mouse monocytic tumor. *Cell* 55: 1115–1122

Seiser C, Teixeira S, Kühn LC (1993): Interleukin-2-dependent transcriptional and post-transcriptional regulation of transferrin receptor mRNA. *J Biol Chem* 268: 13074–13080

Shaw G, Kamen R (1986): A conserved AU sequence from the 3' untranslated region of GM-CSF mRNA mediates selective mRNA degradation. *Cell* 46: 659–667

Skikne B, Baynes RD (1994): Iron absorption. In: *Iron Metabolism in Health & Disease*, Brock JH, Halliday JW, Pippard MJ, Powell LW, eds. London: W.B. Saunders

Stamler JS, Singel DJ, Loscalzo J (1992): Biochemistry of nitric oxide and its redox-activated forms. *Science* 258: 1898–1902

Stripecke R, Hentze MW (1992): Bacteriophage and spliceosomal proteins function as position-dependent cis/trans repressors of mRNA translation in vitro. *Nucl Acids Res* 20: 5555–5564

Stripecke R, Oliveira CC, McCarthy JEG, Hentze MW (1994): Proteins binding to 5' UTR sites: A general mechanism for translational regulation of mRNAs in human and yeast cells. *Mol Cell Biol* 14: in press

Tang CK, Chin J, Harford JB, Klausner RD, Rouault TA (1992): Iron regulates the activity of the iron-responsive element binding protein without changing its rate of synthesis or degradation. *J Biol Chem* 267: 24466–24470

Walden WE, Patino MM, Gaffield L (1989): Purification of a specific repressor of ferritin mRNA translation from rabbit liver. *J Biol Chem* 264: 13765–13769

Weiss G, Goossen B, Doppler W, Fuchs D, Pantopoulos K, Werner-Felmayer G, Wachter H, Hentze MW (1993): Translational regulation via iron-responsive elements by the nitric oxide/NO-synthase pathway. *EMBO J* 12: 3651–3657

Weiss G, Werner-Felmayer G, Werner ER, Grünewald K, Wachter H, Hentze MW (1994): Iron regulates nitric oxide synthase activity by controlling nuclear transcription. *J Exp Med* 180: in press

White K, Munro HN (1988): Induction of ferritin subunit synthesis by iron is regulated at both the transcriptional and translational levels. *J Biol Chem* 263: 8938–8942

Yen TJ, Machlin PS, Cleveland DW (1988): Autoregulated instability of β-tubulin mRNAs by recognition of the nascent amino terminus of β-tubulin. *Nature* 334: 580–585

Yu Y, Radisky E, Leibold EA (1992): The iron-responsive element binding protein. *J Biol Chem* 267: 19005–19010

Zähringer J, Baliga BS, Munro HN (1976): Novel mechanism for translational control in regulation of ferritin synthesis by iron. *Proc Natl Acad Sci USA* 73: 857–861

Index

Combined Index for Volumes 1 and 2

Abducens motor nucleus: (II) 15
Acetylsalicylic acid: (I) 161
Achaete–complex, *drosophila*: (I) 180
Aconitase: (I) 246–247, 257, 259
Acrodermatitis enteropathica: (I) 206
ACTH. *See* Adrenocorticotropic hormone
Actinomycin D: (I) 256
Activating Protein–1 (AP–1)
  basic zipper region and, (I) 220
  c–fos gene and, (II) 170
  dependent genes and, (I) 76
  factor family, (I) 62
  like binding sites, (I) 67
  modifications of, (I) 72–73
  NFκB and, (I) 75
  nuclear receptor and, (I) 220
  sites of, (II) 6
  transcription factor as, (I) 62–84
Activation functions (AFs): (II) 210–212
Acute phase response factor (APRF): (II) 116
Acute promyelocytic leukemia (APL): (II) 223
Acyl CoA thioesters: (I) 160–162
Adenoviruses:
  DRTF1/E2F and, (II), 80–81
  E1A product, (I) 67, 75–76
  NF kB and, (I) 111, 121
  See also specific types
Adenylyl cyclase: (II) 2, 10
Adipate esters: (I) 144
Adipocytes, 3T3 L1 cells and: (I) 154
Adrenal gland: (II) 30
Adrenocorticotropic hormone (ACTH): (I) 31
AFs. *See* Activation functions
Aging systems: (I) 32
Agonist/Antagonist action, nuclear
  receptors: (II) 212–215
Alkylating agents: (I) 62
Alpha chorionic gonadotropin gene: (II) 3
Alpha helix, DNA recognition and: (I) 7–8
Alzheimer's disease: (I) 211
Aminolevulinate synthase: (I) 242
Amyloid A: (I) 120
Androgen receptor (AR): (I) 153; (II) 143, 161, 205
Angiotensinogen: (I) 120

Animal model system, tumor development
  and: (I) 81.
  See also Mammalian cells; *specific studies*
Anisomycin: (II) 52
Ankyrin domains: (I) 98–100, 105, 121; (II) 252
Antagonists, nuclear receptors and: (II) 212–215
Antibodies:
  anti-ERK, (II) 52
  anti-HSP70, (I) 48
  anti-MAPK, (I) 72
  perturbation experiments and, (I) 37
  See also specific types
Antigen presenting cells (APC): (I) 104
Antihormones, nuclear receptors: (II) 212–215
Antioxidant response element (ARE): (I) 79
Antioxidants, NF kB: (I) 109
Antiviral factors: (II) 101. *See also*
  Interferons, *specific types*
Aorta: (I) 31
APC. *See* Antigen presenting cells
APL. *See* Acute promyelocytic leukemia
apo CIII protein: (II) 218
AP-1. *See* Activating Protein-1
ApoAi-RARE, response elements: (II) 168
Apolipoprotein (apo) gene: (II) 217–218
Apoptosis: (I) 121
Apotransferrin/TfR receptor: (I) 242
APRF. *See* Acute phase response factor
AR. *See* Androgen receptor
A-raf, genes: (II) 50
ARE. *See* Antioxidant response element
ARG80, yeast proteins: (II) 44
Arachidonic acid: (I) 51, 160; (II) 104
Arnt forms, dioxin receptor and: (I) 187, 192, 197
ASV17, retrovirus: (I) 81
ATF genes: (I) 73, 75
Atherosclerosis: (I) 168
Autophagocytosis: (I) 103
Autoregulation, hormone mediated: (II) 131
Autosomal dominant disorders: (II) 174
Autosomal recessive disorder: (I) 206
Auxiliary operators: (I) 10
Avian bone marrow cells: (I) 103

Avian erythroleukemia virus: (II) 226
Avian Rel protein: (I) 102
Avian retrovirus, REV–T: (I) 102
Azetidine: (I) 28, 46–47

Bacteria: (I) 93, 122, 143. *See also specific types*
Bacteriophage P22, salmonella: (I) 8
Bandshift analyses: (I) 214–216, 231
Basal promoter, HSP70: (I) 32
Basal transcription machinery: (II) 215–217
Basic–helix–loop–helix (bHLH) factor:
    C/EBP proteins, (I) 117
    dioxin and, (I) 177–199
    twiprotein and, (II) 257
    See also Helix–loop–helix receptor
Basic leucine zipper (bZIP): (I) 117
    AP-1 and, (II) 220
    c-Jun and, (I) 74
    ICER and, (II) 26–27
    Jun/Fos and, (I) 75
    proteins, (I) 7, 66–67
    See also Leucine zipper group
B cells: (I) 101
Bcl-3 gene: (I) 100, 104–105
Beta-oxidation: (I) 143, 160
Beta-turn-beta structure: (I) 96
bFGF, UV response: (I) 76
bHLH. *See* Basic-helix-loop-helix
Binding constant, *lac* repressor: (I) 10
Birth defects, dioxins and: (I) 177
B-*myb* genes: (II) 75
Bone marrow: (I) 102, 154
B-raf, genes: (II) 50
Brain: (II) 173
B-region, thyroglobulin: (II) 47–48
brm/SWI 2 homologue: (II) 144
bZIP. *See* Basic leucine zipper

C1 gene: (I) 15
C437 gene: (I) 248
C56BL enzymes: (I) 178
CAM. *See* Calmodulin-dependent kinases
cAMP: (II) 99
    CREM and, (II) 1–32
    G proteins and, (II) 58–59
    ICER and, (II) 23
    melatonin and, (II) 27
    testes and, (II) 16–17
    transduction pathway and, (II) 2

CAP protein: (I) 5–6, 13–16
Cactus gene: (II) 243–245, 251–253
Cadmium (cd2): (I) 30, 46, 207, 208, 222, 229, 232
Cadystins: (I) 224
Caenorhabditis elegans: (I) 224; (II) 60
Calcineurin: (I) 110; (II) 56
Calcium (Ca2): (II) 56–58
Calmodulin-dependent kinases (CAM): (II) 5 8, 45, 56 58
Calmodulin-dependent protein kinase II, (CaM KII): (II) 45
Calyculin A: (I) 109
CaM KII. *See* Calmodulin-dependent protein kinase II
Cancers, retinoids and: (II) 222 223
Candida glabrata: (I) 224, 226, 227–229, 232
Carbonic anhydrase, zinc and: (I) 206
Carcinogens:
    DNA damage and, (I) 76
    Jun protein and, (I), 62
    mouse models of, (I) 74
    peroxisomes and, (I) 147, 162
    retinoids and, (II) 222
    See also specific substances
Carcinomas: (I) 82, 113, 150; (II) 197. *See also specific types*
Carnitine acyltransferase: (I) 164
Casein kinase II (CKII): (I) 69; (II) 7, 136
Catalase enzyme: (I) 144
CBF promoters: (I) 33
cdc10, yeast proteins: (II) 252
cDNA: (II) 43, 51–52, 105
cDNA libraries: (I) 142; (II) 9, 89
C/EBP proteins: (I) 117–118
CEFs. *See* Chicken embryo fibroblasts
Cell adhesion: (I) 119
Cell cycle, control: (II) 73–92. *See also specific receptors*
Cell death: (I) 121
Cell surface receptors: (II) 99–123. *See also specific types*
Cell transfection assays: (I) 192; (II) 168, 218
Cellular retinoic acid binding proteins (CRABPs),
(II) 167–168, 190
Cellular retinol binding proteins (CRBPs): (II) 190–193
Cellular stress responses: (I) 210

Cerebellar nuclei, motor nucleus: (II) 15
c-fos genes:
  AP-1 and (II) 170
  CRE and, (II) 6
  Ets and, (II) 46
  mitogens and, (II) 100
  proto-oncogene and, (II) 3
  SRF and, (II) 114
  signal uptake of, (II) 39 61
  SRE and, (II) 39 61
  See also Immediate early genes (IEGs)
Chaoptin protein: (II) 246
Chaperones, HSPs and: (I) 25, 184 186
Chelators, iron and: (I) 245
Chick embryos: (I) 103; (II) 213
Chicken embryo fibroblasts (CEFs): (I) 81
Chicken ovalbumin upsteam promoter
    transcription factor (COUP-TF):
  drosophila and, (II) 218
  gene of, (I) 151
  homodimer of, (I) 158
  orphan receptors and, (II) 168
  PPARs and, (I) 164 165
  receptor binding and, (II) 217, 218
  RXR and, (II) 204, 205, 210
Chicken studies:
  F2 element and, (II) 169
  HSF3 and, (I) 39
  pp-40 proteins and, (I) 99
  T3Ralpha and, (II) 211
  vitellogenin II gene, (II) 141
  See also specific factors
Chlorambucil: (I) 79
Cholesterol: (I) 168; (II) 218
Chromatography: (I) 244
Chromosomal puffs, heat shock: (I) 27, 51
Chronic lymphocytic leukemias: (I) 100
Chronic lymphoproliferate disorders: (I)
  151
Chymotrypsin inhibitors: (I) 114
Ciliary neutrophic factor (CNTF): (II) 116
Circadian rhythms: (II) 15, 27–29
CIRE. *See* C-residue from an IRE
Cirrhosis, retinoids and: (II) 226
Cisplatin: (I) 79
c-*jun*, transcription factor: (I) 71, 220; (II)
  170
CKII. *See* Casein kinase II
Clofibrate, peroxisomes and: (I) 144
Cloning, HSFs and: (I) 35

c-Myc, heterodimerizers: (I) 187; (II) 100
CNTF. *See* Ciliary neutrophic factor
Collagenase gene: (I) 63, 68, 72 73, 75; (II)
  145, 221
Complement factor C4: (I) 120
Complementation assays: (I) 186
Copper: (I) 210, 224, 226, 230
Coronary heart disease: (I) 168
Cotransfected cells, Schneider cells: (II)
  248 249
COUP-TF. *See* Chicken ovalbumin
  upsteam promoter
transcription factor
CRABPs. *See* Cellular retinoic acid binding
  proteins
CRBPs. *See* Cellular retinol binding
  proteins
CREB. *See* CRE binding protein
CREB/AFT protein family: (I) 64, 73
CRE-binding protein (CREB): (II) 4, 15, 42
CRE(cAMP reponsive element): (II) 1 4,
  6, 40
C-region, TCF: (II) 48 49
c-Rel, oncogene: (II) 250
CREM protein:
  FSH and, (II) 21 22
  gene structure of, (II) 9 11
  germ cells and, (II) 21
  ICER and, (II) 24 27, 31
  nuclear response and, (II) 1 32
  spermatogenesis and, (II) 16 17
C-residue from and IRE (CIRE): (I) 254
Cross-hybridization: (I) 142
Cross-talk, signaling pathways: (II) 217
  222
Crystallography: (I) 248
CTF, promoters: (I) 33
CUP1, regulatory protein: (I) 30, 226
CyclicAMP. *See* cAMP
Cyclin A: (II) 75, 79, 83
Cyclin–dependent kinase (cdk): (II) 79–80
Cycloheximide: (I) 28–29, 110, 211, 248;
  (II) 27
Cytochalasin B treatment: (I) 78
Cytochrome P-450 genes: (I) 143, 163, 178,
  186, 192
Cytokines:
  AP-1 and, (I) 83; (II) 170
  Bcl-3 protein and, (I) 104–105
  defensive response and, (I) 93

IFN-beta gene and, (I) 117
induction of, (I) 116 118
inflammation and, (I) 106 107
mammalian cells and, (I) 62
receptor for, (II) 41, 53
Cytoplasmic network: (I) 143, 241 259
Cytotoxic metals: (I) 232. *See also* Heavy
metals
Cyt repressor: (I) 5, 13

DAG. *See* Diacylglycerol
DBD. *See* DNA binding domain
ddRA, retinoid receptor: (II) 213
Decapentaplegic (dpp) receptor: (II) 255
Defensive responses, NF-kB: (I) 93 122
Defoliants, pollution and: (I) 177
DEHP. *See* Di(2ethyhexyl) phthalate
Dehydroepiandrostenedione (DHEA) acid:
(I) 161
Deo system: (I) 5, 13
Desferrioxamine: (I) 257
Developmental effects, vitamin A and: (II)
222
Dexamethasone: (II) 23, 139, 148
DHEA. *See* Dehydroepiandrostenedione
acid
DHFR. *See* Dihydrofolate reductase
Diabetes: (I) 146, 168
Diacylglycerol (DAG): (I) 106; (II) 1, 56,
99, 104
Diets, high-fats and: (I) 144
Dif, nuclear receptor: (I) 121
Dihydrofolate reductase (DHFR): (II) 74
75, 83 84
Dimerization: (I) 4, 96, 157
Dioxins:
activation of, (I) 186 190
arnt and, (I) 189 190
contaminants as, (I) 177 199
functional architecture of, (I) 190 192
hsp90 and, (I) 193 196
See also specific compounds
Direct repeat (DR) sequences: (I) 165; (II)
163
Direct signal transduction, tyrosine and:
(II) 99 123
Di(2ethyhexyl) phthalate (DEHP): (I) 167
dl protein. *See* Dorsal protein
DNA binding domain (DBD):
GAL4 and, (I) 47

glucocorticoid receptors and, (II) 131–
134
Jun/Fos and, (I) 65 66
retinoic acid receptor and, (II) 201 202
thyroid receptor and, (II) 160
DNA binding sites:
alpha helix and, (I) 7 8
AP-1 and, (II) 172
CREB protein and, (II) 4 8
DRTF1/E2F and, (II) 74 76
hsp90 and, (I) 185
motifs of, (I) 96
proteins and, (I) 62 64, 68, 212
repressors of, (I) 8 10
RHD and, (I) 95
UV radiation and, (I) 76
zinc fingers and, (I) 142
See also specific studies
DNase, footprinting: (I) 41
Dodecanedioic acid: (I) 160
Dorsal protein (DL), *drosophila*: (II) 243
259
Dorsal ventral (D/V) polarity: (II) 243
DP-1 proteins: (II) 87, 88 89
dpp. *See* Decapentaplegic receptor

DR. *See* Direct repeat sequence
Drosophila:
achaete complex and, (I) 179 180
AF-2 and, (II) 211
COUP-TF and, (II) 218
cactus protein and, (II) 251 253
dioxin and, (I) 179
dorsal protein and, (II) 243 259
E75 gene and, (I) 153
early development of, (I) 2
FTZ-F1 protein and, (II) 206
genetic analysis of, (I) 115
growth temperature of, (I) 29
HSP gene and, (I) 34, 44 45
heat shock and, (I) 26
k enhancer and, (I) 120
melanogaster, species, (I) 26, 34, 37, 60
NF-kB gene and, (I) 94, 113, 121
nuclear transport of, (II) 243 259
Per factor and, (I) 191
protein kinase and, (I) 69
RXR gene and, (II) 166, 195 196
SP1 factor and, (I) 165
sub-families of, (II) 199

SWI protein and, (II) 144
thermotolerance and, (I) 51
See also specific studies
DRTF1-E1F, molecular switch: (II) 73–92
DRTF1/E2F: (II) 76–81, 83–84, 90–92
D-type cyclins: (II) 79

E1A, viral proteins: (I) 75; (II) 80
E2F-1, analysis of: (II) 83–86, 88–89
E7 proteins: (II) 76, 80
eALAS. *See* Erhythroid 5-aminolevulinate
synthase
EAR. *See* erb-a related genes
Early response genes: (I) 67–68
Easter zymogen: (II) 253
EBNA–2 protein: (I) 111
EBV. *See* Epstein–Barr virus
EC. *See* Embryonal carcinoma
Ecdysone receptor (EcR): (II) 196
E. Coli. See Escherichia coli
EcR. *See* Ecdysone receptor
EGF. *See* Epidermal growth factor
Egon, sub-families: (II) 199
Egr, proteins: (II) 121
egr-1 gene: (II) 40
Eicosanoid: (I) 160
Eisosatetraynoic acid (ETYA): (I) 160
ELAM-1. *See* Endothelial leukocyte
adhesion molecule
ELP. *See* Embryonal long terminal repeat
binding protein
Embryogenesis: (II) 195, 243
Embryonal carcinoma (EC): (II) 74, 194,
198, 222
Embryonal long terminal repeat binding
protein (ELP): (II) 200
Embryonic cell lines, HSPs and: (I) 38
Embryonic stem (ES) cell line: (I) 216
Emotions, anatomical circuit: (II) 14
EMS. *See* Ethylmethane sulfonate
Endothelial cells, NF-kB and: (I) 93
Endothelial leukocyte adhesion molecule I
(ELAM-1): (I) 119
Environmental agents: (I) 27–30, 143, 177–
179.
See also Heavy metals; UV radiation
Enzymes, peroxisomal: (I) 143. *See also*
specific chemicals
Epidemiological studies, dioxins and: (I)
177

Epidermal growth factor (EGF):
casein kinase II and, (I) 69
kinase pathway and, (II) 114
mitogen as, (II) 100
nT3RE and, (II) 219
p91 and, (II) 115, 119
TCF domain and, (II) 48
Epidermoid lung cancer cells: (II) 225
Epithelial cells: (II) 226
Epstein–Barr virus (EBV): (I) 111
erg-2 gene: (II) 40, 44
ER/PR synergism: (II) 143
Erucic acid: (I) 160
Erythroid 5–aminolevulinate synthase
(eALAS): (I) 243, 250
Erythroleukemia cells: (I) 37
Erythroleukemia virus, avian: (II) 226
Erythropoietin: (I) 118; (II) 117
ES. *See* Embryonic stem (ES) cell line
Escherichia coli (E. Coli): (I) 1–8, 241; (II)
133
Estrogen receptors (ER):
AP-1 and, (I) 74
cloning of, (II) 157
ERE and, (II) 205
HREs and, (II) 162
PPAR and, (I) 165
TRs and, (II) 165–167
zinc finger, (II), 133
Estrogen response element (ERE): (I) 158;
(II) 141, 205
ETYA. *See* Eisosatetraynoic acid
Ethylmethane sulfonate (EMS): (I) 227
Ets, oncoprotein family: (II) 46–47, 121
Eukaryotic studies: (I) 1–8, 37, 224, 226,
241.
See also Mammalian cells; *specific studies*
Evolution, nuclear receptor family: (II)
199–201
Exonuclease III, footprinting: (I) 34
Expression vector, dl as: (II) 250
Eye development, photoreceptor cell: (II)
219

F9, embryonal carcinoma cells: (I)I, 197–
198
FABP. *See* Fatty acid binding protein
FAP binding site: (II) 42
Fatty acid binding protein (FABP): (I) 161,
166–167

Fatty acids: (I) 144, 155, 160, 165
Fc receptor for IgG (FcgRI): (II) 109
Fedault pathway: (II) 216
Ferritin, regulation of: (I) 249
Ferritin repressor protein (FRP): (I) 244
Fibric acid derivatives: (I) 144
Fibroblasts:
    chicken embryo, (I) 102
    Jun protein and, (I) 80
    rat embryo and, (I) 70
    RelB and, (I) 101
    See also Mammalian cells
Fish oil: (I) 144
FK506 protein: (I) 110
Follicle-stimulating hormone (FSH): (II)
    16, 18, 21–22
Footprinting studies:
    analysis of, (I) 68, 74–75
    AP-1 and, (I) 74
    DNA-binding proteins and, (I) 212
    exonuclease III and, (I) 34
    genomic, (I) 40; (II) 41–42, 49
    HSF1 and, (I) 39–44
    in vivo experiments, (I) 184
    See also specific studies
Forskolin: (II) 27
Fos-Jun proteins: (I) 62–63; (II) 121
Fractionation experiments: (I) 190
FSH. See Follicle-stimulating hormone
Ftz-F1, orphan receptors: (I) 159: (II) 206
Functional analysis, receptor superfamily:
    (II) 200
Fushi tarazu protein: (II) 199

Gal repressor system: (I) 4–6, 14–15
GAF. See Interferon–gamma activated
    factor
GAGA factor: (I) 44–45
GAL4, binding domains: (I) 47–48, 215;
    (II) 45, 47–48
GAL4-SRF fusion proteins: (II) 44
GAPs. See GTPase activating proteins
GAS. See Interferon-gamma activated
    sequence
GAS/p91 complex: (II) 118
Gamma-interferon: (I) 249; (II) 108–109,
    112, 118
Gamma-radiation, NF–kB and: (I) 107–109
Gamma-responsive region (GRR): (II) 109
Gastrulation defective (gd) mutant: (II) 244

GBP. See Guanylate binding protein
GCN4, yeast transactivator: (I) 80
G-coupled serpentine receptors: (II) 53
gd. See Gastrulation defective mutant
GEF. See Guanine nucleotide exchange
    factor
Gel mobility shift experiments: (I) 34, 37,
    48, 187
Gel retardation assay: (II) 101, 109, 115
Gene expression:
    CREM and, (II) 1–32
    growth factor and, (II) 60
    heat shock proteins and, (I) 25–52
    iron and, (I) 241–259
    Jun proteins and, (I) 62–84
    MHC and, (I) 104, 119; (II) 163–164
    MyoD family, (I) 74, 197
    NF-kB and, (I) 93–122
    pp42 marker, (I) 71
    PPAR and, (I) 142–169
    prokaryotic vs. eukaryotic, (I) 1–8
    See also Signaling pathway; Transcrip-
        tion response; specific studies
Generalized resistance to thyroid hormone
    (GRTH), (II) 174–175
General transcription factors: (II) 73
Genetic epistasis studies: (II) 244
Genisteine, protein kinase inhibitors: (II)
    108
Genomic footprinting: (I) 40; (II) 41–42, 49
Germ cells: (II) 16–18, 21
Glial cells, T98G: (I) 31
Glucocorticoid receptor (GR): (II) 131–148
    AP-1 and, (II) 171
    apoptosis and, (II) 147–148
    cloning of, (II) 157
    collagenase gene and, (II) 221
    eukaryotic binding, (I) 17
    gene for, (I) 153
    HIV and, (II) 143
    hsp90 and, (I) 193; (II) 202–203
    phosphorylation of, (II) 135–137
Glucocorticoid response element (GRE):
    (II) 131, 140, 143
Glutamic acid: (II) 210
Glutamine: (II) 8–9
Glutamylcysteinyl-glycine: (I) 224
Glutathione transferase: (I) 79, 198
Glycerol gradient sedimentation analysis:
    (II) 103

Glycogen synthase kinase 3 (GSK-3): (I) 69
Glycoprotein 1b (GP1b): (II) 246
GM-CSF. *See* Granulocyte macrophage colony-stimulating factor
GP1b. *See* Glycoprotein 1b
G proteins: (II) 2, 58–59
GPT. *See* Guanine–phosphoribosyl transferase
GR. *See* Glucocorticoid receptor
Granulocyte macrophage colony-stimulating factor (GM-CSF): (II) 116
GRE. *See* Glucocorticoid response elements
Growth factors: (II) 60, 220. *See also* Nerve growth factor; *specific types*
Growth hormone: (II) 117, 132
Growth modulatory genes: (I) 178
Growth regulated gene, HSP70: (I) 32
GRP78/Bip gene: (I) 30, 52
GRR. *See* Gamma-responsive region
GRTH. *See* Generalized resistance to thyroid hormone
GSK–3. *See* Glycogen synthase kinase 3
GTPase activating proteins (GAPs): (II) 53
Guanine nucleotide exchange factor (GEF): (II) 53
Guanine-phosphoribosyl transferase (GPT): (II) 111
Guanylate binding protein (GBP): (II) 108–109

H2O2 *See* Hydrogen Peroxide
Hair follicles, dioxins: (I) 177
Hamster, CREM expression: (II) 21
Ha-ras oncogenes: (I) 81
HBD. *See* Hormone binding domain
hbrm protein: (II) 144
HBV. *See* Hepatitis B virus
Hbx protein: (I) 111
hCS. *See* Human chorionic somato-mammotropin gene
Heart, PPAR and: (I) 154
Heat shock element (HSE): (I) 33–35
Heat shock factor (HSF): (I) 25–52, 35–39, 48–50
Heat shock protein70 (HSP70): (I) 26, 28, 40, 49
Heat shock protein 90 (hsp90): (I) 184–186, 190, 193–196; (II) 138–139, 202
Heat shock proteins (HSPs): (I) 25–52; (II) 131, 137. *See also specific subtypes*

Heat shock response: (I) 27–33, 233. *See also specific factors*
Heat treatment, SREs and: (II) 39
Heavy metals, metallothionein genes: (I) 206–233
HeLa cells: (I) 28, 30
Helix-loop-helix (HLH) receptor: (I) 177–199. *See also* Basic-helix-loop-helix (bHLH) factor
Helix-turn helix protein: (I) 222
Hematopoietic cells: (I) 101
Heme synthesis: (I) 242, 250
Hemin treatment: (I) 37
Hemoproteins: (I) 242
Hepatic peroxisomes: (I) 144
Hepatitis B virus (HBV): (I) 111
Hepatocarcinogenesis: (I) 144, 147, 167
Hepatocyte nuclear factor4 (HNF–4): (II) 199
Hepatoma cell line: (I) 197, 189, 252; (II) 145. *See also* Liver
Herbicides: (I) 143–144, 177
Herbimycin A: (I) 107
Herpes simplex virus (HSV): (I) 111, 121; (II) 164
Heterodimeric transcription factors: (II) 83–84, 89, 90
Heterodimers, nuclear receptors: (II) 203–204
Hexadecanedioic acid: (I) 160
Hexanucleotide polymerase: (I) 223
Hippocampus: (II) 14
Histone-like protein (HU): (I) 10
HIV. *See* Human immunodeficiency virus
HL60 cells: (I) 116
HLH receptor. *See* Helix-loop helix receptor
HMG-CoA synthase gene: (I) 163
HNF-4. *See* Hepatocyte nuclear factor 4
Homeobox (Hox) containing genes: (II) 197
Homodimers: (I) 103–106; (II) 168–170, 203–204
Homologous down regulation: (II) 131
Homologous recombination: (I) 83
Hormonal cross talk: (II) 167–168. *See also specific studies*
Hormone binding domain (HBD): (II) 131, 134, 138, 139
Hormone receptors. *See also specific types*

Hormone responsive unit (HRU): (II) 141
Hox. *See* Homeobox containing genes
HRU. *See* Hormone responsive unit
HSE. *See* Heat shock element
HSF. *See* Heat shock factor
HSPs. *See* Heat Shock proteins
HSV. *See* Herpes simplex virus
HTH repressors, alpha helix and: (I) 7–8
HTLV-I. *See* Human T-cell leukemia
    virus: (I)
HU. *See* Histone-like protein: (I) 10
Human chorionic somatomammotropin
    (hCS) gene: (II) 164
Human collagenase, promoter: (I) 63
Human epidermoid, lung cancer cells: (II)
    225
Human immunodeficiency virus (HIV): (I)
    93; (II) 147, 164
Human leukemia cell lines: (I) 154; (II) 223
Human MAD-3, proteins: (I) 99
Human metallothionein: (I) 211
Human Na,K-ATPase beta1-subunit gene:
    (II) 164
Human papilloma virus (HPV): (I) 74; (II)
    76
Human platelet, glycoprotein 1b: (II) 246–
    248
Human promyelocytic leukemia: (II) 223
Human T-cell leukemia virus (HTLV-I): (I)
    111–112; (II) 44
Human tissues, arnt and: (I) 197. *See also*
    Mammalian cells; *specific types*
Hybridization, in situ: (I) 27; (II) 13, 28
Hydrogen peroxide: (I) 109; (II) 158
Hypoglossal motor nucleus: (II) 15
Hypolipidemic drugs: (I) 143–144, 168
Hypothalamic-pituitary axis: (II) 17
Hypothalamus: (II) 14

ICER factor:
    bZip factor and, (II) 26–27
    cAMP and, (II) 23
    CREM and, (II) 31
    pineal gland and, (II) 27–31
    transcripts of, (II) 24
ICSBP. *See* Interferon consensus sequence
    binding protein
Idiopathic pulmonary fibrosis: (II) 226
IEGs. *See* Immediate early genes
IFN-beta gene, cytokine: (I) 117

IkB proteins: (I) 95, 98 100, 113 116; (II)
    251
IL-1. *See* Interleukin 1
IL-2. *See* Interleukin 2
IL-6. *See* Interleukin 6
Immediate early genes (IEGs): (I) 67–78;
    (II) 39–40. *See also* c-fos gene
Immune system: (II) 173. *See also specific*
    components
Immuno-chemical experiments: (I) 179
Immunocytochemical analyses: (I) 155
Immunofluorescence studies: (II) 246
Immunoglobulins: (I) 100, 113
Immunoprecipitation experiments: (I) 187
Immunoreceptors, induction of: (I) 118–
    120
Immunosuppression, dioxins: (I) 177
Indolo[3,2-b]carbazole: (I) 196
Inflammatory mediaters: (I) 106–107; (II)
    220
Injury, defensive response: (I) 93
Inositol triphosphate (IP3): (II) 56
Insecticides, pollution and: (I) 177
Insects: (I) 93, 121
In situ hybridization: (I) 27; (II) 13, 28
Interferon alpha/beta stimulated genes
    (ISGs): (II) 100–104, 112
Interferon-beta: (I) 111
Interferon consensus sequence binding
    protein (ICSBP): (II) 118
Interferon-gamma: (I) 249; (II) 108–109,
    112
Interferon-gamma activated factor (GAF):
    (II) 108–109, 122
Interferon-gamma activated sequence
    (GAS): (II) 108–109, 116, 118
Interferon Regulatory Factor (IRF): (II)
    105, 117–118
Interferons: (II) 100–101, 111. *See also*
    specific types
Interferon stimulated response element
    (ISRE): (II) 100–104
Interleukins: (I) 76, 210. *See also specific*
    subtypes
Interleukin-1 (IL-1): (I) 106, 178, 252; (II)
    248–249, 253
Interleukin-2 (IL-2): (I) 104, 107, 253
Interleukine-6 (IL-6): (II) 116, 118
Intracellular signaling. *See* Signaling
    pathway; *specific studies*

Inverted palindrome (IP): (I) 74; (II) 163
Iodide ions: (II) 158
Iodoacetamide: (I) 248
Ionizing radiation: (I) 76
IP3. *See* Inositol triphosphate
IP. *See* Inverted palindrome
IPTG, induction: (I) 16
IRE-flanking sequences: (I) 251
I-Rel gene: (I) 97
IRF. *See* Interferon regulatory factor
IRP. *See* Iron regulatory protein
Iron, gene regulation: (I) 241–259
Iron regulatory protein (IRP): (I) 243–245,
    245–249, 252
Iron-responsive elements (IREs): (I) 243
ISGF3: (II) 100–104, 119, 122
ISGs. *See* Interferon alpha/beta stimulated
    genes
ISRE. *See* Interferon stimulated reponse
    element
Isoforms: (II) 173, 193
Isoproterenol (Iso): (II) 29–30
J774, macrophage cell line: (I) 249
Jacob Monod repression theory: (I) 7, 14
Jak family, kinases: (II) 113, 122
JNKs. *See* June N-terminal kinases
June N-terminal kinases (JNKs): (I) 72, 78
Jun proteins gene: (I) 7, 54 67, 70 72, 80;
    (II) 40
Jurkat T cells: (I) 109, 116

K562, erythroleukemia cells: (I) 37, 45
kB elements: (I) 105, 120
Keratin gene family: (II) 220
Keratinocytes, human: (I) 192
KID. *See* Kinase inducible domain
Kidney: (I) 154, 196, 207
Kinase inducible domain (KID): (II) 6
Kinase/receptor complex: (II)108
Kinases: (I) 68 70; (II) 99. *See also specific*
    enzymes
Kluyveromyces lactis: (I) 47
Knirps, sub families: (II) 199
Kozak ATG codon: (II) 24
Kruppel family, transcription factor: (II) 225

Labeling studies, dioxin: (I) 179
Lac operon system: (I) 1 10, 12 16; (II) 177
Lambda repressor system: (I) 1–2, 7–8, 12,
    14 16

LBD. *See* Ligand binding domain
Leucine zipper group: (I) 46, 48, 66;
    (II) 4–8. *See also* Basic leucine zipper
    (bZIP)
Leucine-zipper-like motif: (I) 97; (II) 85
Leukemia cell lines: (I) 37, 45, 100, 154;
    (II) 223
Leukemia inhibitory factor (LIF): (I) 107;
    (II) 116
Leukogenesis: (II) 224
Leukotrienes: (I) 144, 161
LexA, binding domains: (I) 2: (II) 48
Leydig cells: (II) 16–17
LH. *See* Lutenizing hormone
LIF. *See* Leukemia inhibitory factor
Ligand binding: (I) 151, 158, 178; (II) 114–
    117
Ligand-binding domain (LBD): (II) 160,
    206
Ligand-independent regulators: (I) 142–143
Linker scanning mutation analyses: (I) 211
Lipid metabolism: (I) 143
Lipopolysaccharides (LPS): (I) 110, 249
Liver: (I) 143, 153–154, 177; (II) 196, 217.
    See also Hepatoma cell lines
Liver regenerating factor (LRF): (II) 26
LMP protein: (I) 111
Long terminal repeat (LTR) sequence: (II)
    141, 147
LRF. *See* Liver regenerating factor
LTR. *See* Long terminal repeat
Lung cells: (I) 154: (II) 225
Lutenizing hormone (LH): (II) 16, 18, 21
Lymphocytes: (I) 101. *See also* T cells
Lymphoproliferate disorders: (I) 105, 151.
    See also Leukemias
MAD-3 protein: (I) 99
MADS-box: (II) 58
Magnesium (Mg2): (I) 222
MAP. *See* Mitogen activated protein
MAP kinase kinases (MAPKK): (I) 71; (II)
    51–53
MAP kinases (MAPKs): (II) 48–50, 52, 58,
    121
MAPKK. *See* MAP kinase kinases
MAPKs. *See* Mitogen-activated protein
    kinases
Macrophage cell line: (I) 249
Macrophage-induced gene (MIB): (II) 109
Malic enzyme (ME): (II) 163

Mammalian cells:
  HSP and, (I) 34
  IL-1 receptor, (I) 115
  lung cancer cells, (II) 225
  MAPK and, (II) 49–50, 52
  Ras protein and, (II) 53–55
  retinoids and, (II) 188–190
  See also Eukaryotes; *specific cells*
Mammillary body: (II) 14
Maternal genes: (II) 243, 259
MCM1, yeast proteins, (II) 44
McR. *See* Mineralocorticoid receptor
ME. *See* Malic enzyme
MEKK genes: (II) 49, 58–59
MEK proteins: (II) 52
MEL. *See* Mouse erytholeukemia cells
Melanin, tyrosinase and: (I) 230
Melatonin: (II) 27
Memory, anatomical circuit: (II) 14
Mercuric ion reductase: (I) 222
Mercury, operon of: (I) 222–224
Messenger RNAs: (I) 153–154
Metal responsive elements (MREs): (I) 211,
  214
Metallothioneins (MT):
  AP-1 and, (I) 78–79, 82
  heat shock and, (I) 30
  human cells, (I) 211
  physiological functions, (I) 229–232
  promoter, (I) 63
  safeguard system, (I) 241
  transcriptional regulation, (I) 206–233
Metals. *See* Heavy metals
Metastatic cells: (I) 104. *See also*
  Carcinomas
Met repressor: (I) 8
MHC. *See* Myosin heavy chain genes
MIB. *See* Macrophage-induced gene
Milk heat, shock and: (I) 26
Mineralocorticoid receptor (McR): (II)
  161, 205
Mitochondria, aconitase and: (I) 246–247
Mitochondrial electron transport: (I) 107
Mitogen activated protein (MAP): (I) 71,
  106
Mitogens:
  inducible genes and, (II) 39
  kinases and, (I) 71
  NF-kB and, (I) 93
  SREs and, (II) 39

Mitogen-activated protein kinases
  (MAPKs): (II) 40
Mitomycin C: (I) 76
MLV. *See* Moloney leukemia virus
MMTV. *See* Mouse mammary tumor virus
Molecular chaperone, hsp90: (I) 25, 184–
  186
Molecular switch, DRTF1-E1F: (II) 72–92
Moloney leukemia virus (MLV): (II) 164
Monocytoid cells, HIV and: (II) 147
Monomers, nuclear receptors: (II) 203–204
Morphalan: (I) 79
Mos gene: (II) 49
Mouse cells:
  E. coli and, (I) 2
  homologous recombination of, (I) 83
  lymphomas and, (II) 137
  metallothionein and, (I) 212–214
  MGR and, (II) 132
  pituitary and, (II) 9
  PPARs and, (I) 154
  transcription of, (I) 2–6
  transgenic, (I) 81–82; (II) 15
  tumor formation and, (I) 74
  See also specific studies
Mouse erythroleukemia (MEL) cells: (II)
  145
Mouse mammary tumor virus (MMTV):
  (II) 141
MREs. *See* Metal responsive elements
mRNA, tranferrin and: (I) 253–256
MT. *See* Metallothionein
MT11a, UV-induced factor: (I) 76
MTF-1, binding studies: (I) 220
MTFZ-1, zinc finger protein: (I) 214–215
Mucous metaplasia, (II) 226
Multiple transactivation functions: (II)
  210–211
Mutant cell lines: (I) 216; (II) 111. *See also*
  Drosophila; *specific types*
Mutation analysis: (I) 44, 64–66, 211
Myb, transcription factor: (I) 73
Myc-Max, transcription factors: (I) 7
Myc oncoproteins: (I) 179
Mycobacteria tuberculosis: (I) 110
Myeloblastic leukemias: (II) 223
Myeloid gene: (II) 223–226
Myelomas: (I) 105
MyoD gene family: (I) 74, 197
Myogenesis: (I) 74, 180, 187

Myogenin: (I) 192
Myosin heavy chain (MHC) genes: (I) 104,
    119; (II) 163–164

N-acetyl-L-cysteine (NAC): (I) 73, 78, 109
N-acetyl transferase: (II) 30
NAC. See N-acetyl-L-cycteine
Nafenopin-binding protein: (I) 147
Nak1, nuclear receptor: (II) 210
NBRE. See Nerve growth factor I-B
    repsonsive element
Negative GRE (nGRE): (II) 133, 219
Negative RARE (nRARE): (II) 219–220
Negative thyroid response elements
    (nT3RE): (II) 219
NEM. See N-ethyl maleimide
Nerve growth factor I-B responsive element
    (NBRE): (II) 207
Nerve growth factor (NGF): (I) 159: (II)
    114, 199
Nervonic acid: (I) 160
N-ethyl maleimide (NEM): (II) 102
Neuroendocrine systems: (I)CER and:
    (II)23
Neurospora crassa: (I) 207, 230
Newcastle disease virus: (I) 111
NFGI-B protein: (II) 207
NF-IL6 proteins: (II) 49
NF-kB proteins:
    activation of, (I) 110–111
    binding sites of, (II) 250
    dimers of, (I) 100–101
    dl protein and, (II) 255
    DNA binding, (I) 78
    genes induced, (I) 120
    IKB subunit and, (II) 252
    IL-1 and, (II) 249
    rapid cellular response and, (I) 93–122
    Ref-1 and, (I) 73
    signalling pathways of, (I) 106–107
    transcription factor, (I) 73, 78, 93–122
NGF. See Nerve growth factor
nGRE. See Negative GRE
NIH 3T3 cells: (II) 146
Nitric oxide (NO): (I) 120, 248–249, 259
Nitroquinolineoxide: (I) 76
NLS. See Nulcear localization sequence
N-methyl-N-nitrosourea: (I) 79
NO. See Nitric oxide
Nonreceptor tyrosine kinases: (II) 113

Nonsteroid receptors: (II) 206. See also
    specific types
Nonstressful inducers, HSP and: (I) 32
Non-zinc finger residues: (II) 206
NQO. See Quinone oxidoreductase gene
nRARE. See Negative RARE
nT3RE. See Negative thyroid response
    elements
Ntera-2, carcinoma cells: (I) 113
Nuclear localization sequence (NLS): (I) 99;
    (II) 110, 139–140, 155, 202–203, 249
Nuclear receptors:
    activation function of, (II) 212
    agonist/antagonist action, (II) 212–215
    AP-1 signaling and, (II) 220
    crosstalk and, (II) 217–220
    Dif and, (I) 121
    dioxin and, (I) 177–199
    evolution of, (II) 199–201
    Nak I, (II) 210
    Nur77, (II) 210
    PPAR and, (I) 142–169
    proto-oncoprotein family, (I) 64–67
    RA and, (II) 192
    RNA polymerase and, (I) 66
    thyroid hormone and, (II) 157–177
    See also specific types
Nuclear response, CREM and: (II) 1–32
Nuclear translocation: (I) 66; (II) 139–140
Nuclear transport, drosophila: (II) 243–259
Nucleosome: (I) 5
Nudel (ndl) subtype: (II) 244
Nur77, nuclear receptor: (II) 210
Nutrients, PPAR and: (I) 142–169

Occulomotor, motor nucleus: (II) 15
Okadaic acid: (I) 109: (II) 80
Oleic acid: (I) 161
Oncogenes:
    co-expression of, (I) 81
    c-rel type, (II) 250
    Fos-Jun type, (I) 62–63
    Ha-ras type, (I) 81
    Src type, (I) 81
    tumor cells, (II) 76
    v-erbA type, (II) 157, 170–171, 226
    v-rel type, (II) 102, 250
    See also specific types
Oncoproteins: (I) 179, (II) 46–47, 82, 121,
    160. See also specific types

Oncostatin M (OSM): (II) 116
Ontogenesis, nervous system: (II) 195
Oogenesis, *drosophila*: (II) 244
Operators: (I) 14–16. *See also specific types*
Operons: (I) 1–12, 222–224; (II) 177. *See also specific genes*
Orphan receptors: (I) 142–143, 158–159; (II) 162, 168, 199–200. *See also specific types*
OSM. *See* Oncostatin M
Osteocalcin genes: (I) 74
Ovaries, PPARs and: (I) 153–154; (II) 244
Oxidation reactions: (I) 144, 259
Oxidative stress: (I) 93, 167

pp42 marker gene: (I) 71
p48 proteins and: (II) 103, 105, 111
p50 homodimers: (I) 103–106
p50/RelA gene: (I) 101–103
P52, homodimers: (I) 103–106
p52/54 factor: (I) 70–71
p65, subunit NFkB and: (I) 66, 75
p91 proteins: (II) 111, 112, 115, 119
p91/84, subunits: (II) 104–105
p100 proteins: (I) 115
p105 proteins: (I) 99
p107 proteins, (II) 90
p113 proteins: (II) 104–105, 111
p130 proteins: (II) 82, 90
P450IVA1 activity: (I) 161
PAGE. *See* Polyacrylamide gel electrophoresis
Palindromes, inverted: (I) 157; (II) 2–3, 168
Pancreatic islet cell: (II) 6
Papillomas, AP-1 activity and: (I) 82
Parasites, defensive response: (I) 93
Parietal endoderm (PE) cells: (II) 74
Pathogen response: (I) 93–122
PC-PLC. *See* Phosphatidylcholine-specific phospholipase
PCR. *See* Polymerase chain reaction
PDGF. *See* Platelet-derived growth factor
PDTC. *See* Pyrolidinedithiocarbamate
PE. *See* Parietal endoderm cells
Pelle (pll) gene: (II) 244
Peptide maps: (I) 68
Perivitelline space: (II) 244–245
Permease, *E. coli* and: (I) 1
Peroxidase: (II) 158

Peroxisome proliferator receptors (PPARs):
    activation of, (I) 158–162
    fatty acid metabolism, (I) 162–164
    gene interactions and, (I) 142–169
    messenger RNAs and, (I) 153–154
    structure of, (I) 151
    types of, (I) 148–151
Pertussis toxin (PTX): (II) 58
Phorbol esters: (I) 62–84; (II) 220
Phosphatases: (I) 68–72
Phosphatidylcholine-specific phospholipase (PC-PLC): (II) 51
Phosphatidylinositol: (II) 146
Phosphatidylinositol (4,5)-diphosphates (PIP2): (II) 56
Phosphoamino acid analysis: (I) 68
Phospholipase: (I) 106
Phosphopeptide analysis: (I) 69
Phosphorylation: (I) 68; (II) 5–8, 45–46, 251
Phosphotyrosine residues: (II) 105
Photoreceptor cell: (II) 219, 246
Phox1, protein: (II) 44, 49
Phthalate esters: (I) 144
Phylogenetic tree, PPARs: (I) 149
Phytochelatins: (I) 224
Pineal gland: (II) 15, 23, 27–31
pip. *See* Pipe protein
PIP2. *See* Phosphatidylinositol (4,5)-diphosphates
Pipe (pip) protein: (II) 244
Pituitary gland: (II) 9, 30–31
Pituitary-specific transcription factor: (II) 3
PKA. *See* Protein kinase A
PKC. *See* Protein kinase C
PLZF. *See* Promyelocytic leukemia zinc finger
Plants, peroxisomes: (I) 146
Plasma membrane: (I) 77–78; (II) 246. *See also specific receptors*
Plasmids: (I) 222; (II) 11
Plasminogen activator: (I) 120
Plasminogen activator inhibitor-2: (I) 178
Plasticizers: (I) 143. *See also specific types*
Platelet-derived growth factor (PDGF): (II) 100, 114–115, 119
Platelets, glycoprotein 1b: (II) 246–248
Pleckstrin homology: (II) 53
Pleiotropic functions, thyroid hormones: (II) 157–177

pll. *See* Pelle gene
PMA: (I) 62, 68
  c-jun promoter and, (I) 68
  collagenase and, (I) 74
  tumor promoter and, (I) 62–63, 74
Polyacrylamide gel electrophoresis
  (PAGE): (I) 214
Polymerase chain reaction (PCR): (I) 216;
  (II) 24
POMC. *See* Pro-opiomelanocortin gene
Pontine motor nucleus: (II) 15
Portal vein: (I) 143
Positive control (PC), mutant Lambda: (I)
  14–15
Posttranslational modifications, Jun: (I)
  68–70
Post-transcriptional regulation, iron and:
  (I) 241–259
PPARs. *See* Peroxisome proliferators
  receptors
PP–1. *See* Protein phosphatase-1
Prazosin: (I) 31
pRb. *See* Retinoblastoma tumor
  suppressor gene product
Prm promoter: (I) 15
Progesterone: (I) 153; (II) 136, 161
Prokaryotic control, of transcriptions and:
  (I) 1–8
Prolactin: (II) 21, 118
Proliferative diseases: (II) 226. *See also*
  specific types
Promyelocytic cell line: (II) 213, 223–224
Promyelocytic leukemia zinc finger
  (PLZF): (II) 225
Prostaglandins (PGA2): (I) 51
Protein kinase A (PKA):
  CREB and, (II) 2–8
  glucocorticoid receptor, (II) 137
  ICER and, (II) 31
  Ser103 and, (II) 45
  testis and, (II) 18–21
Protein kinase C (PKC):
  activation of, (I) 77
  Ca_2 and, (II) 56
  CREM and, (II) 7
  down regulation of, (I) 192
  glucocorticoid receptor and, (II) 137
  G proteins and, (II) 58–59
  IFN and, (II) 104
  inhibitors of, (I) 107

  isoforms of, (II) 55–56
  NF-kB and, (I) 110
  phosphorylation and, (II) 148
  signaling pathway of, (II) 249
  TPA and, (II) 70
Protein phosphatase I (PPI): (II) 80
Proteolysis: (I) 114
Pro-opiomelanocortin gene: (II) 219
Proto-oncogene, c-fos: (I) 167; (II) 3, 40–44.
  See also specific genes
Psuedogenes, metallothionein: (I) 208
PTX. *See* Pertussis toxin
Pulmonary fibrosis: (II) 226
Purines: (II) 74
Puromycin: (I) 256
Pyrolidinedithiocarbamate (PDTC): (I) 109

Quail, fibroblast cell line: (II) 48
Quercetin: (I) 51
Quinone oxidoreductase (NQO) gene: (I) 79

RAB-9 cells, rabbit: (I) 246
RACE-PCR cloning strategy: (II) 24
Radiation: (I) 62, 76, 93
RAF. *See* Receptor accessory factor
Raf genes: (I) 71, 81, 106: (II) 49
Raf-1 kinase: (I) 77
raf/mos family: (II) 251
Rana esculenta: (I) 147
RAREs. *See* RA responsive elements
RA responsive elements (RAREs): (II) 192
RARs. *See* Retinoic acid receptors
RAR-RXR heterodimers: (II) 166
Ras protein, mammalian: (II) 53–55
Ras-Raf pathway: (II) 115
Rat growth hormone gene (rGH): (II) 132,
  163
Rat studies: (I) 70, 80, 163
RBP. *See* Retinol-binding protein
Rb-related cells: (II) 80, 82
RD4, human cells: (I) 245
Receptor accessory factor (RAF): (II) 143
Receptor models: (I) 142–169, 177–199. *See
  also specific types*
Receptor tyrosine kinase (RTK): (II) 60
Recombinant MTF-1: (I) 215–216
Red nucleus, motor nucleus: (II) 15
Redox state, iron and: (I) 259
Rel homology domain (RHD): (I) 102, 121;
  (II) 249

Rel proteins: (I) 95–96, 115, 117
Rel/NF-kB family, polypeptides: (I) 94–98;
    (II) 249
Renal peroxisomes: (I) 144
Repressor genes:
    cyt repressor, (I) 5, 13
    DNA binding sites and, (I) 8–10
    Gal repressor system, (I) 4–6, 14–15
    Lac and, (I) 13
    Lambda and, (I) 1–2, 7–8, 12–16
    met repressor, (I) 8
    molecular mechanisms of, (I) 12–18
    Tet system, (I) 16
    TR isoforms and, (II) 173–174
    Trp type, (I) 8
    YY1 and, (I) 75
    See also specific types
Retinoblastoma cells, Y79: (I) 31
Retinoblastoma tumor suppressor gene
    product (pRb): (II) 76, 79, 90
Retinoic acid, (RA):
    9-Cis type, (II) 167
    DR and, (II) 164
    HREs and, (II) 162
    ligands of, (I) 158–159
    PPAR and, (I) 153
    X receptors and, (I) 165
    See also Cellular retinoic acid binding
        proteins
Retinoic acid receptors (RARs): (II) 187–
    228
    dimerization and, (I) 157
    PPARs and, (I) 142, 149–151, 166
    TRs and, (II) 158, 160
Retinoid X receptors (RXRs):
    complex of, (I) 158
    C-terminal finger region and, (II) 208
    dimerization of, (II) 208–210
    drosophila and, (II) 166, 195–196
    hormonal cross talk and, (II) 167–168
    HREs and, (II) 162
    RAREs and, (II) 192–193
    RARs and, (II) 187
    receptor binding and, (II) 217
    retinoic acid and, (I) 165
    TRs and, (II) 168
Retinol: (II) 187
Retinol-binding protein (RBP): (II) 187
Retrovirus: (I) 80–81, 102. *See also specific*
    types

Rev-ErbAalpha gene: (I) 153
rGH. *See* Rat growth hormone gene
RHD. *See* Rel homology domain
Rheumatoid arthritis: (II) 226
Rhomboid (rho) factor: (II) 255
Ribosomal S6 kinase (RSK): (II) 52
RNA polymerase:
    cell cycle and, (II) 73
    lac repressor and, (I) 13
    promoter of, (I) 4–5
    sigma subunit, (I) 15
RNA polymerase II: (I) 44, 52, 70, 74, 232–
    233
RNA polymerase transcription factor
    (TFIIIA): (I) 231
RNA synthesis, thyroid hormone
    receptors: (II) 157
ROIs: (I) 109, 113
Rodents, arnt and: (I) 197. *See also* Mouse
    cells; Rat studies
Rous sarcoma virus: (II) 164, 169
RSK. *See* Ribosomal S6 kinase
RTK. *See* Receptor tyrosine kinase
RU 486, glucocorticoid: (II) 147
RXRs. *See* Retinoid X receptors

Saccharomyces cerevisiae: (I) 26, 34–35, 37,
    44, 45, 47, 224, 226, 227, 229, 232, 241
Salicylates: (I) 46–47, 51
Salmonella, bacteriophage P22: (I) 8
SAP–1b protein: (II) 48
Schizosaccharomyces pombe: (I) 35
Schneider cells:
    cactus gene, (II) 252
    cotransfected cells, (II) 248–249
    dl and, (II) 257
    drosophila, (II) 246
SCN. *See* Suprachiasmatic nucleus
SDS-PAGE analysis: (I) 46, 48; (II) 102,
    109, 132, 251
SEA. *See* Staphylococcus entertoxins A
SEB. *See* Staphylococcus entertoxins B
Second messenger systems, Toll: (II) 249–
    251. *See also specific chemicals*
Seminiferous epithelium: (II) 19–22
Sendai virus: (I) 111
Septic shock: (I) 117
Sequence-specific transcription factors:
    (II) 73
Serine proteases, dl proteins and: (II) 245

Serine/threonine kinases: (II) 99–100
Sertoli cells: (II) 16
Serum response element (SRE): (II) 39–61
Sf-1. *See* Steroidogenic factor
SH2 domain: (II) 99–123
Shaggy, *drosophila* protein kinase: (I) 69
Shigella flexneri: (I) 110
SIE-binding complex: (II) 40, 114, 121
SIF, transcription factor: (II) 114–115, 119
SIV. *See* Simian immunodeficiency virus
Signaling pathways:
   cAMP and, (II) 1–32
   CREM and, (II) 1–32
   c-fos gene and, (II) 39–61
   cross-talk and, (II) 220–222
   dioxin and, (I) 177–199
   dl protein and, (II) 243–259
   DRTF1/ETF and, (II) 73–92
   growth factors and, (I) 77
   hormones and, (I) 142
   hypothesis for, (II) 119
   metals and, (I) 206–233
   protein kinase C and, (II) 249
   thyroid hormone receptors and, (II) 157–177
   tyrosine and, (II) 99–123
   See also Gene expression; Transcription response; *specific receptors*
Simian immunodeficiency virus (SIV): (I) 121
Skin, retinoids: (II) 226
Small intestine, receptor binding: (II) 217
Snail (sna), *drosophila* gene: (II) 255
Sodium fluoride: (II) 102
Somatomammotrophs: (II) 16
Somatostatin gene: (II) 6
SOS response: (I) 62
Southern blot analyses: (I) 216
Southwestern blot analyses: (I) 214
SP1 factor, *drosophila*: (I) 165
Spatzle (spz) protein: (II) 244, 253
Spermatogenesis: (II) 16–18
Spleen cells: (I) 101, 102, 154, 196
Squamous metaplasia: (II) 226
src, oncogenes: (I) 81
SRE. *See* Serum response element
STAT-3, protein family: (II) 116
Staphylococcus entertoxins A (SEA): (I) 110

Staphylococcus entertoxins B (SEB): (I) 110
Starvation, peroxisomes and: (I) 146
Staurosporine: (II) 104, 108
Steroid hormone receptors:
   bZIP and, (I) 74
   glucocorticoid receptors, (II) 131–148
   Jun protein and, (I) 66
   TRs and, (II) 158, 160–161, 165–167
   See also Nuclear receptors; *specific types*
Steroid hormone: (I) 142, 196; (II) 199
Steroidogenic factor (SF-1): (II) 200
Stress response: (I) 28, 93–122
Stromelysin I genes: (I) 75, 82
Sunlight, melanin and: (I) 230
Superactivation pathway, RAR and: (II) 216
Superoxide dimutase gene: (I) 227
Suprachiasmatic nucleus (SCN): (II) 27
Supraoptic neurons: (II) 13–14
Suramin: (I) 77
SV40 virus: (II) 76, 249
SW16. yeast prtoteins: (II) 252
SWI-proteins: (II) 144
Synergism, glucocorticoid receptor: (II) 141–142
S. pombe: (I) 224

T cells:
   auto regulation of, (II) 131
   Jurkat cells, (I) 109, 116
   leukemias and, (I) 112
   NF-kB and, (I) 93
   p50 homodimers, (I) 104
   TPA treatment, (II) 146
T3 responsive elements (TREs): (II) 158
T3. *See* Triiodothyronine
T4. *See* Thyroxine
T98G, glial cells: (I) 31
TAFs. *See* TBP associated factors
Tailless mutant genes: (II) 199
Target response elements: (II) 206
TATA binding protein (TBP): (I) 98: (II) 93, 215
TATA box: (I) 16
Tax protein: (I) 111–112; (II) 44
TBP. *See* TATA binding protein
TBP-associated factors (TAFs): (II) 93, 215
TCDD. *See* Tetrachlorodibenzo-p-dioxin
TCF. *See* Ternary complex factor

Teratogenesis, RA–induced: (II) 191. *See also* Carcinogens

Ternary complex factor (TCF): (II) 40, 46–51, 59

Terpenes: (II) 200

Testis:
cAMP and, (II) 16–17
CREM and, (II) 12, 21–22
degeneration of, (II) 197
hormonal control in, (II) 16–17
PKA and, (II) 18–21

Tetrachlorodinenzo-p-dioxin (TCDD): (I) 177–199

Tetradecanoylphorbol-13-acetate (TPA): (I) 69, 192; (II) 23–48, 170

Tet repressor/operator system: (I) 16

TFIIIA. *See* RNA polymerase transcription factor

TfR. *See* Transferrin receptor

TG. *See* Thyroglobulin

TGFbeta. *See* Transforming growth factor beta

Thalamic nuclei: (II) 14

Thermotolerance, *drosophila*: (I) 51

6-Thioguanine: (II) 111

Thioredoxin: (I) 96

Thrombin receptor: (II) 246

Thymic involution, dioxins and: (I) 177

Thymidylate, synthesis of: (II) 74

Thymosin promoter: (II) 16

Thyroglobulin (TG): (II) 158

Thyroid hormone receptors (TRs): (II) 157–177
AP-1 and, (II) 170–173
homodimers and, (II) 168–170
isoforms of, (II) 173–174
mechanism of action, (II) 165–167
NSL proteins and, (II) 140
PPARs and, (I) 142, 149, 153, 157, 166
subtypes of, (II) 160–161

Thyroid stimulating hormone (TSH): (II) 165

Thyroxine (T4): (II) 157

Thyroxine binding protein: (II) 159

TIC. *See* Transcription-initiation complex

TK gene: (II) 101

TNF-alpha gene: (I) 106, 108

TO. *See* Tryptophan oxygenase gene

Toll (T1) system: (II) 244–251

Tolloid (tld), drosophila: (II) 255

Toxic metals: (I) 207. *See also* Heavy metals

Toxic shock syndrome toxin-1 (TSST-1): (I) 110

TPA. *See* Tetradecanoylphorbol-13-acetate

TRAP, general factors: (II) 166

TREs. *See* Thyroid hormone response elements

TRs. *See* Thyroid hormone receptors

Transactivating complex: (I) 99, 100, 104

Transcription–initiation complex (TIC): (II) 141

Transcription:
activation of, (II) 109–111
AP1 factor and, (I) 62–84
cell cycle and, (II) 73–92
COUP-TF and. *See* Chicken ovalbumin upstream promoter transcription factor
direct signal transduction and, (II) 99–123
dl and, (II) 255–259
DNA binding proteins and, (I) 62–64
general factors, (II) 73
heat shock proteins and, (I) 25–52
Kruppel family, (II) 225
ligand-bound receptors and, (II) 114–117
metallothionein gene and, (I) 206–233
MTF-1 and, (I) 215
Myb factor, (I) 73
Myc-Max factor, (I) 7
NF-kB and, (I) 93–122
PPARs and, (I) 155–158
prokaryotic vs. eukaryotic, (I) 1–18
repression of. *See* Repressor genes
SRF and, (II) 44–45
synergism and, (II) 142–144
UV radiation and, (I) 62, 78–80
YY1 repressor, (I) 75
See also Gene expression; Signaling pathways; *specific studies*

Transduction pathway, cAMP: (II) 2

Transfection studies: (I) 103; (II) 143

Transferrin receptor (TfR): (I) 241–242, 253

Transforming growth factor beta (TGFbeta): (II) 221

Transgenic mice: (I) 81–82; (II) 15. *See also* Mouse cells

Transition protein 1: (II) 16–17

Trichlorophenoxyacetic acid: (I) 144

Trigeminal nucleus: (II) 14
Triglycerides, fatty acids and: (I) 168
Triiodothyronine (T3): (II) 157
Trochlear, motor nucleus: (II) 15
Trp repressor gene: (I) 8
Tryptophan oxygenase (TO) gene:
     (II) 141
TSH. *See* Thyroid stimulating hormone
TSST-1. *See* Toxic shock syndrome
     toxin-1
Tube (tub) gene: (II) 244
Tumor promoters: (I) 62, 74, 81, 177;
     (II) 170
Tumor suppressor gene: (II) 76
Twist (twi), *drosophila* genes: (II) 255
Tyrosinase, melanin and: (I) 230
Tyrosine, direct signal transduction: (II)
     99–123
Tyrosine kinase receptors: (I) 79, 99, 109;
     (II) 53, 60, 113
Tyrosine phosphate: (II) 111

U1A cells: (II) 113
U2A, mutant cell line: (II) 112
U3, cell line: (II) 115
U4 cells: (II) 122
U4A, mutant cell lines: (II) 113
UAScup1. *See* Upstream activator
     sequences
Ultraspiracle (usp) locus: (II) 195–196
Untranslated regions (UTRs): (I) 243
Upstream activator sequences (UAScup1):
     (I) 226
Urokinase: (I) 82, 120
UV radiation:
     cross-linking experiments and, (I) 214,
          244; (II) 103, 109, 119
     direct signal transduction and, (II) 103,
          109, 119
     DNA and, (I) 76
     E. coli and, (I) 2
     iron and, (I) 244
     Jun proteins and, (I) 62–84
     NF-kB and, (I) 107–109
     transcriptional response of, (I) 62, 78–80

Vascular cell adhesion molecule 1
     (VCAM-1): (I) 119

VCAM-1. *See* Vascular cell adhesion
     molecule 1
VD3R. *See* Vitamin D3 receptor
Ventral repression element (VRE): (II) 255
V-erbA oncogene: (II) 157, 166–167, 171,
     226
Viruses:
     adenoviruses: (I) 67, 75–76, 111, 121;
          (II) 74, 80–81, 88
     antiviral factors: (II) 101
     defensive response of: (I) 93
     erythroleukemia virus, (II) 226
     E7 proteins and, (II) 76, 80
     hepatitis B and, (I) 111
     HSV and, (I) 93, (II) 147, 164
     HPV and, (I) 74, (II) 76
     HTLV-1 and, (I) 111–112, (II) 44
     induction of: (I) 120–121
     kB elements and: (I) 120
     NF-kB and: (I) 111
     retroviruses: (I) 80–81, (II) 102
     See also specific types
Vitamin A: (II) 187–188, 191, 197, 199, 222.
     See also Retinoic acid receptors
Vitamin D3, HREs and: (II) 162–164
Vitamin D3 receptor (VD3R): (II) 196
Vitellogenin II gene, chicken: (II) 141
v-jun gene: (I) 82
von Willebrand factor: (II) 246
VP16 activators: (I) 52
VRE. *See* Ventral repression element
v-Rel, oncogene: (II) 102, 250

Wasting syndrome, dioxins and: (I) 177,
     198
Windbeutel (wind): (II) 244

Xenobiotic response elements (XREs):
     (I) 183–184, 186
Xenobiotics: (I) 143, 160
Xenopus laevis:
     clofibrate and, (I) 147
     MAPK pathway of, (II) 60
     Mos protein and, (II) 51
     PKC and, (II) 55
     PPARs and, (I) 148
     SRF and, (II) 43
     zinc and, (I) 206

Xeroderma pigmentosum (XE): (I) 76
X-ray analysis: (I) 8, 107–108, 181;
    (II) 206
XREs. *See* Xenobiotic response elements
Y79, retinoblastoma cells: (I) 31

Yeast studies:
    centromere binding and, (I) 180
    GCN4 transactivator and, (I) 80
    gene control and, (I) 143
    GRP78/Bip gene and, (I) 30
    heavy metals and, (I) 222
    hsp90 and, (I) 186
    MAPK and, (II) 49–50
    MCM1 protein, (II) 44
    metallionein and, (I) 227–229
    peroxisomes and, (I) 146

protein types and, (II) 44, 252
    See also specific types
YY1, transcriptional repressor: (I) 75

zen promoter: (II) 257
Z gene, *lac*: (I) 9
Zinc: (I) 206–222, 231
Zinc finger protein:
    A20 type: (I) 120
    DNA binding: (I) 142
    glucocorticoid receptor: (II) 133
    MTFZ-1 and: (I) 214–215
    PLZF and, (II) 225
    PPAR gene and, (I) 151
    transcription factors: (I) 206
Z motifs: (I) 181
Zymogens, dl proteins: (II) 245